This is a professional educational service
from
Searle Laboratories
P.O. Box 5110
Chicago, Illinois 60680

Industrial Pharmacology

Edited By

Stuart Fielding, Ph.D.

Volume I: Neuroleptics 1974
Volume II: Antidepressants 1975

Antidepressants

edited by

STUART FIELDING, Ph.D.

Manager, Psychopharmacology Research, Pharmaceuticals Division, CIBA-GEIGY Corporation; Summit, New Jersey; Adjunct Assistant Professor, Psychology Department, Fairleigh Dickinson University, Madison, New Jersey

and

HARBANS LAL, Ph.D.

Professor of Pharmacology, Toxicology, and Psychology, University of Rhode Island, Kingston, Rhode Island.

FUTURA
PUBLISHING COMPANY
1975

Published by
Futura Publishing Company, Inc.
295 Main Street
Mount Kisco, New York 10549

L.C. #: 74-33237
ISBN #: 0-87993-061-6

To Our Families
and
Friends in Science

Preface

Though less than twenty years have been invested in serious efforts to develop antidepressant drugs, the number of new chemicals which have been investigated is enormous and the variety of approaches to evaluate them are many. Also, the spectrum of activity with which each new drug has been allegedly associated is widespread, encompassing a number of scientific specialties. Because of this vastness of the investigation of antidepressants, the available information on the activity or inactivity of the known antidepressants is often rather confusing. It is this confusion that has motivated us to organize the available data on antidepressant drugs in the form of this book.

The important aspects of research on antidepressants are presented along with descriptions of the usefulness of each agent, particularly to scientists in the area of drug development. Following a brief overview of the disease state in the introductory chapter, aspects of experimentation with new antidepressants are described in the subsequent portions. As in the preceding volume on neuroleptics, we have again selected contributors who have devoted a considerable portion of their scientific endeavors to the search for drugs with antidepressant potential and who have agreed to impart their knowledge and experience.

During the compilation of this book, we paid particular attention to its relevance to newcomers in the field, as well as established investigators. To the former a step-by-step introduction is provided, while the latter will find particular value in its integrated compilation of data.

We have attempted to emphasize the approaches used to distinguish the antidepressants from other psychoactive agents in order to make this book a useful tool for all professionals in the pharmaceutical industry. For those scientists engaged in one particular aspect of drug development, whether it be chemistry, pharmacology, legal regulatory agencies, etc., we have attempted to provide some insight into the intersection between various disciplines. Thus, perhaps, it will help these scientists acquire an overall appreciation of the work of their colleagues in other areas.

This information compiled here may be an aid to teachers of pharmacology, toxicology, and psychology who are concerned with making their students aware of the various approaches successfully employed in the development of new antidepressants. Practicing physicians should benefit from the varied approaches in this book and find it a handy reference. Similarly, for graduate students in pharmacology, psychology, or psychobiology, this monograph will be a useful text to which they can go when in need of comprehensive data on various drugs or the procedures used to generate those data.

The above professionals, researchers, and practitioners were kept in mind as we sought to provide a ready source of the methodology of today and an addition to the armamentarium of tools needed to understand antidepressant drugs. We hope this book will be a stepping stone in the development of new and unique antidepressant drugs.

Foreword

More than twenty years have passed since Dr. Schindler of the Geigy Research Laboratories first synthesized imipramine with the aim of discovering a psychopharmacological agent with properties superior to or different from chlorpromazine. The initial biological profile of imipramine did suggest some differences but the methodology employed in the mid-1950's did not suggest that an agent was in hand with extraordinary properties. It remained for Professor Kuhn, Head of the Psychiatry Clinic in Munsterlingen, Switzerland, to establish that this compound was not just another modification of other tricyclic agents, but indeed was a new therapeutic agent for the treatment of endogenous depressions. This was unquestionably a milestone in chemotherapy in psychiatry. What had been so long considered a difficult disease entity to control and also one which accounted for so much suffering and despair for millions of depressed patients, suddenly became a chemotherapeutic reality with a drug in hand for the treatment and cure of severe depression. Although this discovery by Professor Kuhn has been referred to as clinical serendipity, I prefer to refer to it as an application of a fundamental process of medicinal research, namely, the astute observation of a scientist in assessing the effect of a medicinal agent on a patient undergoing treatment. *Professor Kuhn's mind was prepared to observe the unexpected.* Although regulatory requirements today do not permit the clinical study of new chemical agents in a liberal fashion, nevertheless, the basic fundamentals associated with drug discovery still remain. Presently it is more necessary than ever that the unexpected and unusual effect be observed by astute biologists working on new animal models in the laboratory rather than at the later stage, namely, in man.

Finally, and particularly in the area of psychopharmacology, a study of the biochemical parameters associated with the disease entity has become of paramount importance. The specific effects that various potential antidepressants will have to a varying degree will depend on biochemical evaluations in various brain centers. As a consequence, the opportunity for rational design of new drugs in this area of medicinal research is most promising. I believe that this monograph will stimulate new concepts which will permit scientists working in medicinal research to bring to the patient novel and improved antidepressants.

George deStevens, Ph.D.
Executive Vice-President and
Director of Research
Pharmaceuticals Division
CIBA-GEIGY Corporation
Summit, New Jersey

Acknowledgements

We would like to express our appreciation and gratitude to Dr. Jeffrey K. Saelens, Dr. William C. Govier, Dr. Albert J. Plummer, Dr. Robert Gaunt and the entire Editorial Policy Committee (CIBA-GEIGY Corp.) for many helpful suggestions, criticisms and careful reading of portions of the manuscript.

Miss Susan Edwards, Mrs. Linda Florio, Mr. Michael Cornfeldt, Mr. Bob Outwater, Miss Nancy Howie and the rest of the CIBA-GEIGY Psychopharmacology staff, Mr. Gerald Gianutros (University of Rhode Island), for their editorial assistance. Mrs. Betty Dooley (CIBA-GEIGY Corp.), Mrs. Katherine McGovern, Mrs. Lucille Johnson (University of Rhode Island) for the careful typing of portions of the manuscript, and to numerous friends who interacted in many ways in perceiving and organizing concepts undertaken in the manuscript. The editors wish to express special appreciation to the contributing authors who have provided excellent material and have strived to achieve the objectives of this book.

Finally, especial thanks are due Futura Publishing Company for their patience and helpful collaboration.

Contributors

Michael J. Antonaccio, Ph.D.
Manager, Cardiovascular Research
Pharmaceuticals Division
CIBA-GEIGY Corporation
Summit, New Jersey

Ronald G. Babington, Ph.D.
Head, CNS Group
Sandoz Pharmaceuticals Division of Sandoz Inc.
East Hanover, New Jersey

Jonathan O. Cole, M.D.
Director of Research
Commonwealth of Massachusetts
Department of Mental Health
Boston State Hospital
Boston, Massachusetts

Emanuela I. Dobrin, M.S.
Scientific Liaison
Regulatory Affairs Department
Searle Laboratories Division
G. D. Searle & Co.
Chicago, Illinois

Stuart Fielding, Ph.D.
Manager, Psychopharmacology Research
Pharmaceuticals Division
CIBA-GEIGY Corporation
Summit, New Jersey
Adjunct Assistant Professor, Psychology Department
Fairleigh Dickinson University
Madison, New Jersey

Neville Finch, Ph.D.
Executive Director of Chemical Research

Research Dept., Pharmaceuticals Division
CIBA-GEIGY Corporation
Summit, New Jersey

John H. Gogerty, Ph.D.
Director of Pharmacology and Biochemistry
Sandoz Pharmaceuticals Division of Sandoz Inc.
East Hanover, New Jersey

Turan M. Itil, M.D.
Research Professor and Director
Division of Biological Psychiatry
New York Medical College
New York, New York

Paul A. J. Janssen, M.D.
Janssen Pharmaceutica
Research Laboratoria
Beerse, Belgium

Claude I. Judd, Ph.D.
Merrell-National Laboratories
Division of Richardson-Merrell Inc.
Cincinnati, Ohio

John Karkalas, M.D.
Chief of Psychiatry
Rhode Island Institute of Mental Health
Rhode Island Medical Center
Cranston, Rhode Island

Theodore O. King, Ph.D.
Director, Drug Safety Evaluation
Drug Safety Evaluation Department
Pfizer Central Research
Pfizer Inc.
Groton, Connecticut

B. Kenneth Koe, Ph.D.
Senior Research Investigator
Department of Pharmacology
Medical Research Laboratories
Pfizer, Inc.
Groton, Connecticut

Harbans Lal, Ph.D.
Professor of Pharmacology, Toxicology, and Psychology
University of Rhode Island
Kingston, Rhode Island

Steven L. Malish, Ph.D.
Research Scientist—Toxicology
Drug Safety Evaluation Department
Pfizer Central Research
Pfizer Inc.
Groton, Connecticut

Carlos J. E. Niemegeers, D. Sc.
Janssen Pharmaceutica
Research Laboratoria
Beerse, Belgium

W. Joseph Potts, Ph.D.
Associate Director of Research
Searle Laboratories Division
G. D. Searle & Co.
Chicago, Illinois

Ronald D. Robson, Ph.D.
Director of Pharmacology
Pharmaceuticals Division
CIBA-GEIGY Corporation
Summit, New Jersey

Richard C. Ursillo, Ph.D.
Merrell-National Laboratories
Division of Richardson-Merrell Inc.
Cincinnati, Ohio

John R. Vogel, Ph.D.
Central Nervous System Section
Department of Pharmacology & Toxicology
William H. Rorer, Inc.
Fort Washington, Pennsylvania

Max Wilhelm, Ph.D.
Vice President, Exploratory Research
Pharmaceuticals Division
CIBA-GEIGY Corporation
Summit, New Jersey

Contents

Antidepressants

Introduction

STUART FIELDING, PH.D.
and
HARBANS LAL, PH.D.

The most challenging area of treatment and research in psychiatry today is depression. This is because both the nature of the disease and its treatment have been intriguing and have for centuries defied attempts at understanding. Also, depression is not bounded by any one social stratum and this widespread distribution makes it morally and commercially attractive to design drugs against it.

In contrast to the earlier treatment of other psychiatric disorders such as schizoprenia for which head surgery and physical methods of immobilization were applied, our forefathers often resorted to pharmacotherapy to obtain relief from depression. However, the ancient drugs for depression included a diverse variety of active and inactive ingredients ranging from purgatives to extracts of opium.

Introduction of MAO inhibitors in the U.S.A. in 1957 followed six months later by imipramine introduced in Switzerland was a most fortunate coincidence by way of stimulating the search for discovery of new drugs to fight depression. Both early discoveries were accidental and the drugs belonged to two diverse pharmacological classes. This diversity was crucial in opening multiple areas of research for developing new drugs and for understanding of the disease process. It was fortunate that both drugs were not from the same class because no easy theory could be assumed to account for both types of action and therefore researchers were forced to look beyond the apparent simplicities. What was triggered as a result of these discoveries is well illustrated throughout the pages of this book.

Even though we have come a long way since the days of ancient medicine and more recent convulsive treatments, three interrelated factors were primarily responsible for retarding our progress in developing newer drugs which are significantly different from those earlier prototypes. Uncertainties of clinical features of depression and inability to appropriately classify the illnesses of many depressed patients was one factor. Lack of tangible theories as to the biochemical basis of depression was another factor. Also, there are no provisions to test drugs in humans in the absence of satisfactory animal models of depression.

Depression has meant different things to different people. For the neurophysiologists, depression refers to any decrease in electrophysiological activity such as cortical depression. To a pharmacologist, depression means a state of drug-induced reduction in CNS-mediated activity of various organs. The psychologists have invariably considered any decrement in optimal performance of psychological functions as depression. For the practicing psychiatrist, depression covers a wide range of changes in affective state ranging from usual mood swings to severe melancholic psychosis.

In terms of mood changes, depression is a part of normal living. Feelings of sadness, disappointment, and frustration are experienced by all of us in many life situations. Beyond this, depression often occurs as a symptom secondary to other illnesses such as prolonged infectious attacks as hepatitis, nutritional deficiencies including anemia, degenerative changes such as those associated with senility and chronic neoplastic diseases. This sort of depression has not been recognized as such and is usually not even classified as depression. A more appropriate term to describe such syndromes may be neuroasthenia. Specific chemotherapy of neuroasthenia is not known. Recently, a drug, Levamizole® whose effectiveness was accidently discovered in a patient suffering from depression that was associated with a neoplastic disease, drew some attention and may well be found useful in cases of neuroasthenias. The pharmaceutical industry may come up with more such drugs in the future as neuroasthenia is common and patients often are treated by general physicians with vitamins, etc., in the absence of a specific drug.

Most often, the term depression refers to one or more syndromes in which there are abnormal and persistent affect changes associated with feelings of worthlessness, guilt, helplessness and hopelessness, anxiety, crying, suicidal tendencies, loss of interest in work and other activities, impaired capacity to perform everyday social functions, and hypochondriasis, accompanied by such physical alterations as anorexia, weight changes, constipation, psychomotor retardation, or agitation, headache, and other bodily complaints. Depending on conditions and syndromes that are present, pathological depression is differentiated between reactive and endogenous, between neurotic and psychotic, and endogenous depression has been subdivided into periodic or unipolar or monopolar depression as opposed to manic depression or bipolar depression. A common feature of most classifications has been to separate, on the basis of clinical evaluation, endogenous depression from the rest. The endogenous depression constitutes only 10-20% of all depressed disorders and is generally unresponsive to psychological treatment or administration of placebo, but is relatively responsive to pharmacological treatment, or E.C.T. Further subtyping of the endogenous depression is based on the history of a prior manic or hypomanic episode and is designated as the manic-depression or bipolar disorders. The manic-depressive reactions constitute the most homogenous clinically defined subgroup of the depressive disorders and are distinguished from the unipolar depressions which are characterized by the absence of a prior episode of mania or hypomania and are very heterogenous. To effectively undertake development of new drugs it is essential that all categories of depression are well-defined or placed in other disease categories if uniformity cannot be obtained under a global title of depression. Thereafter it will be less difficult to develop animal models to correspond to each clinical entity which is homogenous.

In the pathogenesis of depressive syndromes, clusters of causes have been implicated. They have been usually investigated for reactive, neurotic and endogenous forms of depression. For reactive depression, distressing experiences in the environment of a susceptible patient are said to be specific causes. It has not yet been demonstrated on a convincing scale that equally specific environmental causes are also involved in the etiology of endogenous depression. Whereas investigations into the families of patients suffering from reactive depression have yielded negative findings, researchers have by and large succeeded in proving that hereditary factors do contribute to causation of endogenous depression.

For rational development of animal models for drug screening it is usually necessary to have an experimental criteria of depression. For this purpose it is required that reliable criteria for this separation of homogenous subgroups of depressed patients be established. Also, it is equally necessary to be able to reliably measure changes in the intensity of depressive pathology due to drug treatments. At present the diagnosis is established by clinical evaluaticn and changes in pathology are measured through the use of rating scales. Although clinical diagnosis as well as rating scales, if used to their best advantage and with expert skill, are of considerable value for clinical practice, both methods depend greatly on subjective factors, and subjective factors are hard to translate into animal models. Encouragingly, attempts are constantly made to employ objective criteria for the assessment of a depressive syndrome. Work is in progress in several laboratories to develop biological criteria as well as behavioral and clinical criteria to define depression. The biological criteria under present investigations include study of metabolites of the important biogenic amines such as MHPG in urine as well as CSF and HVA and 5HIAA in CSF. Also under investigation is activity of several enzymes such as MAO, COMT, DOPA in blood and blood constituents. Recently, attention has been given to the use of drugs to diagnose depression. In this regard, clinical response to acute doses of amphetamine and L-DOPA have been found noteworthy. In addition, pharmacokinetic relationships with different types of depressive illness are being considered for diagnosis. Among the physiological functions that are under scrutiny are thyroid functions, sleep characteristics and electrolyte metabolism. In the clinical field, besides improving rating scales, psychophysiological testing of perceptual, cognitive and psychomotor performances as well as responses to conditional stimuli and alterations in various reflexes are being considered for their reliability in predicting a clinical diagnosis of depression.

In the absence of an objective definition of the disease state, understanding of the neurobiological basis of the disease state can provide directions toward developing new biological models of depression. In this respect, previously discovered effects of known antidepressants on the biogenic amines have been amply considered for application in drug screening. Since these drugs alter biogenic amines (synthesis, release, inactivity and receptor sensitivity) in a significant manner, biochemical differentiation between depressed, manic, and control subjects is being attempted. Methods used entail the utilization of cross-sectional research designs and the examination of biochemical changes that accompany alterations in affective state in depressed or manic patients studied longitudinally. Based upon data available from the best experiments, it is recognized that there are definite alterations in the biogenic amine metabolism related to the affective disorders. Whether or not these alterations ultimately prove to be of etiological importance is not known. However, many of these alterations of biogenic amines found in human depression have already been translated in animals and are readily utilized in the pharmaceutical industry to screen new chemicals for antidepressant potential.

In spite of progress mentioned above, one must concede presently that biological models are not available to discover new antidepressants other than the prototypes of the earlier drugs. This aspect is emphasized appropriately throughout the book. As in the case of the preceding volume on neuroleptics, we invited actively involved investigators to provide whatever recipes are available for drug development to treat depressive disorders.

We have merely attempted here to highlight some of the areas of concern in our efforts to combat depression. In the chapters to follow, each facet will be focused on by authors in their area of expertise.

The first of the fifteen information-laden chapters presents several chemical approaches to antidepressant drug development and emphasizes the communication between chemistry and biological research as a building structure for new chemical compounds. What direction a newly synthesized chemical compound will take is also clearly explained. This is followed by discussion of the preclinical neuropsychopharmacology of antidepressants which is comprised of five chapters in which classical screening procedures are contrasted with designs displaying a more unique methodology. It elaborates upon numerous screening procedures used to elucidate antidepressant activity and from which predictions as to activity in man are made. This leads us to the next section devoted to the effects of antidepressant drugs on brain catecholamines and serotonin. It elucidates the various biochemical hypotheses of depression and how they serve as guides in the search for new drugs. The next chapter discusses the side effects of these compounds on the cardiovascular system such as tachycardia, arrhythmias and hypotension, as well as peripheral findings which may derive from the same fundamental action which is thought responsible for the central effect of these drugs. We now move on to review toxicity which entails a specific testing regimen required by the Food and Drug Administration. The next section relates to the absorption, distribution, excretion, and metabolism of antidepressants. Upon recognition that a compound has potential antidepressant activity with advantages over marketed products, this next section elucidates the developmental process which satisfies F.D.A. regulations for filing an Investigational New Drug Application (INDA). After the completion of necessary preclinical investigation, the next phase of the drug development process involves the clinical evaluation as it relates to their pharmacology, efficacy, and safety in human subjects, as discussed in the chapter entitled "Clinical Evaluation of Antidepressant Drugs". Also included is a detailed discussion on the methodology of clinical trials and the experimental design of efficacy studies and other assessment procedures. The next chapter elucidates how the EEG in man can be used as a useful tool in detecting antidepressant drugs that have lacked effectiveness in classical preclinical screening procedures. Appropriately, our final two chapters devote themselves to a discussion of past accomplishments and future prospects in antidepressant research.

The development of new antidepressant drugs is not a single privilege of chemistry, pharmacology, biochemistry, toxicology, psychology, or psychiatry, but rather the integration of these various disciplines in representing a total picture of drug development. This book has been compiled with the aim of providing a ready source of information on the sequential steps that make up this many faceted process of man's efforts to understand and overcome mental depression.

1

Chemical Approaches to the Development of Antidepressants

NEVILLE FINCH, PH.D.

I. INTRODUCTION

The physicians of the Middle Ages were well aware of the clinical manifestations of depression, and had arrived at a viewpoint of the etiology of the disease similar to that currently held. Namely, that some depressions had a physical cause, i.e. from the black bile or the *atria bilia,* one of the Hippocratic humors, and were susceptible to drug therapy; whereas other depressions arose from the effects of certain circumstances on a person of melancholic temperament. Conceptually, such assignments compare with current diagnosis of endogenous depression and reactive depression. The rather modest progress made in the diagnosis of depressions has limited the development of effective drug therapy. Many clinical trials of potential antidepressants have involved patient groups, which, it will probably ultimately transpire, were too inhomogenous to enable their potential utility against specific forms of depression to be evaluated. The serendipity involved in the discovery of imipramine has been well described by Kuhn (114). Future progress undoubtedly depends on improved classification of depressive illness and the development of understanding of the underlying pathology. Hollister has covered these aspects well in his recent review of the clinical situation from the standpoint of the specialist (92). A less rigorous overview of the clinical problem, directed at the general practioner, has also appeared recently (117).

The most promising developments from the clinical standpoint are the appearance of diagnostic procedures other than patient rating scales, which necessarily retain much subjectivity. Such procedures are, for example, the measurement of the urinary excretion of catecholamines or their metabolites, e.g. 3-methoxy-4-hydroxymandelic acid. These procedures are harbingers of improved diagnoses, the development of more relevant animal models, and, hopefully, better drugs. The methodology for estimating CNS catecholamine levels has been reviewed recently by Schildkraut (156, 157).

The biochemical theories of depression explain not only the clinical effectiveness of the well established tricyclic compounds, imipramine **20a** and amitriptyline **la,** but also the effects on depression seen with monoamine oxidase (MAO) inhibitors. The inhibition of MAO is believed to elevate the levels of norepinephrine in the storage granule by decreasing the destruction of the norepinephrine taken up again from the synaptic cleft. Catecholamine levels in the brain are elevated by treatment with MAO inhibitors (104), and the antidepressant effects of these drugs have been well described (92). The side effects of the MAO inhibitors limit their wide spread utility, but in a hospitalized setting with dietary control, these effects can be minimized (150).

Whether deficiencies in the levels of other biogenic amines, e.g. serotonin, are involved in the etiology depression seems less clearly defined (42). The effects of serotonin on the CNS have recently been reviewed, but only brief mention given to its role in affective disorders (33). Nevertheless, clinical studies have described the utility of tryptophane, either alone, (113) or in combination (109). Furthermore, there has been a report that free tryptophane plasma levels are lower in depressed patients (41).

Several other hypotheses for the causes of endogenous depression are extant, e.g., involving the cholinergic system (100) or modifications of previous biogenic amine hypotheses (6). In addition, other synaptic transmitters in the CNS have been proposed, e.g., glutamic acid, GABA (103), and cyclic AMP have been implicated in anxiety and depression (94).

Thus, while there is a definite move from the clinical standpoint towards more objective measurements of depression, there are differences of opinion about what should be measured and technical limitations about what can be measured. Therefore, it is not too surprising that there are differences of opinions among biologists as to the relevance of various animal tests for depression. Thus, the task of a chemist reviewing this particular field of medicinal chemistry is especially complex, as it is clearly a field in which major advances will be made in the near future, yet it is still too early to exactly identify the type of compound which will achieve prominence. Therefore, this review follows, very much, the lines of a recent excellent review by Kaiser and Zirkle (107), and the reader is urged to refer also to the updates these authors provide in their annual chapters in the Annual Reports in Medicinal Chemistry (108).

II. LINEAR TRICYCLIC ANTIDEPRESSANTS

This broad class of compounds presently dominates the market for the treatment of endogenous depression and hence deserves special attention, both for its obvious efficacy and its shortcomings. Structurally, these compounds, such as imipramine **20a** and amitriptyline **la,** superficially resemble the neuroleptics like chlorpromazine **34a,** yet pharmacologically they are very different. An important difference becomes evident when molecular models of these compounds are inspected. The tricyclic framework of the antidepressant is much further from planarity than that of the phenothiazines such as chlorpromazine. These differences have been discussed in detail by Wilhelm (191). The angle of flexure, that is the angle between the planes containing the aromatic rings, is 55° for imipramine **20a** whereas it is 25° for chlorpromazine **34a.** In design of further drugs of this type, the geometrical parameters defined by Wilhelm should certainly be taken into consideration. Unfortunately, as is almost the rule in medicinal chemistry, by the time the mechanism of drug action is understood and the molecular configurations required to achieve such an effect are defined, there is less interest in such compounds by the clinician and the biologist.

A. 6-7-6 Linear Tricyclics

1. Carbocyclic

a. Amitriptyline and Related Compounds

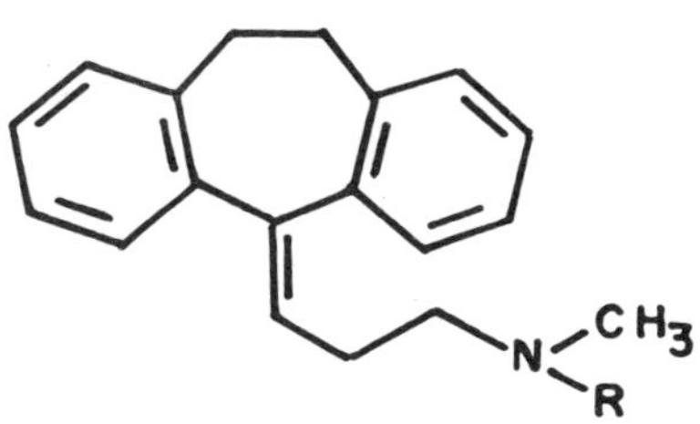

1a R = CH_3

1b R = H

The structure activity relationships for amitriptyline **1a** have been well described (107). The most significant variant is nortriptyline **1b.** Evidence has accumulated which suggests that many of the CNS effects of amitriptyline **1a** are due to the primary metabolite nortriptyline **1b** (82). However, the more recently investigated effects on asthma may be due principally to the unchanged drug, based on results from *in vitro* studies (130).

Other variants of amitriptyline **1a** which have been described recently are keto compounds.

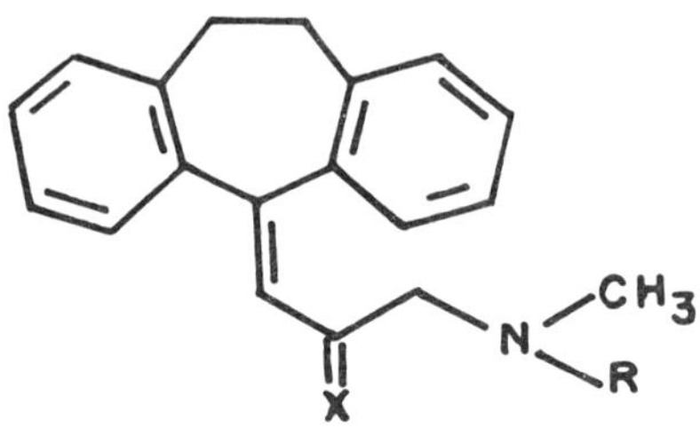

2a R = CH_3 X = O

2b R = H X = $<^{H}_{OH}$

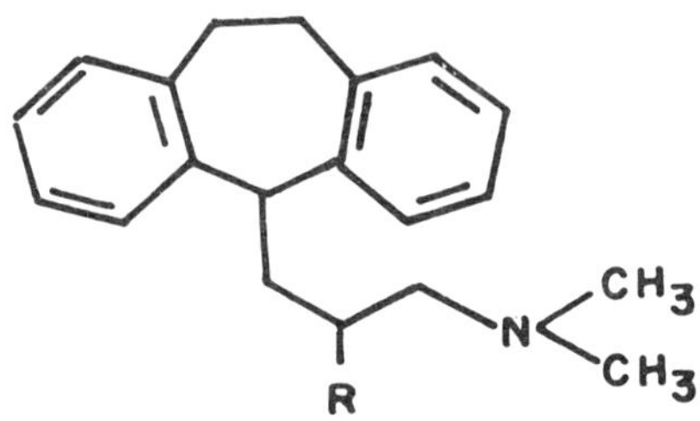

3a R = H

3b R = CH_3

Compound **2a** identified as SD 2203-01 is claimed, on the basis of animal tests, to be less anticholinergic than amitriptyline **1a** (21).

An interesting route to the related compound **2b** was recently described (115), but no clinical evidence has been presented to demonstrate that these variants represent an advance over the parent compound.

While dihydro amitriptyline **3a** has been regarded as a less potent compound (53) than the parent, Ayerst investigators have described clinical studies with a similar compound **3b** having a branched side chain (11). The pharmacology of this compound, butriptyline **3b,** has been previously described (187). Butriptyline, from the available data, does not seem to offer any substantial advantages over amitriptyline **1a.** It is more sedating and may have an anxiolytic effect, but the antidepressant effect is probably achieved via inhibition of reuptake of norepinephrine by the presynaptic terminal, as with amitriptyline **1a.** Also, the onset of the antidepressant effect in man takes several days, which is in accord with this hypothesis.

b. Protriptyline and Related Compounds

Protriptyline **5** is another clinically important tricyclic antidepressant although its share of the U.S. market is less than that of imipramine **20a** or amitriptyline **1a.** It is a more potent compound on a mg/kg basis, but the claim that it is more effective, in the sense that patients who fail with other tricyclic compounds will respond to protriptyline **5**, is still not substantiated. It is, however, less sedating in man than amitriptyline **1a** and is therefore especially useful for apathetic and withdrawn depressed patients.

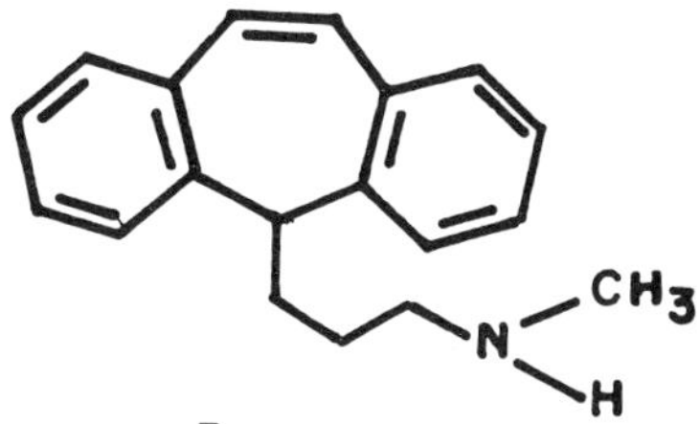

5

The structure activity relationships in the protriptyline **5** series have been reviewed by Kaiser and Zirkle (107) and also by the original workers (53). The criteria for activity are not, surprisingly, similar to those of amitriptyline **1a.** Substitution in the aromatic rings reduces activity. Interestingly, introduction of the additional double bond into protriptyline **5** as it is in amitriptyline to give **6a**

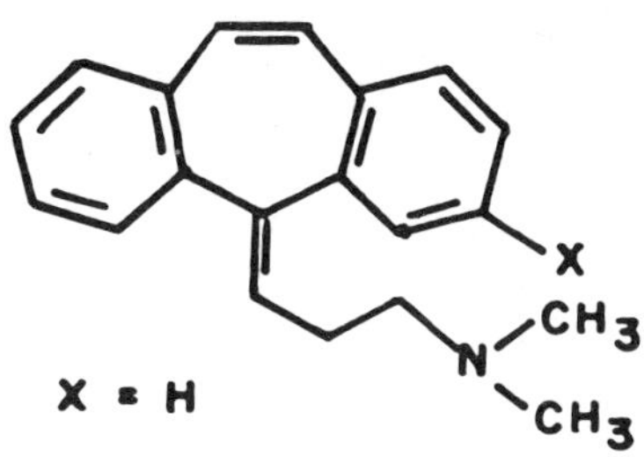

6a X = H

6b X = SO_2CH_3

reduces the antidepressant effects, as measured by antagonism of tetrabenazine ptosis in mice, but introduces neuroleptic properties. Thus, a substituted compound **6b** is comparable to chlorpromazine **34a** in blocking conditioned avoidance responding in monkeys (171).

This change in the pharmacological profile can be related to the change in the angle of flexure between the planes of the aromatic rings as outlined previously (191). A compound of this type, which may be undergoing clinical investigation, is intriptyline **7** (44). No details, pharmacological or clinical, have been published.

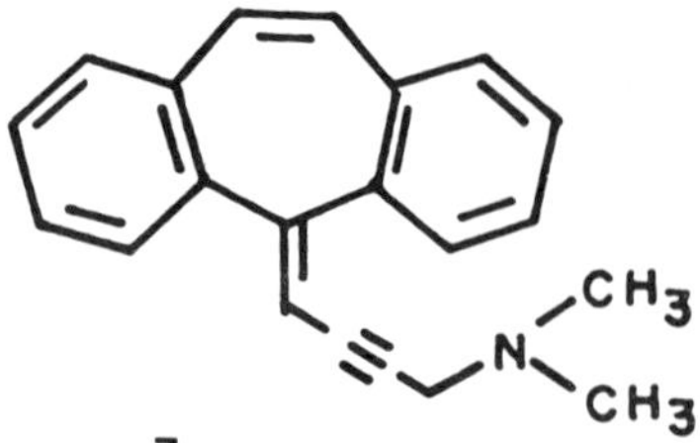

7

c. Noxiptiline and Related Compounds

Noxiptiline **8a** is the most recent of the carbotricyclic antidepressants on which a large body of pharmacological and clinical data have been obtained (16).

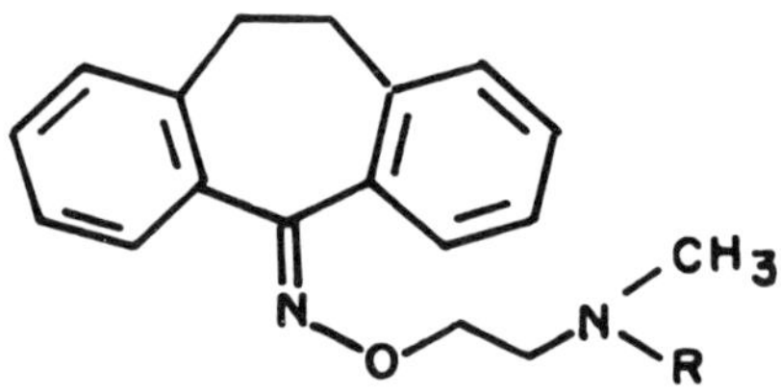

8a R = CH_3

8b R = H

This compound **8a** was also described independently by a Swedish group as CD 37B (Pharmacia) (152, 50).

Noxiptiline **8a** does not really represent a major advance in the therapy of depressive illness, but it is, nonetheless, an interesting addition to the physician's armamentarium. It is claimed to have a more favorable effect upon mood than amitriptyline **1a.** From a commercial standpoint, noxiptiline **8a** has captured only a modest share of the market in its country of origin, West Germany. As with all successful compounds, there have been many imitations bearing the unusual oxime dimethylaminoethylether side chain. For the purpose of this review, mention will be made only of those compounds which are related directly to noxiptiline **8a.**

The scope of the Bayer work on noxiptiline **8a** covers many ring types and sizes, e.g. as in **9a** through **9i** (2). One of these **9b** has been investigated by other groups (186, 153). From the work of Villani (186), it would seem that this particular change with noxiptiline **8a** was developed with the knowledge of the relationship between imipramine **20a** and desimipramine **20b,** amitriptyline **1a** and nortriptyline **1b,** the desmethyl analog of noxiptiline **8b** was also tested clinically, even though, surprisingly, it was less active than noxiptiline **8a** (18) in some tests, e.g. reserpine antagonism. One presumes that these clinical trials confirmed the

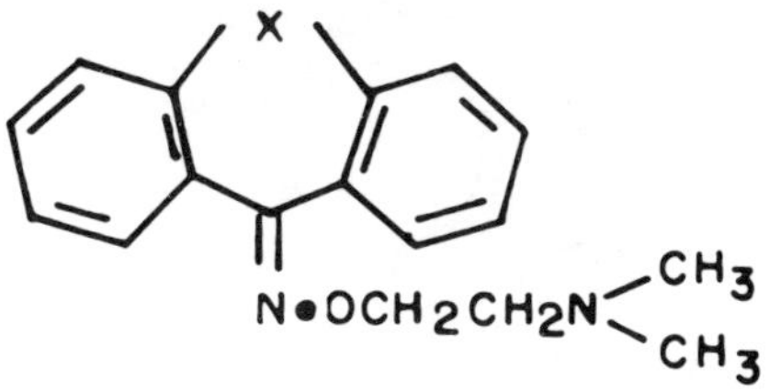

9a X = $-CH_2-O-$	**9d** $-C(CH_3)_2-$	**9g** $-S-$
9b X = $-CH=CH-$	**9e** $-N(CH_3)-$	**9h** $-CH_2-S-$
9c X = $-(CH_2)_3-$	**9f** $-SO_2-$	**9i** $-C(=O)-NH-$

pharmacology. This is because the tertiary base noxiptiline **8a** was selected for introduction as the antidepressant Agedal® rather than the secondary base **8b,** as one might have anticipated from structure activity relationships of the other clinically established tricyclic antidepressants.

d. Bridged Compounds

Although strictly speaking such compounds are tetracyclic, they are best considered for review purposes here because they are closely related, pharmacologically, to amitriptyline **1a.** The most extensively studied compound of this type is MK 940 **10.**

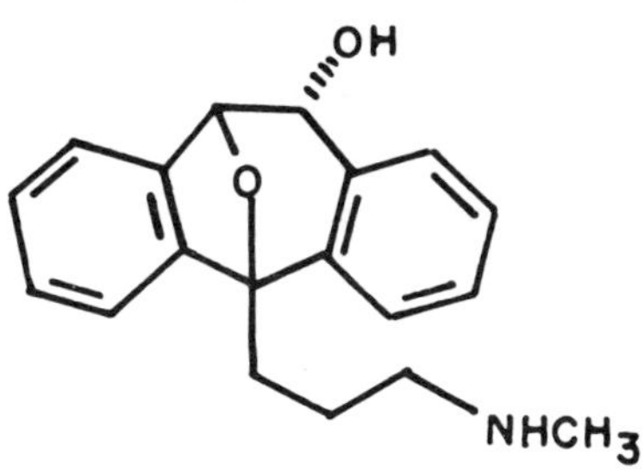

10

This compound **10** was exceptionally potent in the antagonism of tetrabenazine ptosis in mice (37). Interestingly, the stereochemistry of the hydroxyl group was very important for this activity. The epimer with the hydroxyl group *cis* to the bridge was a hundred times less active. Clinical investigation of MK 940 **10** suggested that it resembled the tricyclic antidepressants, but the E.E.G. characterization demonstrated that it may have central stimulant activity (70). No further clinical studies with this compound have been noted so one may presume that this overt stimulating effect may have limited utility.

Another bridged compound **11**

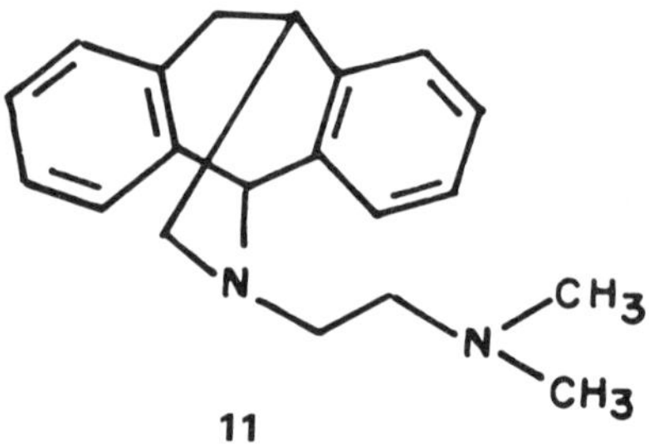

11

was completely devoid of tetrabenazine antagonism activity in mice (78). It did, however, inhibit the uptake of norepinephrine in the rat vas deferens preparation, *in vitro*.

There have been several other chemical efforts in the area of bridged compounds, e.g. **12** (188), **13** (40), and **14** (131).

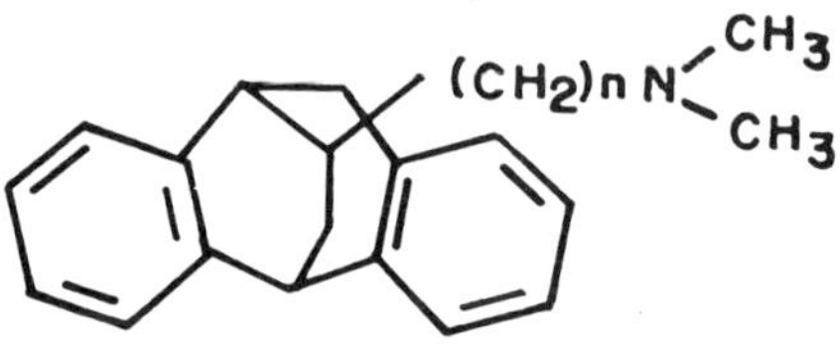

12

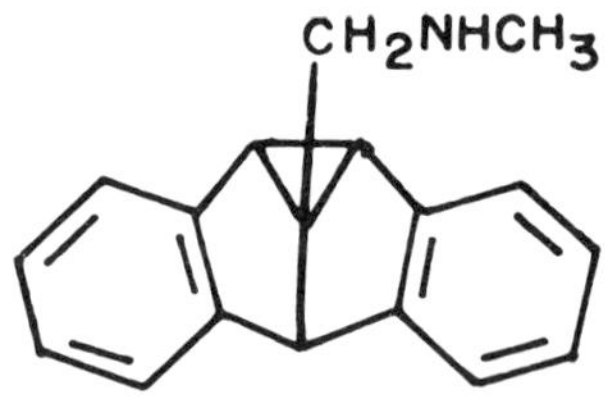

13

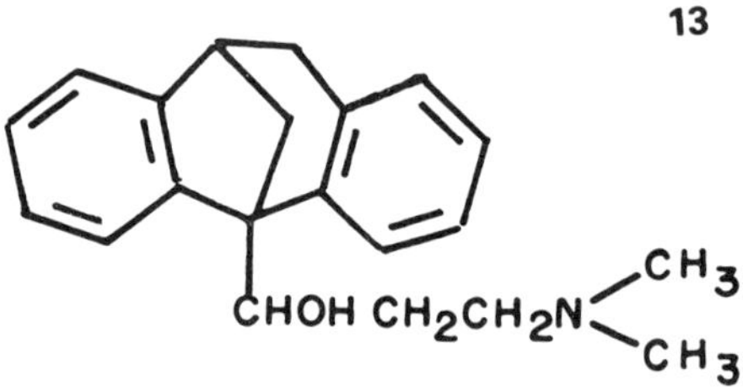

14

However, there are no published clinical or pharmacological data by which to appraise the significance of these developments.

e. Miscellaneous

As amitriptyline **1a** represents such an important target compound, it is not surprising that medicinal chemists still make novel compounds which incorporate the basic skeleton. Some of these have been reported with only minimal pharmacological data, so, mention will be made only of recent examples.

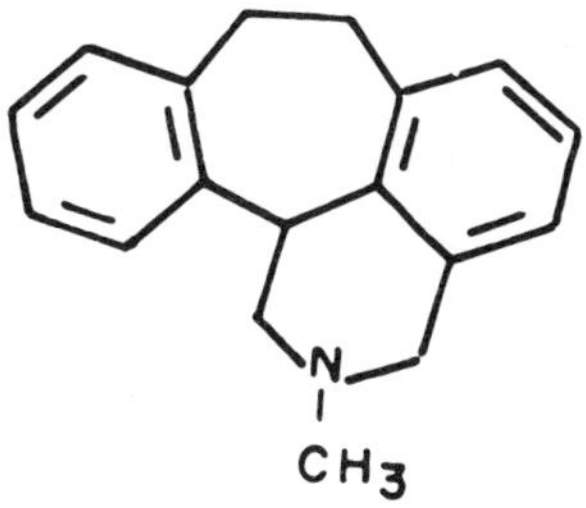

15

The tetracycle **15** has been reported to have an activity profile similar to amitriptyline **1a** (95). Other tetracyclic compounds related to amitriptyline **1a** are compounds **16** (135) and **17** (7).

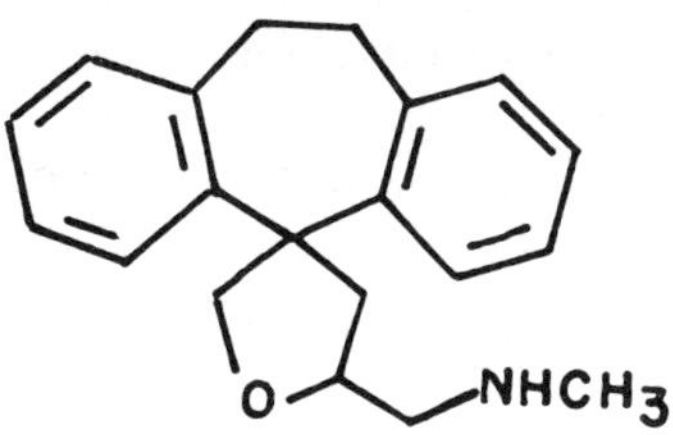

16

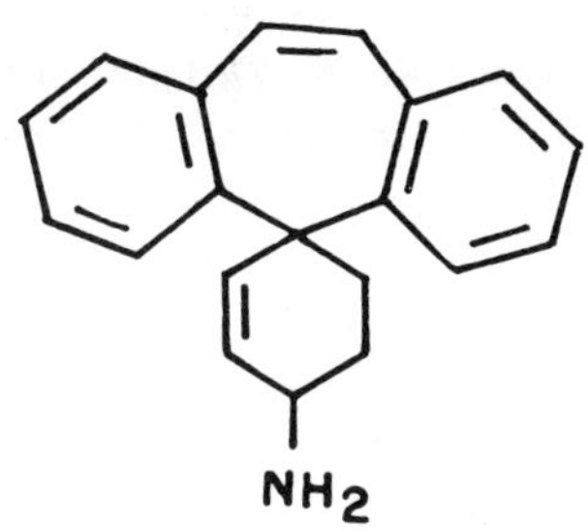

17

The Astra compound **17** (CGP 186) inhibits uptake of serotonin as well as norepinephrine and is devoid of anticholinergic effects in animal studies. This suggests that useful differences from the amitriptyline type may be observed in the clinic.

2. *Heterocyclic*

a. Doxepin and Related Compounds

Doxepin **18**

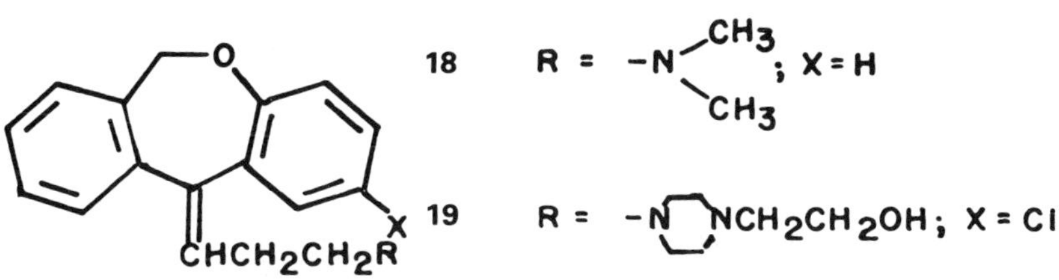

is an interesting drug in that it is inhomogenous. The marketed product Sinequan ® (Pfizer) is a mixture of *cis* and *trans* forms. In the U.S., this compound **18** is the most recently introduced antidepressant. It was launched in 1969 with a vigorous promotion and made some inroads into the market. It is claimed to combine an antianxiety effect comparable to chlordiazepoxide (52) with the antidepressant effects of amitriptyline **1a.**

Other analogs have been investigated, e.g. Pinoxepin **19** (81) and the appropriate variants made by other groups, e.g. Bayer, have prepared the noxiptiline analog **9a** (2). Nevertheless, this particular heterocyclic variant of the amitriptyline skeleton has not attracted as much attention as the carbocyclic parent, e.g. bridged compounds do not appear to have been described.

b. Imipramine and Related Compounds

Imipramine **20a** is the prototype tricyclic antidepressant. The serendipitous discovery of its clinical activity in 1956 has been referred to previously (114), and a complete account of subsequent work, both clinical and biological, has been published (3).

The structure activity relationships in the imipramine series have been described by Kaiser and Zirkle (107), and they resemble those for amitriptyline **1a.** For example, the desmethyl compound desimipramine **20b** is more active in several biological tests than the parent substance **20a.**

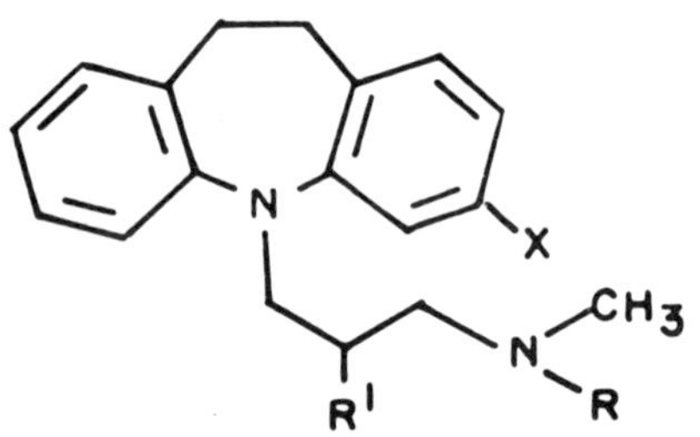

20a	$R = CH_3$; $R' = X = H$
20b	$R = R' = X = H$
20c	$R = R' = CH_3$ $X = H$
20d	$R = CH_3$ $R' = CH_3$ $X = Cl$
20e	$R = CH_2\overset{O}{\overset{\|}{C}}C_6H_4Cl$ $R' = X = H$

This is in contrast to the tricyclic neuroleptics such as chlorpromazine where removal of one of the methyl groups from nitrogen greatly reduces the biological activity (80). The chain length between the nitrogen atoms is important. A three-carbon chain is present on the most potent antidepressant compounds although compounds with a two-carbon chain do retain some activity. A branched three-carbon chain, as in trimipramine **20c** confers good antidepressant activity, although a sedative or antianxiety effect is also seen. A recent sleep study compares the effects of these three imipramine analogs **20a, 20b,** and **20c** (111).

One very important analog of imipramine **20a** is chlorimipramine **20d,** the pharmacology of which has been described (173). This compound **20d** structurally resembles both imipramine **20a** and amitriptyline **1a.** There are, however, important biochemical differences in that it appears that chlorimipramine **20d** may be more effective in blockade of serotonin than norepinephrine reuptake from the neuronal synapse. This may be the reason for the effects on mood and anxiety seen clinically with chlorimipramine (173, 27, 145).

The tricyclic antidepressants in clinical use have peripheral anticholinergic properties. These are evident in the side effects reported by patients, e.g. dry mouth and urinary retention. A new compound lopramine **20e** is claimed to have less peripheral anticholinergic activity in animal studies (54). Some clinical work has been reported but is insufficient to form a good impression of whether lopramine **20e** has achieved the goal of retaining the clinical efficiency of imipramine **20a,** yet with an improvement in tolerability (165, 176).

Many other analogs of imipramine **20a** have been described, e.g. Carpipramine **21.**

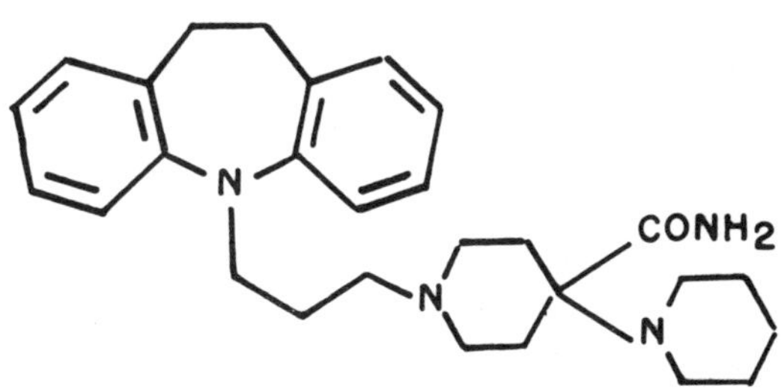

21

Carpipramine **21** (137) shows many of the biological properties of imipramine, e.g. potentiation of amphetamine, but a difference is that carpipramine **21** is much less effective in antagonizing reserpine. Clinical investigation has shown that carpipramine is not antidepressant in man.

Several analogs involving a replacement of one or both of the aromatic rings of imipramine **20a** by pyridyl rings have been described in papers by Villani (185), but no clinical accounts of useful antidepressant activity have been reported. Based on the limited data available, these changes seem to introduce greater toxicity.

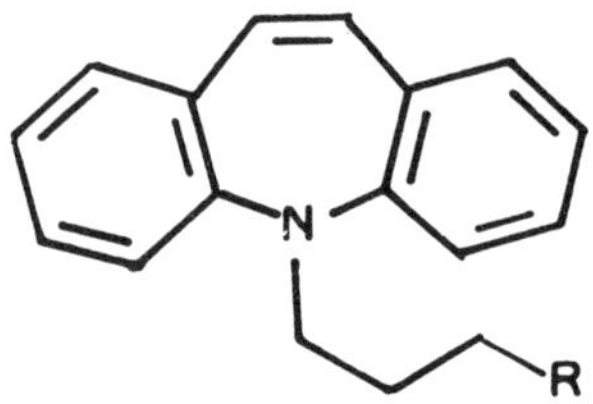

22a $R = -N\quad NCH_2CH_2OH$

22b $R = N(CH_3)_2$

c. Opipramol and Related Compounds

Opipramol **22a** is a member of the imipramine family of compounds. It bears a structural relationship to imipramine **20a** of the same type that amitriptyline **1a** bears to **6a**, i.e. a change of ethylene bridge to an ethylidene bridge. In the case of imipramine, however, the presence of a nitrogen atom between the aromatic rings rather than an sp^2 carbon, introduces sufficient conformational flexibility for the aromatic rings to retain the antidepressant angle of flexure (191). Therefore, G 31406 **22b** is more appropriately compared with protriptyline 5, which has antidepressant properties, than with **6a**, which does not. A detailed comparison of the biological properties of opipramol **22a** and G31406 **22b** with those of imipramine **20a** and desimipramine **20b** has been published (174.)

Opripramol **22a** was much less effective than imipramine **20a** in antagonizing the effects of reserpine and tetrabenazine in acute studies in the rat, yet it did antagonize apomorphine induced emesis in the dog, whereas imipramine **20a** does not. In this regard, one can see the emergence of some biological properties associated with neuroleptics, such as chlorpromazine (i.e. antagonism of apomorphine emesis) and the diminution of some properties associated with antidepressants (i.e. antagonism of tetrabenazine and reserpine). Nevertheless, in man opipramol **22a** does show significant antianxiety and antidepressant effects (136).

An interesting development has been that with some antidepressants there is a marked difference in their central anticholinergic effects relative to their peripheral effects. It may be possible to utilize this property for the treatment of Parkinson's disease. Several compounds derived from tricyclic antidepressant research programs are being evaluated clinically in Parkinson's disease, e.g. MK 130 **6a** (134) and elantrine (178).

d. Ketipramine

One other analog of imipramine **20a,** which has received some clinical attention is Ketipramine **23** (145, 164).

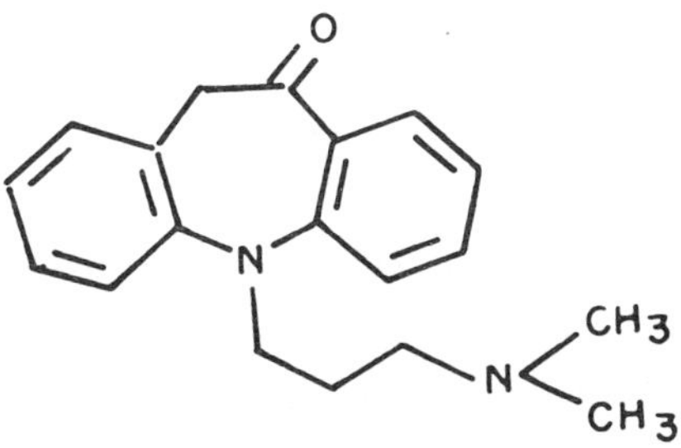

23

The interesting background of the selection of Ketipramine **23** for clinical trial has been described by Kuhn (114). Emphasis was placed on the absence of certain biological effects, and on peripheral anticholinergic properties. Thus, in this regard Ketipramine **22** resembles lopramine **20e.** Ketipramine **23** does possess clinically useful antidepressant properties, but there is presently no evidence to suggest that it has a special place in therapy over imipramine **20a.**

e. Polycyclic Analogs of Imipramine

Various bridged and cyclized versions of imipramine **20a** have been reported. None of these have demonstrated clinically useful antidepressant effects. One interesting example is **23a** (89), but there does not appear to

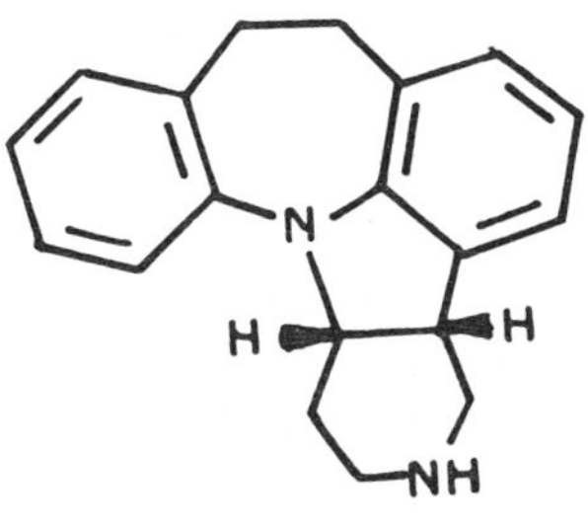

23a

have been any biological data reported on this compound.

f. Mianserin and Related Compounds

Mianserin **24a,** developed by Organon,

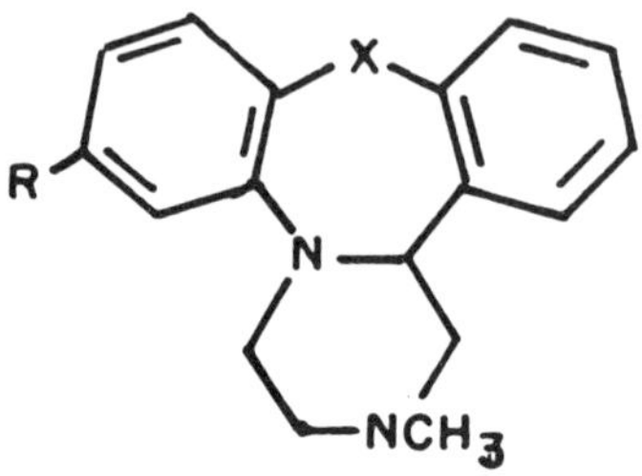

24a	X = $-CH_2$	R = H
24b	X = -O-	R = H
24c	X = -O-	R = CH_3
24d	X = $\cdot CH_2CH_2\cdot$	R = H
24e	X = $\cdot CH{:}CH\cdot$	R = H

possesses a dibenzoazepine tricyclic ring system isomeric with that of imipramine **20a.** The pharmacological profile of this compound (155, 184) did not suggest antidepressant potential in man. It seemed more likely that mianserin would be an antihistamine. Nevertheless, as an outcome of E.E.G. studies in man, which showed that mianserin **24a** induced changes similar to those caused by amitriptyline **1a** (99), Mianserin **24a** has been further investigated clinically for its antidepressant potential (56).

Mianserin **24a** seems free of the peripheral anticholinergic effects of other tricyclic antidepressants. It does, however, cause marked sedation, although some tolerance to this effect is seen on continued treatment.

Other analogs of mianserin, **24b** and **24c,** have been evaluated clinically (97), but mianserin **24a** was preferred for further study based on a more potent antiserotonin and a weaker antihistaminic effect (56).

Other mianserin analogs have been described by the Organon group (180), e.g. **24d** and **24e,** but these compounds were essentially inactive in rat uterus test for antiserotonin activity and do not seem to have been pursued further.

g. Dothiepin

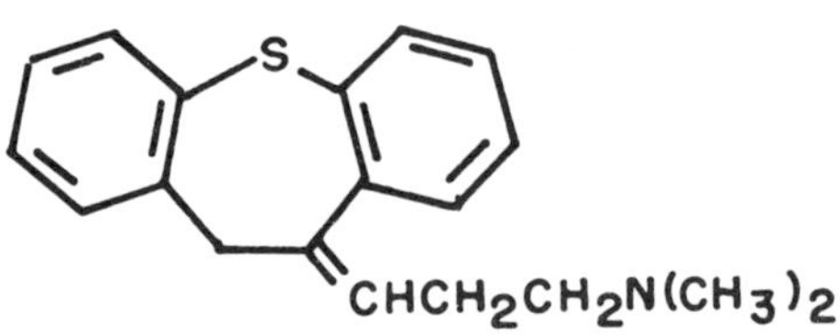

25

Dothiepin **25** has been compared in a double blind controlled study against amitriptyline **1a** (123). It was found in this patient population to be as effective and better tolerated than amitriptyline **1a.** Nevertheless, no further studies on this compound seem to have been reported.

Structurally, this compound is unique among the tricyclic antidepressants of the 6.7.6 type in that a three-carbon basic side chain is attached to the two-atom bridge between the aromatic rings.

3. *6-7-6 Heterocyclic With Two Heteroatoms in the Central Ring*

a. Amoxapine and Related Compounds

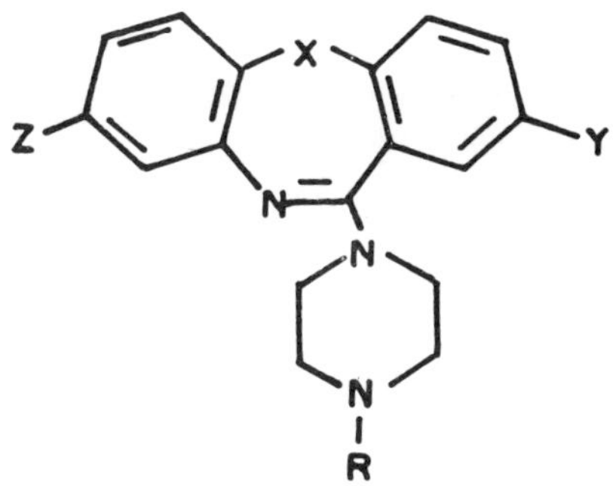

26a	X = O	Y = Cl	Z = R = H	
26b	X = NH	Y = H	Z = Cl	R = CH_3
26c	X = S	Y = Cl	Z = H	R = CH_3
26d	X = O	Y = Cl	Z = H	R = CH_3
26e	X = S	Y = R = CH_3	Z = H	

Amoxapine **26a** is perhaps the "overlap" antidepressant from a family of neuroleptics, just as the protriptyline analog **5** might be described as a neuroleptic from a family of antidepressants. The simple structural change between amoxapine **26a** and loxapine **26d** causes a major change in the biological profile (116).

Although opinions differ about the clinical value of loxapine **26d** as a neuroleptic (73, 192), there is no evidence that it has antidepressant properties in man. On the other hand, amoxapine **26a,** in a double blind study, showed good antidepressant properties with relatively mild side effects (69). Interestingly though, these side effects seem to be mainly of an anticholinergic nature, and this has been reported in other studies of amoxapine **26a** (32). This is in contrast to the animal studies which were reported to show that amoxapine **26a** was devoid of anticholinergic properties. The position of amoxapine **26a** in the future therapy of depression is unclear; it may be of special benefit for only a specific target population, perhaps mixed psychosis and depression. The structure activity relationships in this area have been more thoroughly investigated from the neuroleptic standpoint, i.e. as analogs of clozapine **26b** (46), clothiapine **26c** (126), and metiapine **26e** (66), and a review from the chemical standpoint has been presented (159).

b. Dibenzepin and Related Compounds

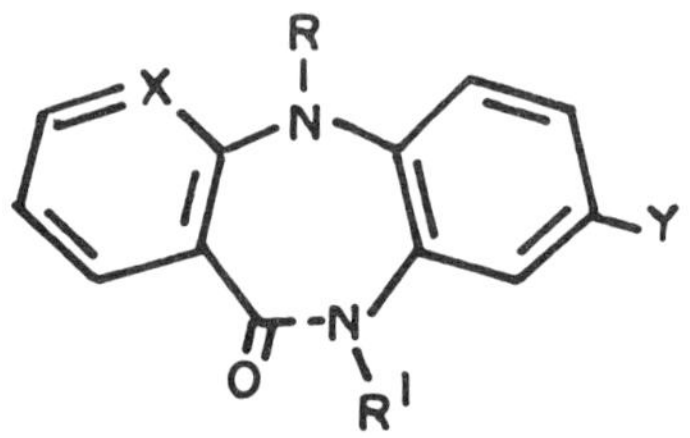

27a R = CH_3	R'	$-(CH_2)_2N(CH_3)_2$	X = CH	Y = H
27b R = CH_3	R'	$-(CH_2)_2N(CH_3)_2$	X = CH	Y = $SO_2CH_2CH_3$
27c R = H	R	$CH_2CH(CH_3)N(CH_3)_2$	X = N	Y = H

Dibenzepin **27a** represents a major structural departure from the amitriptyline **1a**/imipramine **20a** type of tricyclic antidepressant in that it has only a two-carbon basic side chain which is attached to the two atom bridge between the aromatic rings. Dibenzepin **27a** is a relatively old compound (96) and it has not supplanted imipramine **20a** or amitriptyline **1a** in the markets where it has been introduced. Nevertheless, clinical studies still appear which claim comparability with the established compounds (57).

Apart from work by the original developers of dibenzepin **27a**, the Wander group, it has been the target of only few efforts. Two compounds which have been described recently are SM-307 from Tanabe Seiyaku **27b** (140) and UP 106 **27c** (124).

The claim for SM-307 **27b** is fewer peripheral anticholinergic and antihistamine effects. It remains to be seen whether these results presage improved tolerability in man.

c. Other Compounds

In this general category of a central heterocyclic ring with two hetero atoms, the other significant compounds have been discussed as an integral part of the structure activity relationships of the compound with one hetero atom to which they were related, e.g. Mianserin analogs **24b** and **24c** (see section 2.1.2.5).

B. 6-6-6 Tricyclics

1. 6-6-6 Carbocyclic

By definition, this class of compounds is derived from anthracene. Therefore, some provision structurally is usually made to block any metabolic process which would cause conversion to the planar anthracene derivative. Such a flat tricyclic structure is presumed to be devoid of antidepressant activity (191).

a. Melitracen

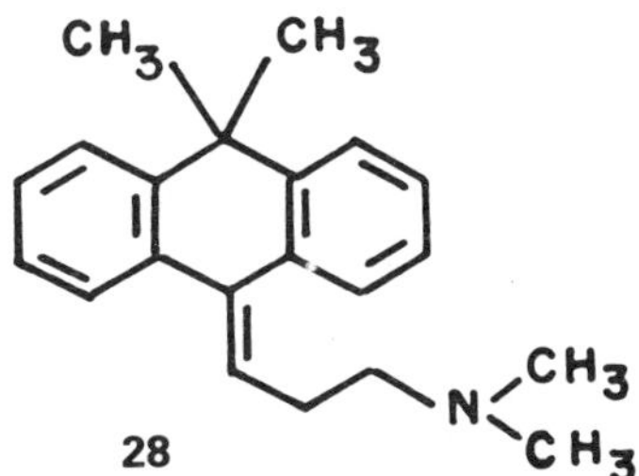

28

Melitracen **28** is blocked to metabolic aromatization by the gem dimethyl group. It is a relatively old compound (93). In double blind studies versus established compounds, e.g. imipramine **20a,** melitracen **28** appears to be less effective, but better tolerated (20).

b. Maprotiline

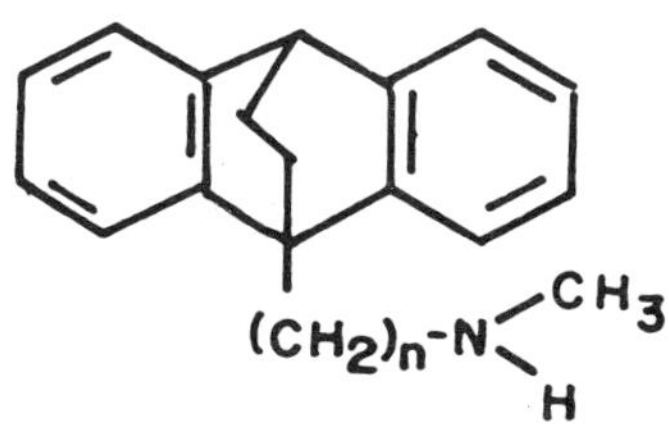

29a	n = 3
29b	n = 2
29c	n = 1

Maprotiline **29a** is blocked to aromatization by an ethano bridge between positions 9 and 10. This compound represents one of the most interesting new types of antidepressant. It was the subject of a major symposium in St. Moritz, Switzerland, in 1972, which was sponsored by CIBA-GEIGY, the developers of maprotiline **29a.** The proceedings of this symposium have now been published, and, as well as providing a source of many interesting biological and clinical details of maprotiline **29a,** it is also an excellent status of the art report with regard to evaluation of antidepressants generally (112).

An evaluation of maprotiline **29a** by a reviewer other than the developer, describes it as an "effective safe antidepressant that possesses properties different from the tricyclics" (10).

Several points from the review are deserving of mention. Maprotiline **29a** is less sedative and causes fewer anticholinergic side effects than amitriptyline **1a.** Tricyclic antidepressants are, however, associated with problems other than the patient inconveniences of a dry mouth; EKG changes have been noted on prolonged administration (45). The package inserts for amitriptyline **1a** and imipramine **20a** both contain warnings when these compounds are used in patients with cardiovascular disorders. The preliminary evidence suggests that maprotiline **29a** has less effect on the cardiovascular system, and may be quite safe to use in such patients. Maprotiline **29a** does not represent the "rapid onset of effect compound," which has been sought by most clinicians. Two to four weeks treatment is still needed to see the maximum clinical response.

One of the most interesting structure activity relationships with maprotiline **29a** is variation of the length of the side chain. This has been well described by Bein (17). If the side chain of maprotiline **29a** is reduced by one methylene group to give **29b,** essentially all of the biological properties are lost. If the chain is reduced by a further methylene group to give benzoctamine **29c,** biological properties appear which are quite different from maprotiline **29a.** The biological profile of benzoctamine **29c** may be described as that of a minor tranquilizer. This dramatic change in biological profile by variation in the side chain length is reminiscent of that seen in the change of the ethano bridge of imipramine **20a** for sulfur to give chlorpromazine **34a.** The differences in the structure-activity relationships between maprotiline **29a** and the other tricyclic antidepressants further emphasizes that maprotiline **29a** represents a significant new development in antidepressant drug design.

c. SKF 28175

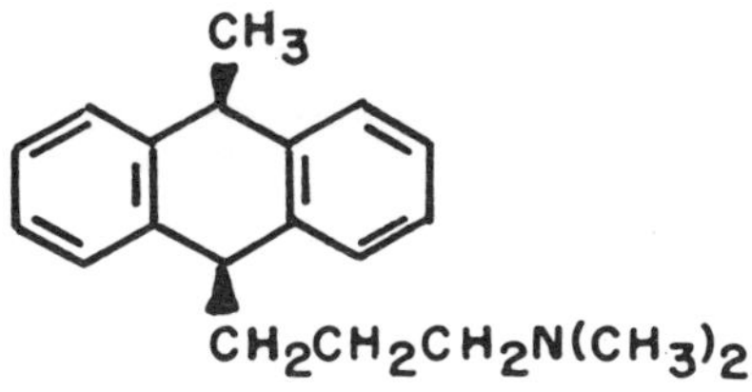

30

A member of this class, which is not blocked to aromatization, has been described, SKF 28175 **30** (63). If aromatization by a metabolic process does take place it would convert SKF 28175 **30** from a molecule, where the aromatic rings are oriented to one another, as in a tricyclic antidepressant, to an anthracene where the rings are coplanar, i.e. closer to the orientation in a neuroleptic (191). This might explain the unusual combination of pharmacological properties, e.g. that SKF 28175 **30** potentiates the norepinephrine pressor response in the dog like amitriptyline **1a,** yet it also antagonizes amphetamine induced stereotypy in the rat, like chlorpromazine **34a.** No clinical reports have appeared on this compound, so its effects in man cannot be evaluated.

d. Other Bridged Compounds

As the importance of maprotiline **29a** has become evident, there have been several bridged compounds described. Unfortunately, most of these references are to the patent literature or only to a description of the synthetic procedure. Reference has already been made to two such cases **12** and **14** (188, 131). Other examples falling within the scope of the 6:6:6 ring system are **31a** (39) and **31b** (72).

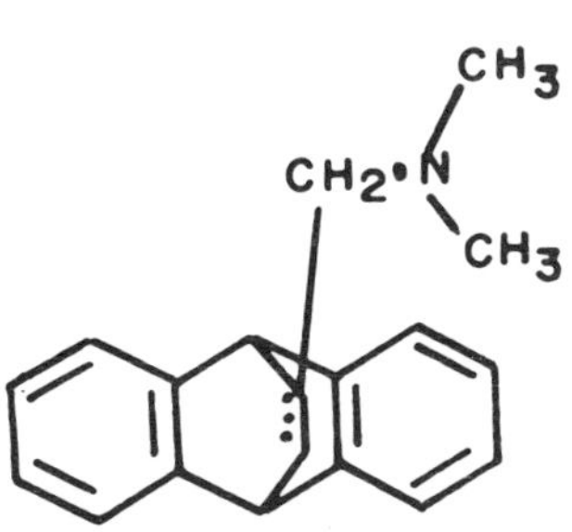

31a WITH A DOUBLE BOND IN THE BRIDGE

31b WITHOUT A DOUBLE BOND IN THE BRIDGE

2. *6-6-6 Heterocyclic. One Heteroatom in the Central Ring*

a. Thioxanthenes

Structural modification, in a given series, usually gives compounds with similar biological profiles. Nevertheless, as has been emphasized at several points in this review, there is always the possibility of encountering "an overlap compound" in a given series. As has been mentioned previously, modification of amitriptyline **1a** to compound **6b** gave a substance with a neuroleptic profile. The reverse situation has been encountered in the thioxanthenes, a series which has usually provided neuroleptics (47).

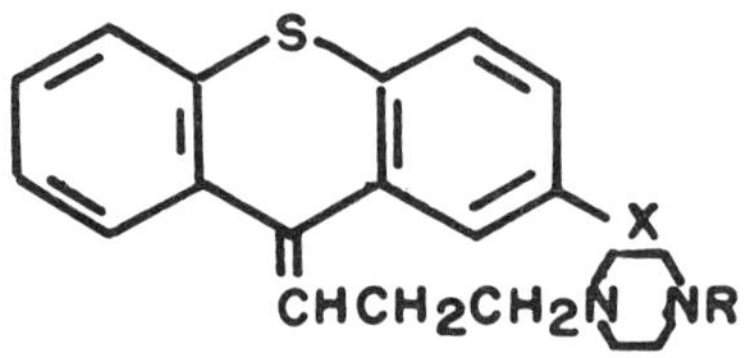

32a	X = $SO_2N(CH_3)_2$	R = $\cdot CH_3$
32b	X = $-CF_3$	R = $\cdot CH_2CH_2OH$

Thus, thioxthixene **32a** is a potent neuroleptic, whereas flupentixol **32b** has demonstrated a good antidepressant effect, with only minimal side effects, in a large open label study of depressed patients (151).

b. Acridones

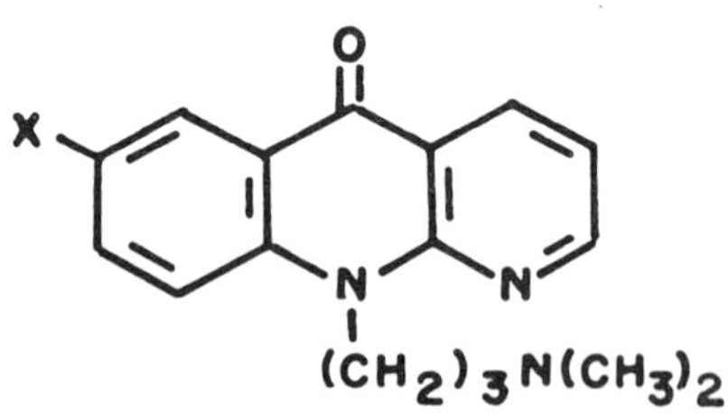

33a	H
33b	OCH_3
33c	Cl

A family of substituted acridones **33a, 33b** and **33c,** has recently been described as potential antidepressants (58), but no clinical results have been described.

c. Other Compounds

One other compound **9g** in this group has been previously described as part of the structure activity work done on noxiptiline **8** (15).

3. 6-6-6 Heterocyclic Two Hetero atoms in the Central Ring

a. Phenothiazines

As with the thioxanthenes (Section 2.2.2.1), structural modifications of the phenothiazine type generally yield neuroleptics. Nevertheless, it is possible to synthesize phenothiazine compounds which exhibit biological properties characteristic of imipramine **20a** and amitriptyline **1a.** The pharmacological profile and structure activity relationships of the neuroleptic phenothiazines have been well reviewed (79, 80).

In order to observe biological properties typical of an antidepressant, it seems that, in accord with the hypothesis discussed previously (191), it is necessary to introduce a substituent which causes the ring structure to be further deformed from planarity. This is accomplished by introduction of substituents in the 1 position.

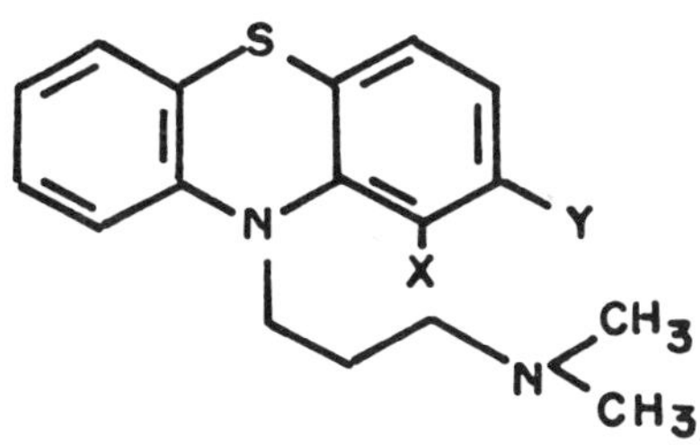

34a X = H; Y = Cl

34b X = Cl; Y = H

Thus, while chlorpromazine **34a** is the classical neuroleptic (79), the isomer **34b** has imipramine-like activity in the biological tests, e.g. antagonism of reserpine ptosis in rodents (106).

b. Azaphen

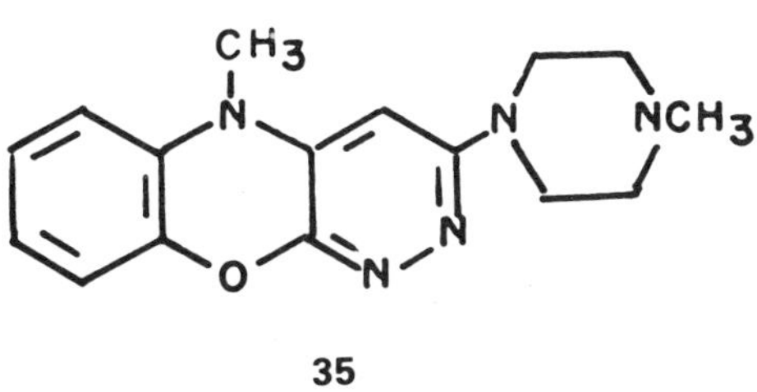

35

Azaphen **35** has been described by Russian workers to be a clinically effective antidepressant (146). Further details of its similarity to imipramine have been published (128).

Structurally, Azaphen **35** represents a major departure from the classical tricyclic antidepressant such as imipramine **20a.** Whether it offers any real advantages over established therapy still remains a moot point, in the absence of objective clinical data.

C. Other Linear Tricyclics

Kaiser and Zirkle have provided an excellent review of other linear tricyclic antidepressants with five and eight membered central rings of various types (107). They concluded that while several of such compounds did have some of the appropriate biological properties, none represented a significant advance from the clinical standpoint. In this reviewer's opinion, nothing has occurred with this type of compound in the past few years to change that conclusion.

One clinically significant compound iprindole **56,** which might be considered under this heading, will be reviewed along with other indoles (Section 6.1.1.).

III. ANGULAR TRICYCLIC ANTIDEPRESSANTS

This group of compounds **37** can be imagined to be perhaps performing a very similar role to that of the linear tricyclic antidepressants **36.**

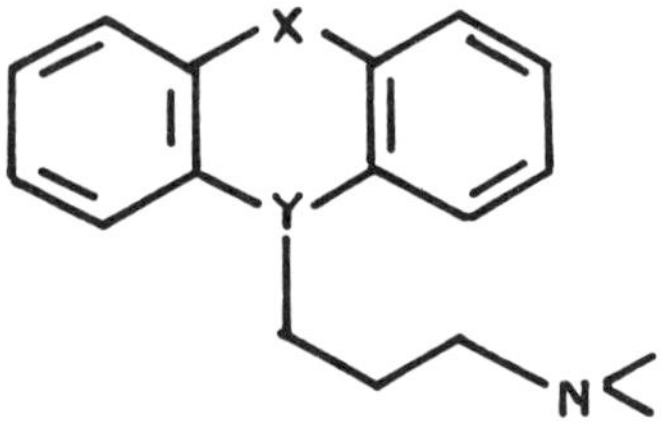

36

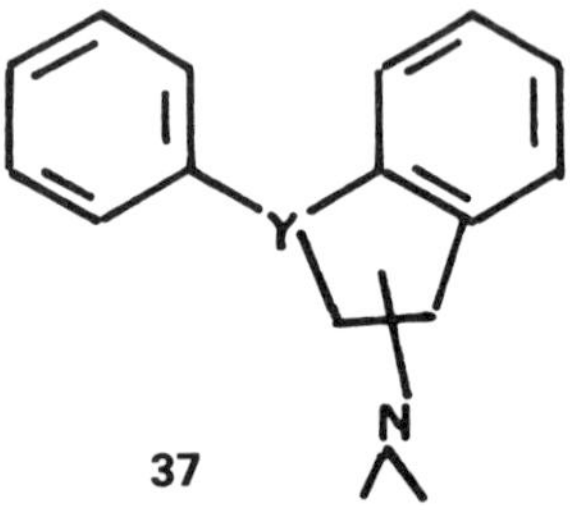

37

Removal of the bridging atom or atoms -x- from **36** would still permit many of the compounds **37** covered in this section to fit the same receptor. There are, however, important differences in biological profiles and tolerability of these compounds, when they are compared with the tricyclics.

A. 6-5-6 Angular Tricyclic

1. 6-5-6 Angular Carbocyclic Tricyclic

By definition this refers to 1-phenyl indane derivatives.

a. Indriline and Related Compounds

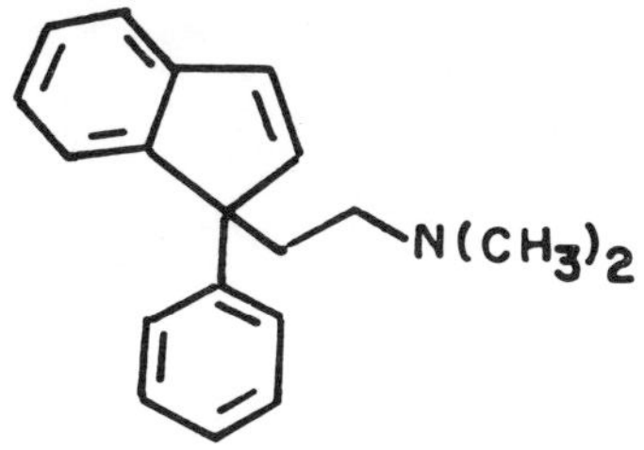

38

Indriline **38** of Mead Johnson, is the best investigated compound of this type. Since the original report (51), a more detailed account of the pharmacology has been published (25).

There do not appear to be published accounts of clinical studies with indriline **38** since the pharmacology appeared in 1968 (25). Therefore, one may conclude that indriline **38** has not proved to be a useful therapy for the treatment of depression, or that toxicological problems precluded clinical trials.

b. Phenindamine Related Compounds

A structure activity study on the antihistamine phenindamine showed the dilhydrodesmethyl analog **39** to be very effective in antagonizing tetrabenazine ptosis in rats and reserpine hypothermia in mice (8).

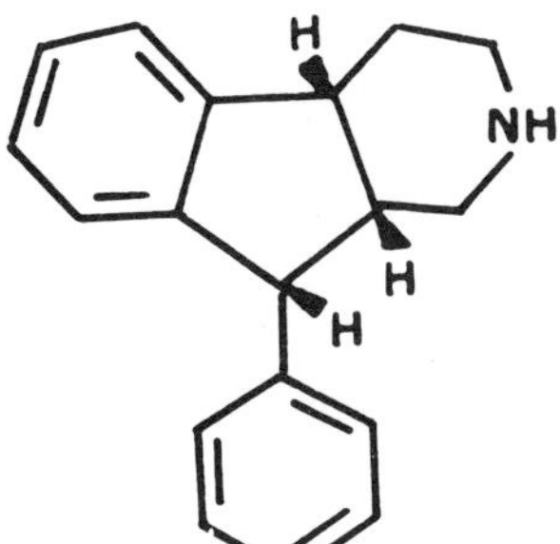

39

Interestingly, the phenyl group can be cis or trans to the ring fusion without affecting the pharmacological profile very much. Unfortunately, in a 90 day rat study testicular damage was observed at 25 mg/kg p.o. Therefore, further clinical studies, one presumes, are precluded from an ethical and regulatory standpoint.

2. 6-5-6 Angular Tricyclic Heterocyclic-One Heteroatom

a. N-Aryl Oxindoles and Related Compounds

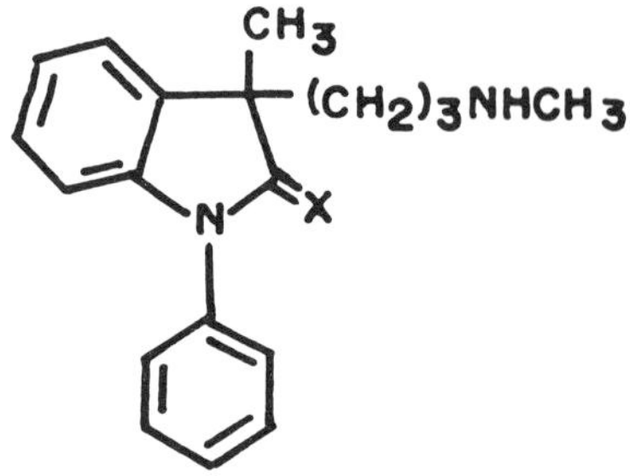

40a X = O

40b = H_2

The first report of these compounds **40a** and **40b** and UK 3540 and UK 3557 described them as possessing the pharmacological profile of the tricyclic antidepressants but without anticholinergic properties (29). Nevertheless, the first clinical report of UK 3540 as amedalin **40a** described extreme difficulty in initiation of urination, an effect usually associated with anticholinergic drugs. Also, there were complaints of scrotal discomfort (68).

It would seem that further clinical development has been directed to daledalin **40b,** although tolerability here may be a problem also. Daledalin **40b** was compared in a crossover double blind study versus amitriptyline **1a** (190). While efficacy was comparable, six of the thirty-eight patients receiving daledalin **40b,** reported headaches. Recently, the full paper on the preparation and structure activity work in this series has been published by the English Pfizer group (28). These authors comment how similar the structural requirements for optimal activity are to those of imipramine **20a** and amitriptyline **1a.**

b. Isobenzfurans and Related Compounds

These compounds can be viewed in an alternative way to that outlined in the beginning of this section, i.e. general formula **37.** Instead one may view LU 3-010 **41a** as being related to the bridged amitriptyline analog MK 940 **10** by the breaking of the bond between the aryl group and the bridge carbon bearing the hydroxyl group.

In fact, LU 3-010 **41a** does possess strong antireserpine activity, and strongly potentiates catecholamines (138). The Lundbeck group also described the thia analog LU 5-003 **41b** in similar terms (142).

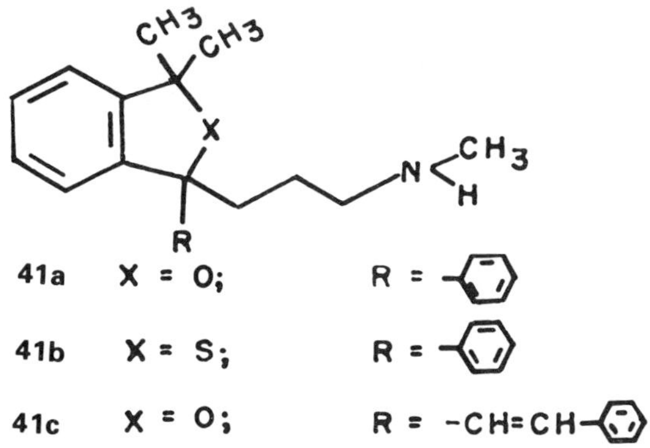

Since these earlier reports, several papers on the pharmacology and biochemistry of these substances have been published (121), but no clinical work has been reported. One, therefore, presumes that there may be some toxicological problems which preclude study in man.

A new analog **41c** was recently reported by a Lederle group (129), and was claimed to be almost as potent as LU3-010 **41a** in reversing tetrabenazine ptosis in mice, but no toxicological data were reported. Yet another variant **42,** from an ICI group, was described in more pharmacological detail (120), but no clinical results have been published.

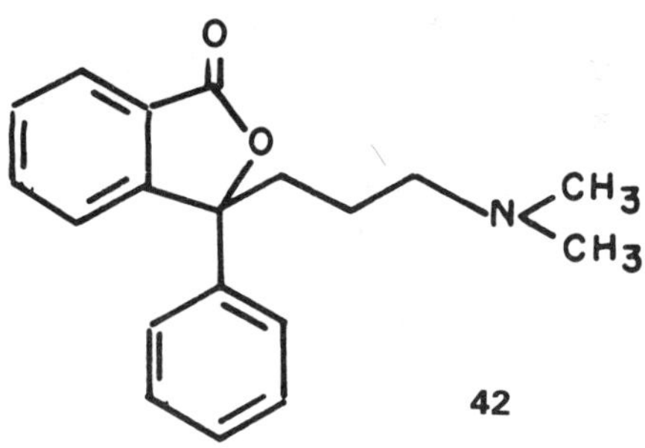

42

3. Angular Tricyclic Heterocyclic - Two Heteroatoms

a. N-Aryl Benzimidazolones

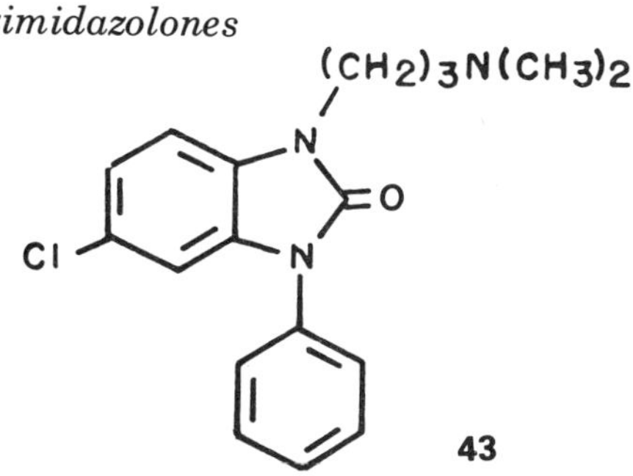

43

Clodazone **43** of Wander is the only compound of significance in this category. It has been tested in a large open label study with moderately good results (4).

Side effects do not seem to have been a problem in this study, so the sponsors of this study must have been discouraged by the moderate response in endogenous depressions, which usually respond well to drug therapy. Some variants of this type, e.g. N-aryl-pyrido imidazolones, have been reported (38), but no biological data have been published.

B. 6-6-6 Angular Tricyclic Antidepressants

1. Angular Tricyclic Carbocyclic

No examples of this class have been reported.

2. Angular Tricyclic Heterocyclic– one Heteroatom

a. 4-Aryl isoquinolines

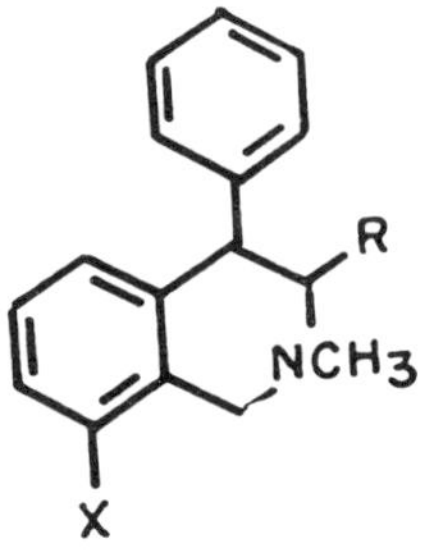

44a R = H; X = NH_2

44b R = X = CH_3

Nomifensin **44a** from Hoechst is an interesting new type of antidepressant. The compound itself is not new (87). The first account of the pharmacology of nomifensin **44a** described studies on the antagonism of reserpine and tetrabenazine effects in rodents and its ability to potentiate the pressor effect of norepinephrine (91). A recent account of nomifensin **44a** (90) describes the absence of cardiovascular and anticholinergic effects, which are typically associated with tricyclic compounds. Although clinical data are not provided, a good antidepressant action with a mild central stimulating effect was reported to have been observed in man. If this profile, and the claims of efficacy and tolerability are substantiated by well controlled studies against imipramine **20a** amitriptyline **1a,** then nomifensin **44a** will become a significant new development in antidepressive therapy.

There have been other analogs reported in the patent literature (88) which may indicate interest by other groups in nomifensin **44a** as a target compound.

A Dow group recently described an analog **44b** (175). The preliminary account of the pharmacology provided in this article suggests that this compound **44b** resembles nomifensin **44a.**

IV. OTHER TRICYCLIC ANTIDEPRESSANTS

A. Phenanthridines

Phenanthridines are the only other class of tricyclic compounds for which are substantiated claims of antidepressant effects.

1. OI-77

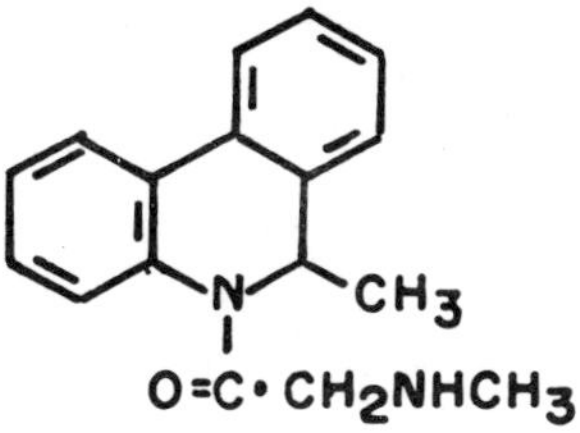

45

A compound from Organon OI-77 **45** was reported to resemble imipramine **20a** in a small open label trial (98). These similarities were in the EEG changes seen in patients on the drug compared to placebo and imipramine **20a** groups, the Global Rating Scales, and also in the side effects, such as dryness of the mouth and drowsiness.

2. Fantridone

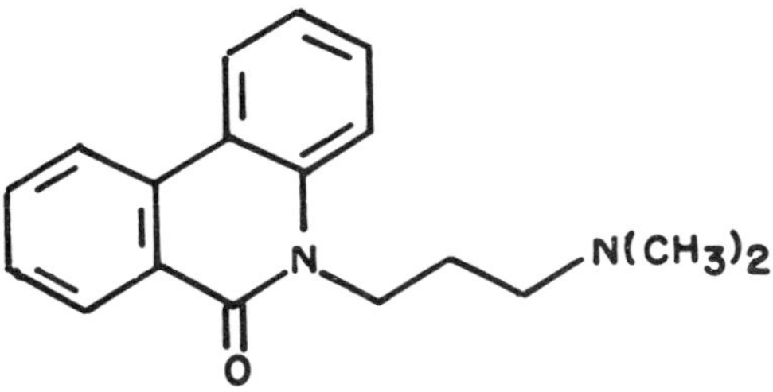

46

Fantridone **46** was mentioned in the Council on Drugs, New Names List No. 78 of the American Medical Association as an antidepressant (43). No details, chemical, biological or clinical, seem to have been published about fantridone **46.**

3. Phenanthridine Analogs of Mianserin

In the broad scope of the structure activity work carried out on mianserin **24,** a phenanthridine analog **47** was prepared.

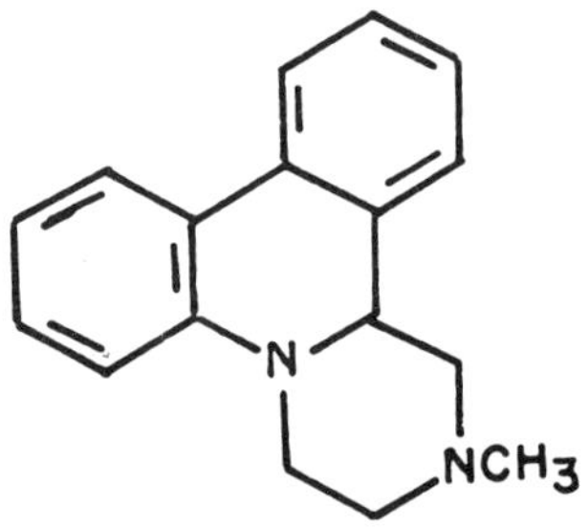

47

This compound **47** had only very low activity in the antiserotonin models used to assay mianserin analogs. This virtual lack of biological activity was attributed to the inappropriateness of the orientation of the planes of the aromatic rings with respect to one another (180).

V. DIPHENYLMETHANE DERIVATIVES

A. Diphenylmethane derivatives. Both aryl rings carbocyclic

1. AHR 1118

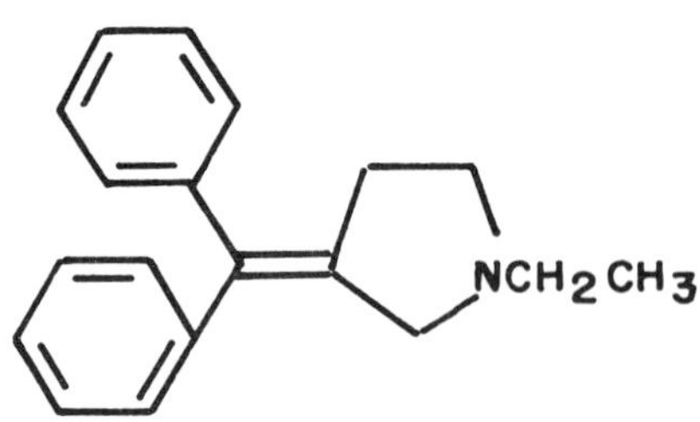

48

AHR 1118 **48** antagonizes reserpine induced hypothermia in mice, but has also been characterized as an antidepressant by EEG studies in cats. But, AHR 1118, **48** did not show the characteristic suppression of paradoxical sleep (101).

2. Tofenacine

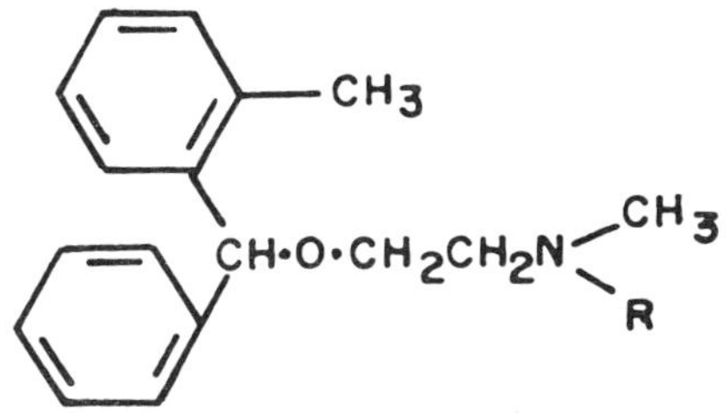

49a R = H

49b R = CH_3

Tofenacine **49a** is related to orphenadrine **49b,** an anticholinergic, which is used in Parkinsonism. Tofenacine **49a,** in an open label study using a rating scale as a measure of efficacy, was regarded as being more successful in neurotic and mixed depressions than endogenous depression (22). Surprisingly, there were no reports of anticholinergic side effects.

3. 1,1 Diphenyl-3-Aminopropanes

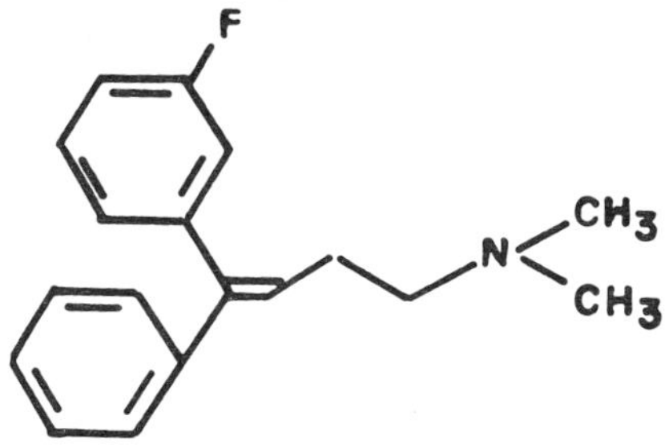

50

Several 1,1 diphenyl-3-aminopropanes were prepared and evaluated by antagonism of reserpine induced hypothermia in the mouse and the inhibition of serotonin uptake by human platelets. Compound **50** was the most active member of the series (105).

This is an old, well investigated, area. The chances that compound **50** will warrant clinical trial seem small.

4. Diphenylaminopropanols

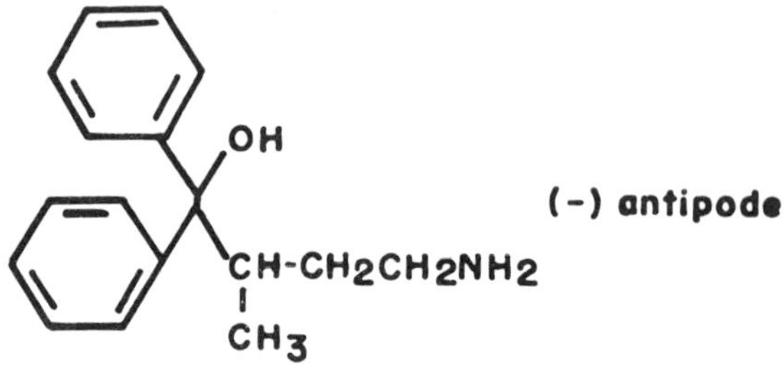

51

U 23807A **51** from Upjohn was described as being inactive in a pilot study in patients with neurotic depression (163). Furthermore, a diverse collection of side effects were recorded from visual hallucinations to episodic dizziness. A full account of the chemical work and some preliminary accounts of the pharmacology have appeared (133, 132, 110).

5. Gamfexine

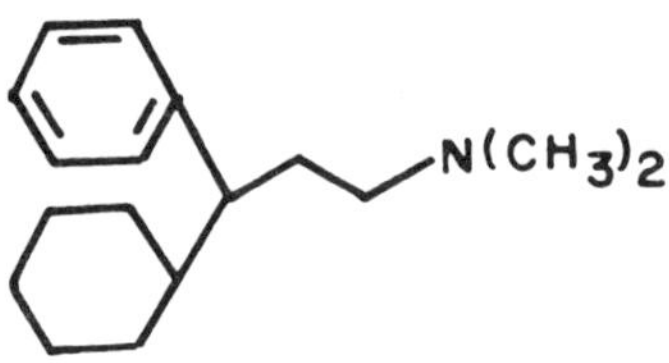

52

Gamfexine **52** from Winthrop was evaluated in a small group of endogenous depressed patients (76).

A comparable group was treated with imipramine **20a** for control purposes. A marked stimulant effect was seen with gamfexine **52** even leading to a worsening of depression in two patients, and side effects in all.

Winthrop apparently does not intend to pursue gamfexine **52** as an antidepressant because a subsequent clinical study described its use in combination with thioridazine in anergic schizophrenia (193).

6. 5.1.6 Cyprolidol

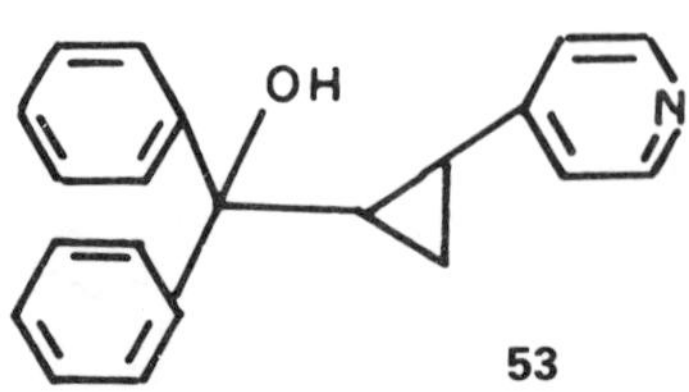

53

Cyprolidol **53** from Neisler was evaluated in a controlled study versus imipramine **20a** in a small group of endogeneously depressed patients (83).

Cyprolidol **53** was well tolerated but, if anything, slower acting and less efficacious than imipramine **20a.**

B. Diphenylmethane derivatives; one ring heterocyclic

1. Sch 12560

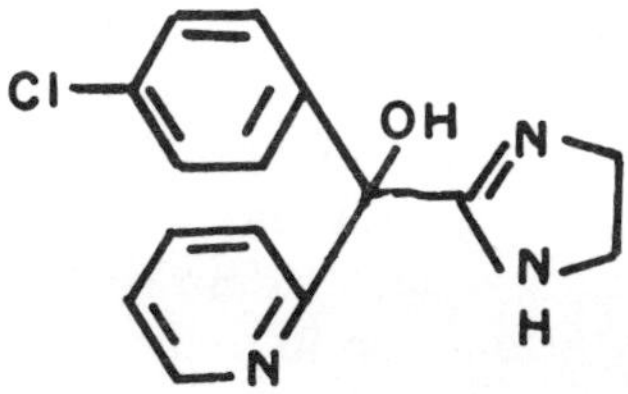

54

Although the preliminary account of the pharmacology of Sch 12560 **54** was published by the Schering group (172), further details have been published by other groups (158, 122).

As the Schering group provided Dr. Lippman of Ayerst with their experimental compound, one presumes that they did not have any further interest in developing it themselves.

No clinical studies have been published with Sch 12560 **54.**

2. Miscellaneous

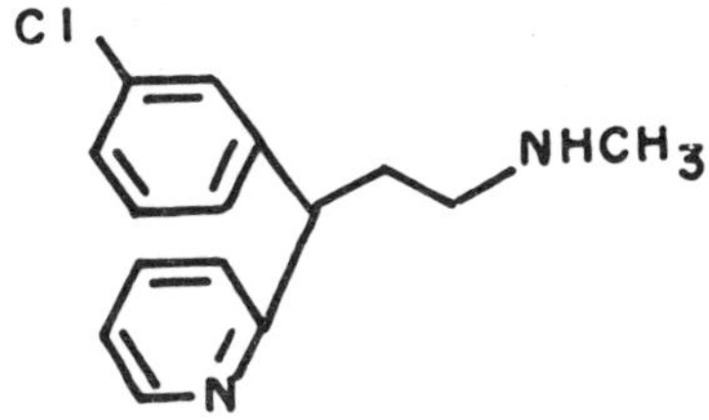

55

A patent disclosed compounds such as **55,** but no biological details have appeared as yet (71).

VI. INDOLES

A. Tricyclic Indoles

1. Iprindole

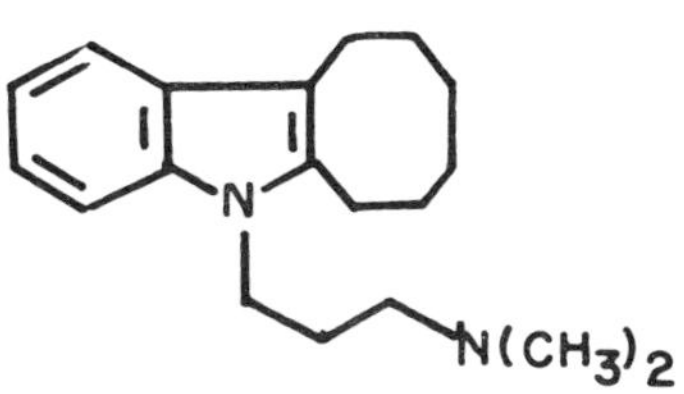

56

Iprindole **56** is the most significant of the indole antidepressants. It has been introduced onto the market in the U.K. by Wyeth. Iprindole **56,** in its biological profile, clearly stands apart from all other antidepressants in clinical usage. Like AHR 1118 **48** (Section 5.1.1.), but unlike imipramine **20a** and amitriptyline **1a,** iprindole **56** does not block REM sleep in cats (14). Interestingly, iprindole **56** is ineffective in antagonizing the effects of tetrabenazine or reserpine in rodents (77). These are the tests which have been used most to help identify potential new antidepressants. One characteristic property that iprindole **56** shares in common with imipramine **20a** and amitriptyline **1a** is the potentiation of the central actions of amphetamine (77). It does this, however, not by blocking reuptake of biogenic amines from the synaptic cleft as the tricyclic antidepressants do, but by inhibition of the para hydroxylation step in amphetamine metabolism (64).

While such biological properties are understood in some detail, their significance, concerning the clinical effects, remain obscure. It may well be that iprindole **56** has some as yet undisclosed effect on serotonergic mechanisms in the CNS, which are more significant for the clinical outcome than the now well understood adrenergic effects (55).

While the commercial success of iprindole **56** in the U.K. appears to be modest, perhaps because of unsubstantiated claims of hepatoxicity, there seems to be little doubt that iprindole **56** is an effective, well tolerated antidepressant in man (9). Iprindole **56** could prove to be a treatment of choice for depressed patients with cardiac problems, alluded to previously, with the classical tricyclic antidepressants (55).

2. WIN 27, 147-2

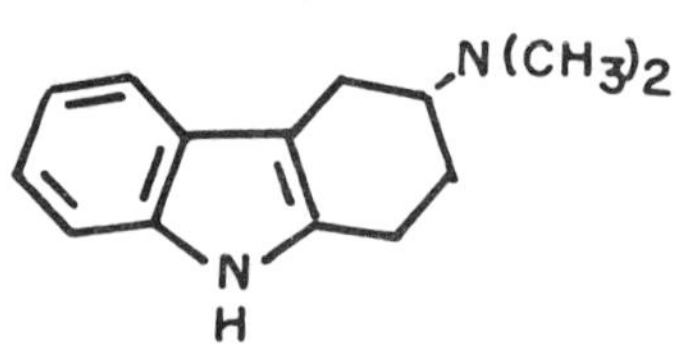

57

Since the first account of WIN 27, 147-2 **57** (167), a description of the biological profile and a small open label uncontrolled study have been published (67). Some degree of improvement was noted in the patients treated, but further studies are needed to give a fair assessment of this compound.

3. Carbidine

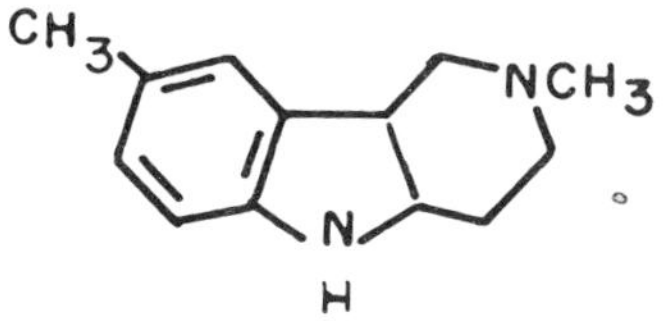

58

A preliminary clinical account of work with carbidine **58** was reported (13). Carbidine **58** seems to be of most use in depressed schizophrenics and its utility in a normal depressed patient group is less clear. A recent account of the pharmacology has appeared and the profile of carbidine **58** suggests a mixture of neuroleptic and antidepressant properties (12).

B. Other Indoles

1. Tetracyclic

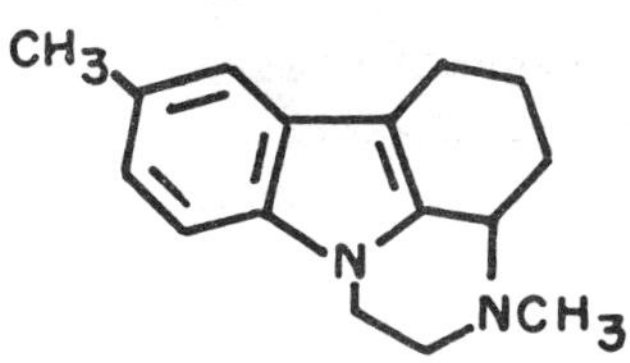

59

A compound **59** was reported as potentiating the effects of amphetamine and antagonizing those of reserpine in animals (127). No clinical reports about this compound have appeared.

2. Tryptophane and Derivatives

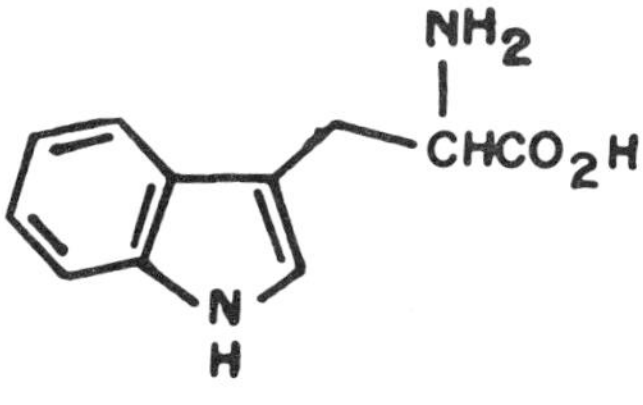

60

With the opinion of some workers in the field that serotonin levels in certain parts of the brain affect mood, considerable attention has been directed to tryptophane **60** (33).The analogy being made is with the treatment of Parkinsonism by administration of

L -DOPA. Efforts in this direction have been referred to in the introductory section (113, 109, 41). These efforts are of considerable importance for developing an understanding of the underlying biochemical defects in specific groups of depressed patients. Nevertheless, in this reviewer's opinion, the development of tryptophane alone or in combination, as established therapy for depression, seems unlikely.

Other developments in this area are the synthesis of small peptides incorporating the tryptophane moiety.

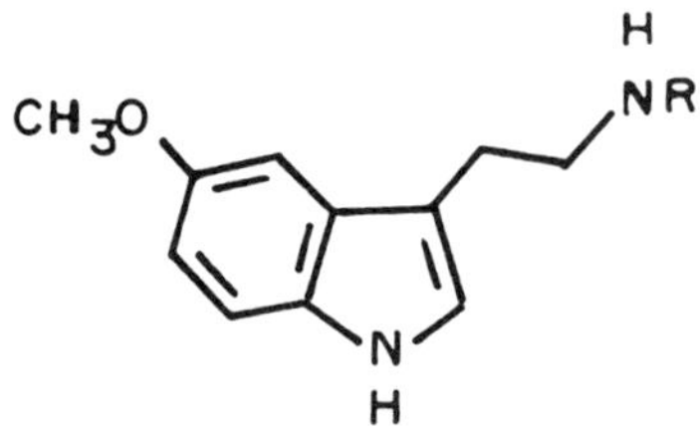

R = Phe-arg

= Arg

= His-phe-arg

61

These compounds **61** were less active than desmethyl imipramine **20b** in antagonizing tetrabenazine and reserpine in mice (160).

VII. MONOAMINE OXIDASE INHIBITORS (MAOI)

The mechanism by which MAO inhibitors influence the depressed state were alluded to in the introductory section. Excellent reviews of the antidepressant effects and the care necessary to achieve relatively side effect free use of the marketed MAO inhibitors have been published (92, 104, 150). This brief review will therefore describe recent efforts with experimental compounds. A complete review of MAO inhibitors with all their effects discussed, has recently appeared (86).

A. Clorgyline

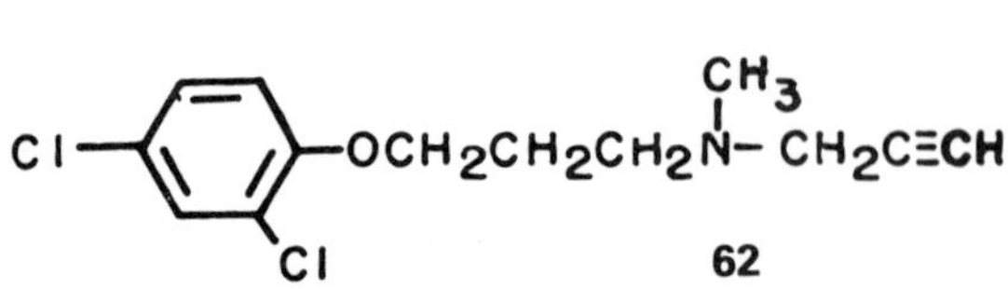

62

Clorgyline (M and B 9302) **62** was originally described in very optimistic terms after preliminary clinical experience (84). A subsequent account describes the same type of difficulties as with other MAO inhibitors, particularly with the requirement of dietary restriction in unsupervised patients (189).

At the biochemical level it has been possible to demonstrate that clorgyline **62** is substrate selective particularly inhibiting the oxidation of serotonin (36). It would seem, from the clinical experience though, that clorgyline **62** is not tissue selective, i.e. it does inhibit MAO in the periphery as well as the CNS.

B. A-25794

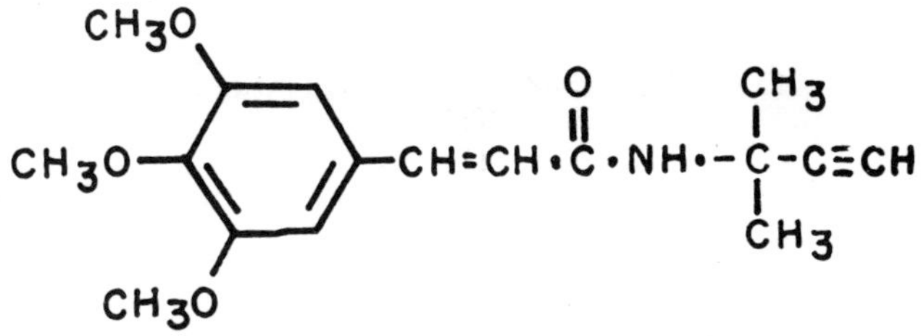

63

A-25794 **63** from Abbot was initially studied in an open label pilot clinical trial (60). The outcome was inconclusive, but further trial was recommended. A more definitive open label study described A-25794 as inactive (154). A full account of the pharmacology of A-25794 **63** has appeared (144).

C. Lilly 51641

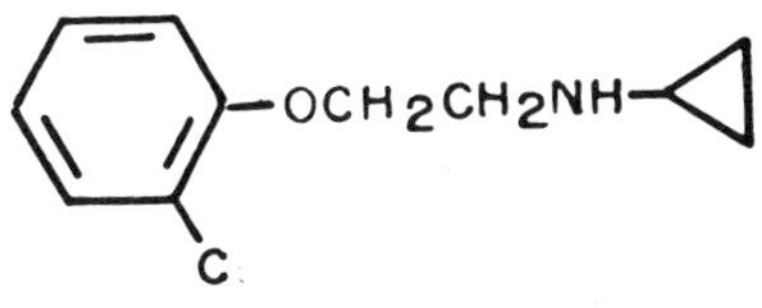

64

Lilly 51641 **64** has been described as both substrate selective and tissue selective in mouse brain versus mouse heart and liver, when compared to pargyline (65). It remains to be seen with Lilly 51641 **64** how these differences will translate into clinical effects.

D. Miscellaneous

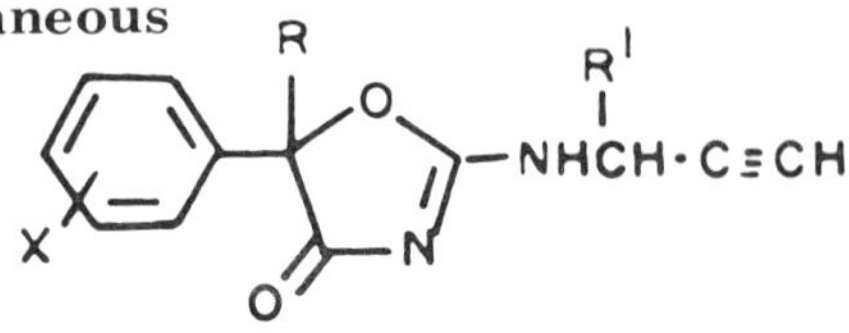

65

66 X = R = R' = H

A series of compounds **65** related to pemoline were described by Abbot to be potential antidepressants based on the DOPA potentiation test in the mouse (118). The most active compound of the series **66** showed an unusually long lasting effect in this test. Further, studies suggested that compound **66** may not be a central MAO inhibitor, despite the structural relationship to pargyline.

VIII. PHENETHYLAMINES AND RELATED COMPOUNDS

Before the advent of the tricyclic antidepressants, amphetamine **67a**

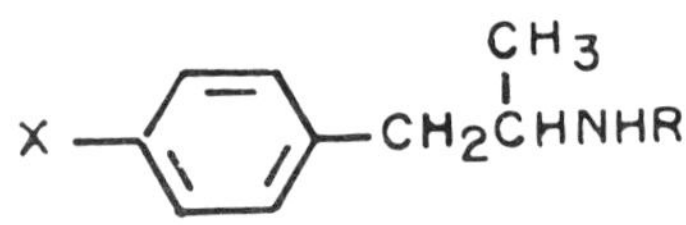

67a X = R = H

67b X = Cl; R = CH_3

67c X = Cl; R = H

67d X = H; R = CH_3

was used in the treatment of depression. It has the advantage of rapid onset of action, but suffers from many limitations, among the more serious being the stimulation of a retarded depressive into suicidal behavior. Amphetamine **67a** does have a place in the treatment of mild self-limiting reactive depressions, but even here it has been replaced by other therapy, e.g. methylphenidate (Ritalin®). Nevertheless, considerable interest still centers on phenethylamine derivatives, more for their role in uncovering the underlying pathology of depression and as biochemical tools rather than as new therapy.

A. Para-substituted amphetamines

Para-chloromethamphetamine **67b** is believed to act biologically by releasing serotonin and inhibiting its synthesis (166). A detailed structure/activity analysis of such serotonin depleting effects in mouse brain with amphetamine analogs was recently described (161). In man administration of para-chloromethamphetamine **67b** caused only slight central stimulation. Clinical improvement was noted in patients who were previously noted to have low levels of urinary 5-hydroxyindole acetic acid. During treatment, urinary excretion of 5-hydroxy indole acetic acid and 5-hydroxy tryptamine increased in all patients (183).

In a further study with para-chloromethamphetamine **67b,** some CNS stimulation was noted but without effects on sleep or appetite (47). In a double blind trial versus placebo, para-chloromethamphetamine **67b** was superior to placebo (182). This study also showed that para-chloramphetamine **67c** was not superior to para-chlormethamphetamine **67b** in treatment of depression (182). Notably, as in the previous studies, there was only mild CNS stimulation and no evidence of insomnia, anorexia, agitation, or hypertension, which are typically associated with amphetamine **67a** administration.

B. Para-methyl-α-ethyl-metatyramine

Para-methyl-α-ethyl-metatyramine **68a** is also capable of releasing serotonin from central stores (31). The related α methyl compound **68b** does not possess this property (30). Work by other groups has confirmed these findings with **68a** (49).

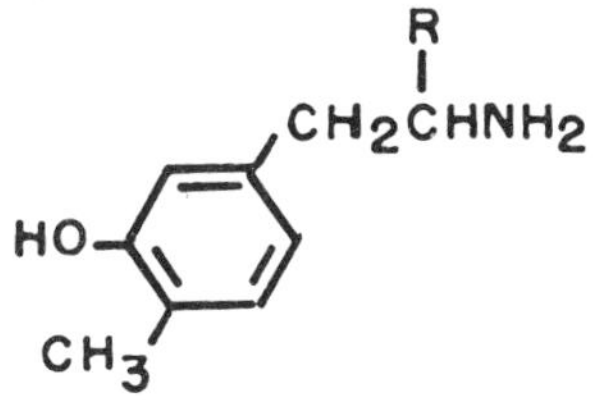

68a R = CH_2CH_3

68b R = CH_3

C. Aletamine

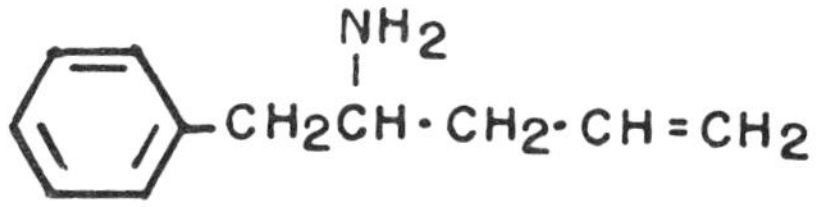

69

Aletamine **69** was originally tested in the clinic by Richardson Merrell as an analgetic. From some evidence of mood elevating effects seen in normal subjects, it was reevaluated pharmacologically as a potential antidepressant (85).

Aletamine **69** may also function by causing serotonin release in the CNS.

IX. PEPTIDES

A. Tryptophane Derivatives

These efforts were reviewed under Indoles (Section 6.2.2.), e.g. compounds **61** (160).

B. Thyrotropin Releasing Hormone (T.R.H.)

It was previously recognized that administration of *l* triiodothyramine had a beneficial effect on certain types of retarded depression (148). These findings encouraged Prange and his colleagues to investigate the use of thyrotropin releasing hormone (pyroglutamyl-histadylproline amide) clinically (147). In a ten-patient study, the effects of i.v. saline were compared to 600 mg of TRH. The effects on the Hamilton Rating System were compared for three successive days. A prompt but brief improvement occurred in all treated patients, without significant side effects. Similar findings were reported almost simultaneously by other groups (109, 181).

In this area the clinical studies seem to have preceded the pharmacological, but now studies in rodents have been published which substantiate the clinical observations. TRH potentiates the effects of DOPA in mice and this occurs also in hypophysectomized mice so that the effect is independent of the release of endogenous TSH (143). Other studies showed that TRH did not affect biogenic amine uptake by rabbit platelets or rat brain synaptosomes, as do the tricyclic antidepressants (177).

C. Miscellaneous Peptides

A patent describes the activity of L-prolyl-L-leucyl-glycylamide in potentiating the effects of DOPA as was reported for TRH (1).

X. DIVERSE STRUCTURAL TYPES

A. A-10749

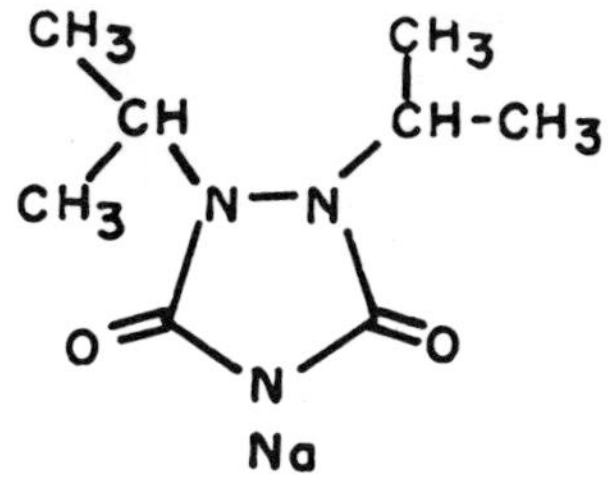

70

Several clinical studies have been reported with A-10749 **70** from Abbot. A preliminary study suggested some activity (74) and this was confirmed in a double blind study versus imipramine **20a** (26). More recent studies show less conclusive results (23).

As Brown points out in his paper (23), it would be of interest to see whether A-10749 **70** has any effect on serotonin reuptake or release. It would also be of interest to see if the metrazole antagonism described in the biological studies is an indicator of any antianxiety effects in man.

B. FI 6654

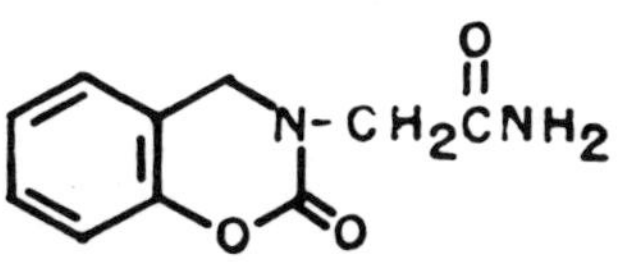

71

FI 6654 **71** has been described as an antagonist of the effects of reserpine (168). This antagonism was demonstrated in rats, cats, and monkeys, as well as in the mouse hypothermia test. FI 6654 **71** was also reported to affect cerebral serotonin levels (170). It has no antihistamine or anticholinergic activity (169). However, since these extensive descriptions of the pharmacology of FI 6654 **71** have appeared, there have been no reports of clinical trials. One concludes that there is some good reason for the absence of human data on an otherwise fully studied compound.

C. L9 152

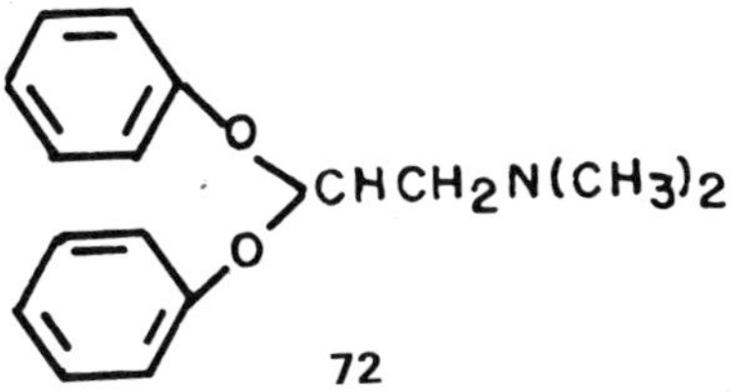

72

L9 152 **72** was described on the basis of animal studies as impraminelike. It is not an MAO inhibitor and was devoid of anticholinergic effects (179). No further reports have appeared on this compound.

D. Tetramisole and Related Compounds

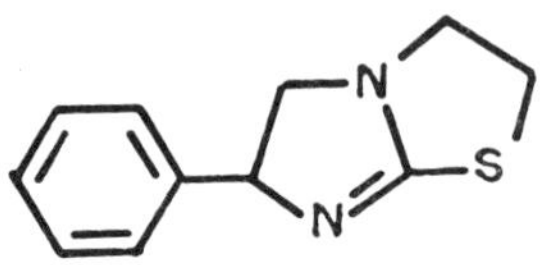

73

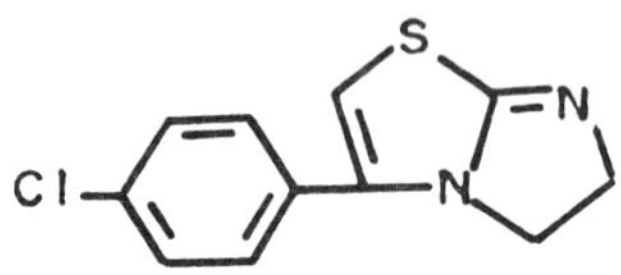

74

Tetramisole **73** was described several years ago and has become established as a broad spectrum anthelmintic (149). Recently, some evidence of a mood elevating effect has been noted in man. A double blind study in depressed schizophrenics has confirmed the initial observation (139, 24). Interestingly, tetramisole **73** has few of the accepted biological attributes of a potential antidepressant, although a related structure type **74** has been reported to antagonize reserpine induced hypothermia and potentiate DOPA in mice (162, 5).

E. Wy 23409

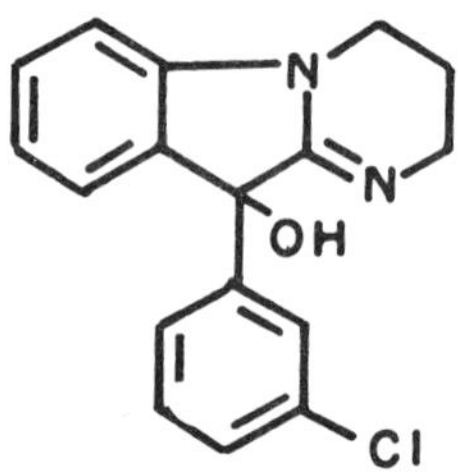

75

Wy 23409 **75** also represents a novel structural type. Only a very brief account of this compound has been published (102). Wy 23409 **75** was claimed to be devoid of anticholinergic and MAO inhibitory activity, yet it antagonized reserpine hypothermia in mice and potentiated the effects of amphetamine in rats.

F. EXP 561

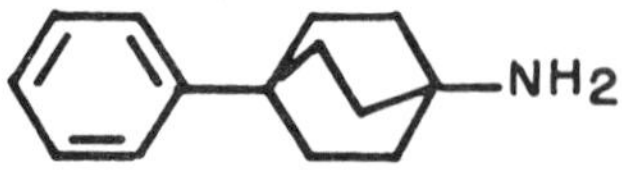

76

A preliminary clinical account of EXP 561 **76** did not give encouraging results. In depressed schizophrenics, a deterioration of their condition was noted (119). In a subsequent paper, a description of the pharmacology of EXP 561 **76** was provided. EXP 561 **76** was equiactive to imipramine **20a** in antagonizing reserpine induced hypothermia in mice, about ten times as potent in antagonizing tetrabenazine induced depression, and about thirty times as potent a potentiation of norpinephrine pressor effects. In an open label trial with ten patients with endogenous depression, only overt stimulation was seen and there was no evidence of an antidepressant effect (75).

G. DH-524

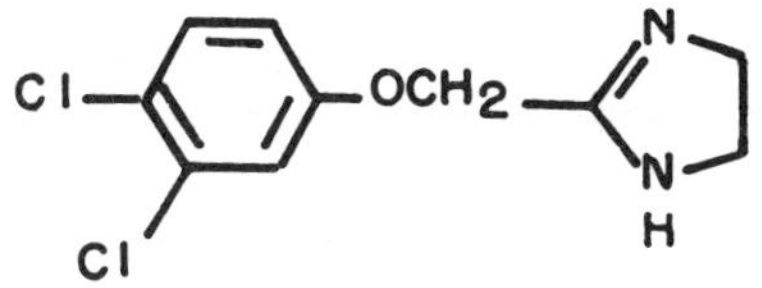

77

A preliminary open label study of DH 524 **77** in five patients suggested some antidepressant potential (34).

The selection of DH 524 **77** for clinical trial appears to have been based principally on its ability to potentiate the effects of amphetamine. A double blind study with DH 524 **77** versus imipramine had to be halted because of marked hypertension in 3 out of 4 patients (35).

The antidepressive effect seen prior to termination was not impressive.

H. Vivalan

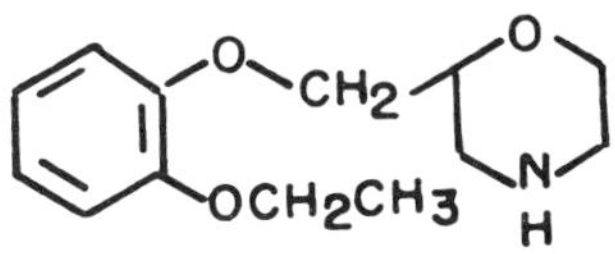

78

Vivalan (ICI 58 834) **78** was reported to reverse reserpine hypothermia in mice, antagonize tetrabenazine induced ptosis, and potentiate several effects of norepinephrine (125).

A brief account of an open label study in a small number of neurotic depressed patients has subsequently appeared (19). It was claimed that Vivalan **78** induced rapid improvement during the first week based on Hamilton rating scores. Two from the nine patient group, however, withdrew from the study because of gastrointestinal upsets, principally nausea.

I. Cyclazocine

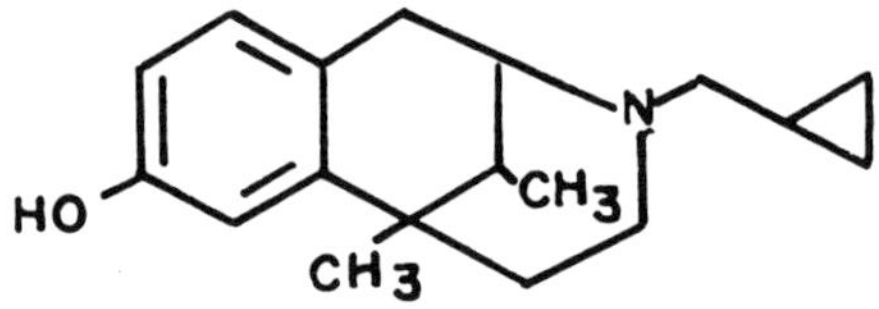

79

Despite the poor tolerability in man on chronic administration, cyclazocine **79** does have a definite antidepressant effect (59).

A recent neuropharmacological study attempted to define what biological parameters were associated with the antidepressant effects seen in man (48). EEG was used as the principal tool and it was concluded that inhibition of the EEG activation produced by physostigmine and, more interestingly, that produced by methamphetamine **67d** was an important property shared by imipramine **20a** and cyclazocine **79**.

J. Steroids

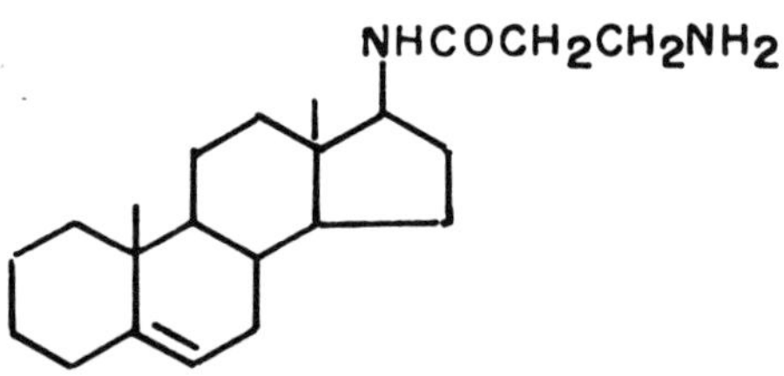

80

Several amides of 17 β amino-5-androsten-3β-ol were described as possessing oral antidepressant activity in mice, yet being devoid of any significant endocrinological effects (61).

A further publication from this group identified compound **80** as one of the most potent compounds in the DOPA potentiation test in mice, with activity about half that of amitriptyline **1a** (62).

K. CP 14368

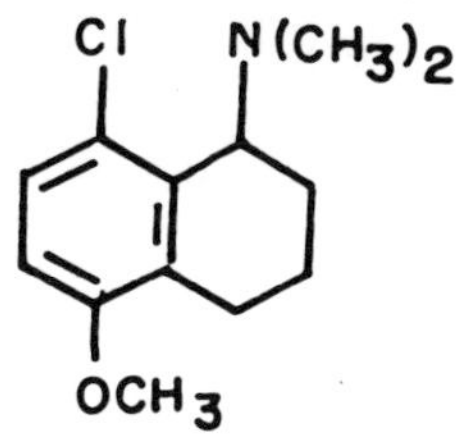

81

An experimental compound of Pfizer CP 14368 **81**, has many of the biological properties of the tricyclic antidepressants, such as, antagonism of tetrabenazine and reversal of the catalepsy induced by haloperidol. However, CP 14368 **81** was devoid of antidepressant properties in a small open label trial (141). Nine out of the ten patients in this trial experienced side effects.

XI. THE SEARCH FOR A NEW ANTIDEPRESSANT

The chemist, who is assigned the task of synthesizing novel antidepressants, should be aware in general terms of what problems exist with the present therapy, e.g. from cardiotoxicity to dryness of the mouth. He should also recognize the limitations of the therapy, e.g. delayed onset of effect and large groups of nonresponders. The awareness of the shortcomings of existing therapy is an important motivating factor for the chemist.

For human depression there is, as was indicated in the introduction (Section 1), considerable subjectivity in the established diagnostic criteria, and differences of opinion exist as to the acceptability or even relevance of more objective ones. It is, therefore, not surprising that, for the biologist, there are serious problems in the assignment of more or less clinical predictability for various animal models (75). Until the ambiguities surrounding diagnosis and the etiology of depression are resolved, it is obviously not going to be possible to be sure whether any of the newer psychopharmacological models involving deprived animals are better prognosticators. Nevertheless, important developments in biological methodology are taking place, based on the biochemical hypotheses of endogenous depression (156, 157). The effects of novel potential antidepressants on the metabolism of norepinephrine in mouse brain can be characterized as to whether they inhibit the reuptake of norepinephrine from the synapse into the nerve terminal, as does imipramine **20a**, or whether they achieve increased levels of norepinephrine in the synapse by some other mechanism. Analogous studies can be carried out to determine the effect a compound has on the serotonergic system (33). The biochemical hypothesis suggests that depression is a consequence of decreased levels of these biogenic amines in the synapse. Therefore any substance, which can increase the concentration of such amines in the synapse without tachyphylaxis developing, should, in principle, be a potential antidepressant, irrespective of its mechanism or combination of mechanisms of action. These detailed mechanistic studies are time consuming and, therefore, necessarily constitute part of the secondary evaluation of a potential antidepressant compound. Another development in biological methodology, which has evolved directly from clinical experience, is the use of the EEG changes induced by administration of antidepressant drugs (98). The changes observed in the EEG's of primates on drug relative to control can be characterized with appropriate computer handling of the data. The procedure presently is quite empirical, providing yet another method of characterizing the compounds known to be clinically effective and then identifying new compounds with similar effects on the EEG. Nevertheless, when the EEG changes between the depressed and the normal state are better understood from the clinical standpoint, it may well be that such methodology will identify significant new compounds with completely novel mechanisms of action. Nevertheless, EEG also constitutes methodology which would be part of a secondary biological evaluation of a potential antidepressant compound rather than a primary screen.

The problem facing the chemist and biologist is, therefore, which new compounds are deserving of such secondary evaluation. The chemist can make his recommendations based partly on intuition, or more objective criteria, such as a structural relationship to clinical effective compounds or potential patentability in a well established chemical series. The biologist identifies those compounds deserving of secondary evaluation based on his views of the significance to be attached to effects the compound exerts on rodent behavior. Such effects may be observed when the compound is administered by itself, or when given prior to or subsequent to administration of other substances, e.g. amphetamine, reserpine, and tetrabenazine, whose effects on rodent behavior have been well defined. The relevance of these effects in rodents to the clinical situation is often called into question (75). For example, high potency in the antagonism of tetrabenazine-induced effects in mice (37) may portend a smaller tolerated dose in man, but does not necessarily ensure a more effective antidepressant action (70). Nevertheless, for the primary evaluation of large numbers of new compounds, no other methodology is extant which seems likely to replace such procedures in the foreseeable future.

When a new compound is identified in these primary screening procedures as causing in rodents one, or preferably several, of the effects associated with clinically effective antidepressants, an important decision point is reached. The choice is essentially whether to evaluate immediately this compound in the secondary screens or merely to consider it a potential lead and recommend synthesis of several related compounds. In the latter case, secondary evaluation of the "best" member of the series then takes place after much of the synthetic work has been undertaken. The dilemma is the definition of "best." It should be again an outcome of joint deliberations between chemist and biologist that decides which is the "best" compound in any given series. Considerations, such as patentability, chemical stability, and synthetic accessibility, have to be included in the evaluation along with potency in the various primary screening procedures and tolerability. There is an understandable tendency in any series to proceed further with the member on which the most biological data has been obtained. This, alas, with benefit of hindsight, often turns out not to have been the "best" member of the series. In a given series, it may well be the wisest course of action to give full secondary evaluation to several members of that series. It is certainly tempting fate to restrict such evaluation to only one member of the series, before being faced with the decision to recommend clinical evaluation in man.

When a lead has been identified based on results from the primary screening procedures, the directions which are taken depend principally on the chemist, but hopefully with regard for suggestions and recommendations of the biologist. The lead compound has to be viewed from all possible aspects, e.g. what structural relationship does it bear to imipramine **20a** or amitryptyline **1a**, what relationships can be perceived to other classes of biological activity compounds. Often structure-activity relationships, which evolve on a further testing in the series, resemble some other indication entirely, e.g. analgesia or antihistamines. Obviously, such an observation should be exploited and other analgetic-like modifications wrought on the parent molecule. Some congeners of the lead compound are, and should be, made on a systematic basis, e.g. if the ethyl compound is biologically active, one should know at least how the methyl, propyl, and isopropyl compounds behave in the same biological tests. Last, but not least, some compounds are made solely on the basis of the chemist's intuition.

The most troublesome problem from the standpoint of the medicinal chemist has been deferred until last. What type of compounds should be made in order to optimize his chances of obtaining a biologically interesting lead in the antidepressant area? The preceding sections are an attempt to provide an up-to-date reasonably comprehensive review of what types of compounds have been reported to have "antidepressant properties." The majority of such compounds have brief clinical reports on their effects in man. Only a few of them have had broadly based controlled clinical trials, which make possible any real evaluation of their potential utility. Unfortunately, by the time a potential antidepressant has reached such a point in its development, work on analogs is hardly likely to yield profitable returns, unless some really significant new synthetic methodology can be employed, which was not available to, or was unlikely to have been considered by the original group. The majority of the compounds cited in the preceding sections 2 through 10 may be regarded as potential target compounds. Nevertheless, before work is initiated based on one of these compounds, it is usually wise to synthesize the compound and evaluate it biologically in-house. When the data is generated, the biologist and chemist can get together and decide, if this were "their compound," how they would proceed. Such a *modus operandi* imposes additional demands on the chemist. Firstly, he must develop the lead in the face of known and potential prior art (many are the chemists who have developed a promising and apparently neglected area, only to see it published subsequently in its entirety by another group). Secondly, he is required to make some really significant improvement in the biological profile to offset the lead in development time held by the original group. Sometimes such an improvement can be defined by the biologist based on the profile of the target compound. But the assumption is that he has "approved" the profile as deserving of further chemical efforts.

The ultimate strategy is to make novel, yet reasonably accessible compounds which, in gross detail, resemble antidepressants, and hope that one of them will be identified by the primary screening procedures as being of potential utility. Such gross detail might be of no more than a new molecular structure containing two aromatic rings attached to each other *via* a single atom. The molecule could then have a nitrogen atom oriented above the convex surface, which could be formed by the two aromatic rings.

This final section has been more philosophical than factual, therefore it might be appropriate to reflect on some important facts with regard to the therapy of depression. Imipramine **20a,** the first effective drug therapy for endogenous depression, was discovered less than twenty years ago by clinical serendipity (114). Since that time, many related compounds have been developed, but essentially the compounds presently dominating medical practice and the market place are of the imipramine, tricyclic antidepressant type, such as were described in section 2.1. Recent developments in the biochemistry of the central nervous system raise the hope that the next quantum leap in the therapy of depression will come from a rational use of new understandings of the etiology of depression, rather than clinical serendipity. Perhaps with the development by the various regulatory authorities of strict clinical guidelines for the evaluation of potential drugs, this may become the only approach possible.

It is to be hoped this will not be the case. Foreclosing the option on clinical serendipity would be a serious handicap for all researchers looking for the next generation of compounds, which can, for some, convert despair to hope. The need for such compounds is all too evident to the medicinal chemist struggling in this difficult area.

REFERENCES

1. Abbot, U.S. Patent 3,708,593 (U.S. Priority 8-24-71).
2. Aichinger, G., Behner, O., Hoffmeister, F., and Schutz, S.: Basische tricyclische oxyiminoather und ihre pharmakologischen eigenschaften, *Arzneim. Forsch.,* **19**:838-845, 1969.
3. Angst, J. and Theobald, W.: *Tofranil®*, Verlag Stampfli & Cie A. G., Berne, Switzerland, 1970.
4. Arnold, O. H. and Guss, O. H.: Klinische erfahrungen mit dem antidepressivum AW 14′2446 (Clodazon), *Wien. Med. Wochenschr.*, **119**:130-135, 1969.
5. Ashford, A. and Ross, J. W.: Phenacylthioimidazolines and 3-Aryl-5, 6-dihydroimidazo [2, 1-b] thiazoles with antidepressant activity, *J. Med. Chem.,* **14**:977-981, 1971.
6. Ashcroft, G. W., Eccleston, D., Murray, L. G., Glen, A. I. M., Crawford, T. B. B., Pullar, I. A., Shields, P. J., Walter, D. S., Blackburn, I. M., Connechan, J., and Lonergan, M.: Modified amine hypothesis for the etiology of affective illness, *Lancet,* **II**:573-577, 1972.
7. Astra, Belgian Patent 784,720 (Swedish Priority 11-6-71).
8. Augstein, J., Ham, A. L., and Leeming, P. R.: Relationship between antihistamine and antidepressant activity in hexahydroindenopyridines, *J. Med. Chem.,* **15**:466-470, 1972.
9. Ayd, Jr. F. J.: Clinical evaluation of a new tricyclic antidepressant iprindole, *Dis. Nerv. Syst.,* **30**:818-824, 1969.
10. Ayd, F. J.: Maprotiline: an effective tetracyclic antidepressant, *Int. Drug Ther. Newslett.*, **8**:17-24, 1973.
11. Ayerst Symposium: Butriptyline Evadyne®, *J. Med.,* **2**:250-343, 1972.
12. Barkov, N. K.: Pharmacological properties of carbidine, *Farmakol. Toksikol.,* **34**:647-650, 1971 (*Chem. Abs.,* **76**: 94788g, 1972).
13. Barkov, N., Geller, A., and Jarvik, M. E.: The behavioral effects of a new psychoactive drug (d-Carbine) on a passive avoidance response and locomotion and its interaction with amphetamine, *Psychopharmacologia,* **21**:82-88, 1971.
14. Baxter, B. L. and Gluckman, M. I.: Iprindole: an antidepressant which does not block REM sleep, *Nature,* **223**:750-752, 1969.

15. Bayer, S. African Patent 667,771 (German Priority 7-1-66).
16. Bayer Symposium: Bericht über das symposium anlaesslich der einführung des antidepressivums Agedal®, *Arzneim. Forsch.,* (5a) **19**:835-912, 1969.
17. Bein, H. J.: Biological research in pharmaceutical industry with reserpine, in *Discoveries in biological psychiatry,* Ayd, F. J. Jr. and Blackwell, B., eds., Chapter 11, J. P. Lippincott Company, 1970.
18. Bente, D., Feder, J., Helmchen, H., Hippius, H., and Rosenberg, L.: Doppelblindprüfung von drei antidepressiva, *Arzneim. Forsch.,* **23**:247-255, 1973.
19. Bereen, F. J.: A new potential antidepressive, *Lancet,* **I**:379-380, 1973.
20. Biros, D., Schiele, B. C., and Ferguson, D.: A comparison of melitracen and imipramine in treatment of depressed patients, *Curr. Ther. Res.,* **II**:289-295, 1969.
21. Boissier, J.-R., Dumont, C., and Ratouis, R.: Etude pharmacologique d'un nouvel antidépresseur tricyclique, *Thérapie,* **26**:459-479, 1971.
22. Bram, G. and Shanmuganathan, N.: An evaluation of tofenacine (Elamol), A new drug for the treatment of depression, *Curr. Ther. Res.* **13**:625-630, 1971.
23. Brown, G. L., Green, Jr., R. L., and Martin, Jr., R. M.: Double-blind, noncrossover study of imipramine and A-10749, *J. Clin. Pharmacol.,* **12**:40-45, 1972.
24. Brugmans, J., Van Lommel, R., and Baro, F.: Clinical aspects of tetramisole, an anthelmintic with antidepressant activity, *Psychopharmacologia,* **26**:85, 1972.
25. Buchel, L. and Levy, J.: Sur les proprietes pharmacologiques centrales et peripheriques du 1-(2 dimethylaminoethyl)-1-phenylindene, *Thérapie,* **23**:1135-1146, 1968.
26. Burke, T. F. and Templar, D. I.: Comparison of Abbott A-10749 with imipramine, *Curr. Ther. Res.,* **10**:335-341, 1968.
27. Campbell, P., Gomez, L., Ananth, J. V., Bronheim, L. A., Klinger, A., and Ban, T. A.: An uncontrolled clinical trial with clomirpramine in the treatment of depressed patients, *Curr. Ther. Res.,* **15**:223-230, 1973.
28. Canas-Rodriguez, A. and Leeming, P. R.: N-phenyl-2-indolinones and N-phenyl-indolines. A new class of antidepressant agents, *J. Med. Chem.,* **15**:762-770, 1972.
29. Canas-Rodriques, A. and Leeming, P. R.: N-phenyl indoline derivatives-A new class of antidepressant agents, *Nature,* **223**:75-76, 1969.
30. Carlsson, A., Corrodi, H., Fuxe, K., and Hokfelt, T.: Effects of some antidepressant drugs on the depletion of intraneuronal brain catecholamine stores caused by 4, α-Dimethyl-Meta-Tyramine, *Eur. J. Pharmacol.,* **5**:367-373, 1969.
31. Carlsson, A., Corrodi, H., Fuxe, J., and Hokfelt, T.: Effect of antidepressant drugs on the depletion of intraneuronal brain 5-hydroxytryptamine stores caused by 4-methyl-α-ethyl-meta-tyramine, *Eur. J. Pharmacol,* **5**:357-366, 1969.
32. Charalampous, J. D.: Amoxapine: A clinical evaluation in depressive syndromes, *Curr. Ther. Res.,* **14**:657-663, 1972.
33. Chase, T. N. and Murphy, D. L.: Serotonin and central nervous system function, *Annu. Rev. Pharmacol.,* **13**:181-197, 1973.

34. Chien, C-P and Kaplan, R. M.: Clinical trial of imidazoline (DH-524) as an antidepressant, *Curr. Ther. Res.,* **11**:471-474, 1969.
35. Chien, C-P and Kaplan, R. M.: Clinical trial of imidazoline (DH-524) as an anti-depressant, *Curr. Ther. Res.,* **13**:350-352, 1971.
36. Christmas, A. J., Coulson, C. J., Maxwell, D. R., and Riddell, D.: A comparison of the pharmacological and biochemical properties of substrate-selective monoamine oxidase inhibitors, *Br. J. Pharmacol.,* **45**:490-503, 1972.
37. Christy, M. E., Boland, C. C., Williams, J. G., and Engelhardt, E. L.: Antidepressants. II.[1] Bridged ring ether derivatives in the dibenzocycloheptene series, *J. Med. Chem.,* **13**:191-195, 1970.
38. Ciba-Geigy U.S. Patent 3,719,683 (U.S. Priority 11-20-70).
39. Ciba-Geigy U.S. Patent 3,767,817.
40. Ciba, Ltd. German Patent 1,957,947.
41. Coppen, A., Eccleston, E. G., and Peet, M.: Plasma total and free tryptophan concentration in female depressive patients and control subjects, *Lancet,* **II**:1415-1416, 1972.
42. Coppen, A. J.: Depressed states and indolealkylamines, *in* Garattini, S. and Shore, P. A., editor: *Advances in Pharmacology, Vol. 6,* Part B, Academic Press, N. Y., 1968, pp. 283-291.
43. Council on Drugs: New names list No. 78, *JAMA,* **208**:680-681, 1969.
44. Council on Drugs: New names list No. 102, *JAMA,* **217**:469-470, 1971.
45. Crane, G. E.: Cardiac toxicity and psychotropic drugs, *Dis. Nerv. Syst.,* **31**:534-539, 1970.
46. DeMaio, D.: Clozapine, a novel major tranquilizer, *Arzneim. Forsch.,* **22**:919-923, 1972.
47. Deniker, P., Peron-Magnan, P., Eliet-Le Guillou, C., and Hanus, M.: Essais cliniques d'une amphétamine anti-dépressive originale, la d-1-para-chloro-N-méthylamphétamine ou Ro 4 6861, *Therapie,* **26**:219-226, 1971.
48. Drew, W. G. and White, R. P.: Neuropharmacological comparison of cyclazocine and imipramine, *Pharmacology,* **9**:65-73, 1973.
49. Dubnick, B., Rucki, E. W., and Salama, A. I.: A comparison of l-p-acetyldeoxyephedrine and 4-methyl-α-ethyl-metatryamine as to lowering of brain serotonin and their antagonism by antidepressants, *Fed. Proc.,* **32**:776abs, 1973.
50. Dureman, I. and Henriksson, B.: Behavioural pharmacology in pigeons and rats of a new tricyclic antidepressant, *Acta Pharmacol. et Toxicol.,* **25**, suppl. 4:71, 1967.
51. Dykstra, S. J., Berdahl, J. M., Campbell, K. N., Combs, C. M., and Lankin, D. G.: Phenylindenes and phenylindans with antireserpine activity, *J. Med. Chem.,* **10**:418-428, 1967.
52. Editorial: Doxepin: a review, *Drugs,* **I**:194-227, 1971.
53. Engelhardt, E. L., Christy, M. E., Colton, C. D., Freedman, M. B., and Boland, C.: Antidepressants. Tetrabenazine-antagonizing activity in a series of 5-H-dibenzo [a, d] cycloheptene-5-propylamines, *J. Med. Chem.,* **11**:325-332, 1968.
54. Eriksoo, E. and Rohie, O.: Chemistry and Pharmacology of a new potential antidepressant, *Arzneim. Forsch.,* **20**:1561-1569, 1970.
55. Fann, W. E., Davis, J. M., Janowsky, D. S., Kaufmann, J. S., Griffith, J. D., and Oates, J. S.: Effect of iprindole on amine uptake in man, *Arch. Gen. Psychiatry,* **26**:158-162, 1972.

56. Fell, P. J., Quantock, D. C., and vanderBurg, W. J.: The human pharmacology of GB 94-a new psychotropic agent, *Eur. J. Clin. Pharmacol.,* **5**:166-173, 1973.
57. Fielding, J. M.: A double-blind comparative trial of dibenzepin and imipramine, *Med. J. Aust.,* **1**:614-616, 1969.
58. Filczewski, M, Oledzka, K., Malecki, I., and Paszek, T.: Pharmacological investigations on the effect of three new benzonaphthyridones on the circulatory system, *Diss. Pharm. Pharmacol.,* **22**:263-74, 1970. (*Chem. Abs.*, 74797q, 1971).
59. Fink, M., Simeon, J., Itil, T. M., and Freedman, A. M.: Clinical antidepressant activity of cyclazocine—a narcotic antagonist, *Clin. Pharmacol. Therap.,* **11**:.41-48, 1970.
60. Flemenbaum, A. and Schiele, B. C.: The antidepressant properties of A-25794: a pilot study, *Curr. Ther. Res.,* **13**:53-56, 1971.
61. Flouret, G. and Cole, W.: 17-aminoacylamido-5-androsten-3β-ols, *J. Med. Chem.,* **11**:.880-885, 1968.
62. Fluret, G., Cole, W. and Biermacher, U.: 17-aminoacylamido steroid antidepressants, *J. Med. Chem.,* **15**:1281-1283, 1972.
63. Fowler, P. J., Tedeschi, D. H., Zirkle, C., and Macko, E.: The unusual pharmacological profile of SK&F 28175, a compound with the combined properties of antidepressants and neuroleptics in animals, *The Pharmacologist,* **13**:235, 1971.
64. Freeman, J. J. and Sulser, F.: Iprindole-amphetamine interactions in the rat: the role of aromatic hydroxylation of amphetamine in its mode of action, *J. Pharmocol. Exp. Thera.,* **183**:307-315, 1972.
65. Fuller, R. W. and Roush, B. W.: Substrate-selective and tissue-selective inhibition of monoamine oxidase, *Arch. Int. Pharmacodyn.,* **198**: 270-276, 1972.
66. Gallant, D. M., Bishop, M. P., and Guerrero-Figueroa, R.: Metiapine: a double-blind evaluation in chronic schizophrenic patients, *Curr. Ther. Res.,* **13**:734-736, 1971.
67. Gallant, D. M., Bishop, M. P., and Guerrero-Figueroa, R.: WIN 27, 147-2: a preliminary evaluation of a potential antidepressant compound: animal and human correlations, *Curr. Ther. Res.,* **14**:61-64, 1972.
68. Gallant, D. M., Bishop, M. P., Guerrero-Figueroa, R., O'Meallie, L., and Moore, B.: UK-3540: a preliminary evaluation of a potential antidepressant compound: animal and human correlations, *Curr. Ther. Res.,* **11**:296-299, 1969.
69. Gallant, D. M., Swanson, W. C., Mielke, D. H., Guerrero-Figueroa, R., and Collins, H.: Amoxapine: a double-blind evaluation of antidepressant activity, *Curr. Ther. Res.,* **15**: 56-59, 1973.
70. Gannon, P., Itil, T., Keskiner, A., and Hsu, B.: Clinical and quantitative electroencephalographical effects of MK 940, *Arzneim. Forsch.,* **20**:971-974. 1970.
71. Geigy U.S. Patent 3,423,510 (U.S. Priority 8-31-66).
72. Geigy U.S., Patent 3,422,104 (U.S. Priority 10-20-64).
73. Gershon, S., Hekimian, L. J., Burdock, E. I., and Kim, SukSik: Antipsychotic properties of loxapine succinate, *Curr. Ther. Res.,* **12**:280-285, 1970.
74. Gershon, S., Hekimian, L. J., and Floyd, Jr. A.: Evaluation of a new antidepressant: A-10749, *J. Clin. Pharmacol.,* **7,** 348-353, 1967.

75. Gershon, S., Hekimian, L. J., and Floyd, A.: Non-correlation of preclinical evaluation of a proposed antidepressant 4-phenyl-bicyclo (2,2,2) octan-1-amine hydrochloride monohydrate (EXP 561), *Arzneim. Forsch.,* **18**:243-245, 1968.
76. Gershon, S, Hekimian, L. J., and Floyd, A.: Preclinical-clinical correlation of anti-depressant activity: controlled study of gamfexine and imipramine, *Curr. Ther. Res.,* **9**:349-354, 1967.
77. Gluckman, M. I. and Baum, T.: The pharmacology of iprindole, a new antidepressant, *Psychopharmacologia,* **15**:169-185, 1969.
78. Gootjes, J., Funcke, A. B. H., and Timmerman, H.: Experiments in the 5H-dibenzo [a, d] cycloheptene series, *Arzneim. Forsch.,* **22**:632-634, 1972.
79. Gordon, M.: Phenothiazines: Gordon, M. ed., *Psychopharmacological Agents,* Vol. 2, Academic Press, New York, 1967, pp 1-198.
80. Gschwend, H.: Chemical approaches to the development of neuroleptics. *in* Fielding, S. and Lal, H. eds: *Industrial Pharmacology*: Vol. *1*, Neuroleptics. Futura Publishing Co., Mount Kisco, New York, 1973, pp. 1-51.
81. Guerrero-Figueroa, R. and Gallant, D. M.: Effects of pinoxepin and imipramine on the mesencephalic reticular formation and amygdaloid complex in the cat: neurophysiological and clinical correlations in human subjects, *Curr. Ther. Res.,* **9**:387-403, 1967.
82. Gyermek, L.: The pharmacology of imipramine and related antidepressants, *Int. Rev. Neurobiol.,* **9**:95-143, 1966.
83. Hekimian, L. J., Gershon, S., and Floyd A.: Cyprolidol and imipramine: a double-blind controlled study in endogenous depression, *Arzneim. Forsch,* **19**:955-956, 1969.
84. Herd, J. A.: a new antidepressant-M&B 9302—a pilot study and a double-blind controlled trial, *Clin. Trials J.,* **6**:219-227, 1969.
85. Hitchens, J. T., Orzechowski, R., Goldstein, S., and Shemano, I.: Pharmacologic evaluation of aletamine (β-allylphenethylamine hydrocloride) as an antidepressant, *Toxicol. Appl. Pharmacol.,* **21**:302-314, 1972.
86. Ho, B. T., Monoamine oxidase inhibitors, *J. of Pharm. Sci.,* **61**:821-837, 1972.
87. Hoeschst, Belgian Patent 698,033 (German Priorities 5-5-66; 12-8-66; 15-4-67).
88. Hoffmann-LaRoche & Co., Ger. Offen. 2,062,001, (*Chem. Abs. 75*: 129683c, 1971).
89. Hoffmann-LaRoche & Co., Netherlands Patent 6506929 (*Chemical Abs. 64*: 17604n, 1966).
90. Hoffmann, I.: 8-amino-2-methyl-4-phenyl-1,2,3,4-tetrahydroisoquinoline, a new antidepressant, *Arzneim. Forsch.,* **23**:45-50, 1973.
91. Hoffmann, I., Ehrhart, G., and Schmitt, K.: 8-amino-4-phenyl-1,2,34-tetrahydroisochinoline, eine neue gruppe antidepressiver psychopharmaka, *Arzneim. Forsch.,* **21**:1045-1046, 1971.
92. Hollister, L. E.: Clinical use of psychotherapeutic drugs, II: antidepressant and antianxiety drugs and special problems in the use of psychotherapeutic drugs, *Drugs,* **4**:361-410, 1972.
93. Holm, T.: Preparation and properties of 1,1-diaryl-1,3-butadienes, *Acta. Chem. Scand.,* **17**:2437-2443, 1963.

94. Horovitz, Z. P., Beer, B., Clody, D. E., Vogel, J. R., and Chasin, M.: Cyclic AMP and Anxiety, *Psychosomatics*, **13**:85-92, 1972.
95. Humber, L. G., Davis, M. A., Beaulieu, G., and Charest M. P.: Chemistry and pharmacology of some benzo (1,2) cyclohepta (3,4,5-d,e) isoquinolines, *Canad. J. Chem.*, **46**:2981-2988, 1968.
95. Humber, L. G., Davis, M. A., Beaulieu, G., and Charest M. P.: Chemistry and pharmacology of some benzo (1,2) cyclohepta (3,4, 5-d,e) isoquinolines, *Canad. J. Chem.*, **46**:2981-2988, 1968.
96. Huñziker, F., Lauener, H., and Schmutz, J.: Zur chemie und pharmakologie von in 10-stellung basisch substituierten 5-dibenzo (b,e) (1,4)-diazepin-derivaten, *Arzneim. Forsch.*, **13**:324-328, 1963.
97. Itil, T. M.: Quantitiative pharmaco-electroencephalography in the discovery of a new group of psychotropic drugs, *Dis. Nerv. Syst.*, **33**:557-559, 1972.
98. Itil, T. M., Cora, R., Hsu, W., Cig, E., and Saletu, B.: Clinical, toxicological and electroencephalographical effects of a new tricyclic antidepressant, (0I-77), *Arzneim. Forsch.*, **22**:2063-2066, 1972.
99. Itil, T. M., Polvan, N., and Hsů, W.: Clinical and EEG effects of GB-94, a "Tetracyclic" antidepressant (EEG model in discovery of a new psychotropic drug), *Curr. Ther. Res.*, **14**:395-413, 1972.
100. Jankowsky, D. S., El-Yousef, M. K., Davis, J. M., and Sekerke, H. J.: A cholinergic-adrenergic hypothesis of mania and depression, *The Lancet*, **II**:632-635, 1972.
101. Johnson, D. N., Funderburk, W. H., and Ward, J. W.: Preclinical evaluation of AHR-1118. a potential antidepressant drug, *Curr. Ther. Res.*, **12**:402-411, 1970.
102. Johnson, E. S., Southgate, P. J., Sugden, R. F., and White, A. C.: The pharmacology of WY-23409, a new antidepressant agent, *Abstracts of Volunteer Papers*, Fifth International Congress of Pharmacology, 1972, p. 116.
103. Johnson, J. L.: Glutamic acid as a synaptic transmitter in the nervous system. A review, *Brain Research*, **37**:1-19, 1972.
104. Jones, A. B. B., Pare, C. M. B., Nicholson, W. J., Price, K., and Stacey, R. S.: Brain amine concentrations after monoamine oxidase inhibitor administration, *Br. Med. J.*, **1**:17-19, 1972.
105. Jones, G., Maisey, R. F., Somerville, A. R., and Whittle, B. A.: Substuted 1,1-diphenyl-3-aminoprop-1-enes and 1,1-diphenyl-3-aminopropanes as potential antidepressant agents, *J. Med. Chem.*, **14**:161-164, 1971.
106. Kaiser, C, Tedeschi, D. H., Fowler, P. J., Pavloff, A. M., Lester, B. M., and Zirkle, C. L.: Analogs of phenothiazines. 3. synthesis and potential antidepressant activity of some phenothiazine derivatives and related compounds containing a carbocyclic basic side chain, *J. Med. Chem.*, **14**:179-186, 1971.
107. Kaiser, C. and Zirkle, C. L.: Antidepressant drugs, *in* Burger, E., editor: *Medicinal chemistry*, Wiley Interscience, New York, 1970, pp. 1470-1497.
108. Kaiser, C. and Zirkle, C. L.: Antidepressives and stimulants, *in* Heinzelman, R. V., editor: *Annual reports in medicinal chemistry*, Vol. 8, Academic Press, New York and London, 1973, pp. 11-19.
109. Kastin, A. J., Ehrensing, R. H., Schalch, D. S., and Anderson, M. S.: Improvement in mental depression with decreased thyrotropin re-

sponse after administration of thyrotropin-releasing hormone, *Lancet,* **II**: 740-742, 1972.

110. Keasling, H. H., and Moffett, R. B.: Central nervous system agents. 3. structure-activity relationship of a series of diphenylaminopropanols, *J. Med. Chem.,* **14**: 1106-1111, 1971.
111. Khazan, N. and Brown, P.: Differential effects of three tricyclic antidepressants on sleep and REM sleep in the rat, *Life Sci.,* **9**: 279-284, 1970.
112. Kielholz, P.: *Depressive illness,* Hans Huber, Bern/Stuttgart/Vienna, 1972.
113. Kline, N. S. and Shah, B. K.:. Comparable therapeutic efficacy of tryptophan and imipramine: average therapeutic ratings versus "true" equivalence. an important difference, *Curr. Ther. Res.,* **15**:484-487, 1973.
114. Kuhn, R.: The imipramine story, *in* Ayd, F. J. Jr. and Blackwell, B., editors: *Discoveries in biological psychiatry,* Lippincott Company, Philadelphia, 1970, pp. 205-217.
115. Lacefield, W. B.: Synthesis of an allylic alcohol and chloride in the nortriptyline series, *J. Med. Chem.,* **14**:82, 1971.
116. Latimer, C. N. and Malone, L. C.: Neuropharmacologic evaluation of a dibenzoxazepine, *Fed. Proc.,* **27**:438, 1968.
117. Labensohn, Z. M., Modlin, H. C., Romano, J., and Sabshin, M.: The pervasive problem of mental depression, *Medical World News,* **14**:42-48, April 20, 1973.
118. Lee, C. M., Horrom, B. W., Michaels, R. J., Rasmussen, R. M., and Plotnikoff, N. P.: Synthesis and antidepressant activity of 5-phenyl-2-(2-propynylamino)-2-oxazolin-4-one and derivatives, *J. Med. Chem.,* **15**:1252-1255, 1972.
119. Lehmann, H. E., Ban, T. A., and Debow, S. L.: A clinical pharmacological study with EXP 561, *Curr. Ther. Res.,* **9**:306-310, 1967.
120. Leonard, B. E.: The effects fo 3-γ-dimethylamino-propyl-3-phenylphthalide (I.C.I. 53,165) on brain monoamines and their precursors, *Arch. Int. Pharmacodyn.,* **199**:94-107, 1972.
121. Lippman, W.: Potentiation of ocular response to adrenaline by 3,3-dimethyl-1-(3-methylaminopropyl)-1-phenylphthalan (Lu 3-010) and a thiophthalan analogue (Lu 5-003): blockers of catecholamine uptake, *Experientia,* **27**:927-928, 1971.
122. Lippman, W.: Blockade of noradrenaline uptake and inhibition of gastric acid secretion by 2-[p-chlorophenyl-2-(pyridyl)-hydroxymethyl] imidazoline maleate (Sch-12650), *J. Pharm. Pharmac.,* **22**:387-388, 1970.
123. Lipsedge, M. S. and Rees, W. L.: A double-blind comparison of dothiepin and amitriptyline for the treatment of depression with anxiety, *Psychopharmacologia,* **19**:153-162, 1971.
124. Lwoff, J. M., LaRousse, C., Simon, P., and Boissier, J. R.: Profile psychopharmacologique d'un antidépresseur potentiel appartenant à la série pyridobenzodiazépine, *Therapie,* **26**:451-457, 1971.
125. Mallion, K. B., Todd, A. H., Turner, R. W., Bainbridge, J. G., Greenwood, D. T., Madinaveitia, J., Somerville, A. R., and Whittle, B. A.: 2-(2-ethoxyphenoxymethyl) tetrahydro-1,4-oxazine hydrochloride, a potential psychotropic agent, *Nature,* **238**:157,1972.
126. Malm, U.: Clothiapin in the treatment of chronic schizophrenia, *Curr. Ther. Res.,* 12:261-270, 1970.

127. Mashkovskii, M. D., Grinev, A. N., Adreeva, N. I., Shvedov, V. I., and Altukhova, L. B.: Psychotropic action of 1,10-trimethylene-pyrazino-[1,2-a]indole, *Farmakol. Toksikol.,* **34**:387-391, 1971 (*Chem. Abs.,* **75**:139240v 1971).
128. Mashkovskii, M. D. and Roshchina, L. F.: Action of azaphen (a new antidepressant) on the bioelectric activity of the brain, *Farmakol. Toksikol.,* **34**:144-8, 1971 (Russ.), (*Chem. Abs.,* **75**:18396s, 1971).
129. McEvoy, F. J., Church, R. F. R., Greenblatt, E. N., and Allen, Jr., G. R.: 1-substituted vinyl-1-phthalanpropylamines as potential antidepressant agents, *J. Med. Chem.,* **15**, 1111-1116, 1972.
130. Meares, R. A., Mills, J. E., Horvath, T. B., Atkinson, J. M., Pun, L. Q., and Rand, M. J.: Amitriptyline and asthma, *Med. J. Aust.,* **2**:25-28, 1971.
131. Merck, Belgian Patent No. 712,160 (U.S. Priority 3-21-67).
132. Moffett, R. B. and Pickering, T. L.: Central nervous system agents. 2. synthesis of diphenyl primary and secondary aminopropanols, *J. Med. Chem.,* **14**:110-1106, 1971.
133. Moffett, R. B., Strube, R. E., and Skaletzky, L.: Central nervous system agents. 1. synthesis of diphenyl-tert-aminopropanols, *J. Med. Chem.,* **14**:1088-110, 1971.
134. Molina-Negro, P., and Illingworth, R. A.: Rapport préliminaire sur l'action de la cyclobenzaprine (MK-130) dans la maladie de parkinson, *Union Med. Can.,* **102**:303-308, 1973.
135. Monkovic, I., Perron, Y. G., Martel, R., Simpson, W. J., and Gylys, J. A.: Substituted tetrahydrofurfurylamines as potential antidepressants, *J. Med. Chem.,* **16**:403-407, 1973.
136. Murphy, J. E., Donald, J. F., and Beaumont, G.: A comparative clinical trial of opipramol and chlordiazepoxide employing a method of patient self assessment, *Clin. Trials. J.,* **8**, No. 2: 28-32, 1971.
137. Nakanishi, M., Tsumagari, T., Okada, T., and Kase, Y.: Pharmacological studies on 5-[3-(4-piperidino-4-carbamoyl-piperidino)-propyl]-10,11-dihydro- 5(H)-dibenz- (b,f)-azepine (Carpipramine) dihydrochloride, a new psychotropic agent, *Arzneim. Forsch.,* **18**, 1435-1441. 1968.
138. Nielsen, I. M.: La 3-olo (3,3 dimethyl-l-phenyl-1-3 methylamino-propylphtahlane): pharmacological profile, *Acta Pharmacol. Toxicol.,* **25**, suppl. 4: 70, 1967.
139. Niemegeers, C. J. E.: On the pharmacology of tetramisole, an anthelmintic with antidepressant activity in man, *Psychopharmacologia,* **26**:84, 1972.
140. Nose, T. and Kowa, Y.: Pharmacological studies of 5-methyl-8-ethyl-sulfonyl- 10-10-(2-dimethylaminoethyl)-5H-dibenzo[B,E] [1,4] diazepine-11 (10)-one (SM-307), an antidepressive substance, *Jap. J. Pharmacol.,* **21**:47-55, 1971.
141. Park, S., Gerson, S., Angrist, B., and Floyd, A.: Evaluation of an aminotetraline, CP 14,368, as an antidepressant, *Curr. Ther. Res.,* **14**:65-70, 1972.
142. Petersen, P. V., Lassen, N., Ammitzboll, T., Nielsen, I. M., Nymark, M., Pedersen, V., and Franck, K. F.: Further pharmacological studies of bicyclic thymoleptics, *Acta Pharmacol. Toxicol.,* **28**: 241-248, 1970.
143. Plotnikoff, N. P., Prange, A. J., Breese, G. R., Anderson, M. S., and

Wilson, I. C.: Thyrotropin releasing hormone: enhancement of dopa activity by a hypothalamic hormone, *Sci.,* **178**: 417-418, 1972.
144. Plotnikoff, N., Will, F., Evans, A., and Meekma, P.: PS-2747: a new antidepressant agent, *Arch. Int. Pharmacodyn.,* **195**:300-342, 1972.
145. Poldinger, W., Gehring, A., Schaublin, A., and Thilges, R.: Vergleichende klinische-erfahrungen mit chlomipramin und ketimipramin, *Arzneim. Forsch.,* **19**:492-493, 1969.
146. Polezhaeva, A. I., Vertogradova, O. P., and Bagreeva, M. R.: New antidepressant azaphene, *Khim.-Farm. Zh.,* **4**:59-61, 1970, (*Chem. Abs.* **73**: 2459n, 1970).
147. Prange, A. J., Jr., Wilson, I. C., Lara, P. P., Alltop, L. B., and Breese, G. R.: Effects of thyrotropin-releasing hormone in depression, *Lancet,* **2**:999-1002, 1972.
148. Prange, A. J., Jr., Wilson, I. C., Lipton, M. A., Rabon, A. M., McClae, T. K., and Knox, A. E.: Use of a thyroid hormone to accelerate the action of imipramine, *Psychosomatics,* **11**:442-444, 1970.
149. Raeymaekers, A. H. M., Allewijin, F. T. N., Vandenberk, J., Demoen, P. J. A., VanOffenwert, T. T. T., and Janssen, P. A. J.: Novel broad-spectrum anthelmintics. tetramisole and related derivatives of 6-arylimidazo (2,1-b) thiazole, *J. Med. Chem.,* **9**:545-551, 1966.
150. Raskin, A.: Adverse reactions to phenelzine: results of a nine-hospital depression study, *J. Clin. Pharm.,* **12**:22-25, 1972.
151. Reiter, P. J.: On flupentixol, an antidepressant of a new chemical group, *Br. J. Psychiat.,* **115**:1399-1402, 1969.
152. Richter, W.: Pharmacological effects of a new antidepressant drug, *Acta Pharmacol. Toxicol.,* **25**: suppl. 4, 67, 1967.
153. Rossi, S., Pirola, O., Fanelli, O., and Maggi, R.: *Il Farmaco Fed. Sci.,* **24**:685-703, 1969.
154. Sathananthan, G., Park, S., Lee, H. K., and Gershon, S.: Clinical evaluation of two proposed antidepressants, *Curr. Ther. Res.,* **14**:711-715, 1972.
155. Saxena, P. R., vanHouwelinger, P., and Bonta, I.L.: The effects of mianserin hydrochloride on the vascular responses evoked by 5-hydroxytryptamine and related vasoactive substances, *Eur. J. Pharmacol.,* **13**:295-305, 1971.
156. Schildkraut, J. J.: Neuropharmacology of the affective disorders, *Annu. Rev. Pharmacol.,* **13**:427-454, 1973.
157. Schildkraut, J. J.: Norepinephrine metabolites as biochemical criteria for classifying depressive disorders and predicting responses to treatment: preliminary findings, *Am. J. Psychiatry,* **130**: 695-698, 1973.
158. Schmitt, H. and Petillot, N.: Propriétés pharmacologiques d'un nouvel antidépresseur potentiel: [le(p-chloro-phényl)-2-(pyridyl)-hydroxyméthyl] imidazoline (SCH 12,650), *Therapie,* **26**: 805-821, 1971.
159. Schmutz, J., Hunziker, F., Stille, G., and Lauener, H.: Constitution chimique et action pharmacologique dún nouveau groupe de neuroleptiques tricycliques, *Chim. Therap.,* **2**:424-429, 1967.
160. Segawa, T., Yajima, H., and Kawasaki, K.: Effects of 5-methoxytryptamine derivatives on reserpine-syndrome in mice, *Arch. int. Pharmacodyn.,* **186**:129-132, 1970.

161. Seifter, J., Friedman, E., Gerson, S., Ventura, D. F., and Seifter, E.: Effect of 2-arylalanines, 2-arylserines, tetraphenylboron and 1,2-dl (2,4-dichlorophenyl)-ethanolamine on levels of serotonin (5HT), Norepinephrine (NE) and dopamine (DM) in whole brain of mice, *Fed. Proc.,* **32**:3367, 1973.
162. Sharpe, C. J., Shadbolt, R. S., Ashford, A., and Ross, J. W.: Phenacylthioimidazolines and 3-aryl-5,6-dihydroimidazo [2,1-b]thiazoles with antidepressant activity, *J. Med. Chem.,* **14**:977-982, 1971.
163. Shipley, G. S., Bishop, M. P., and Gallant, D. M.: A controlled evaluation of U-23,807A in the neurotic depressive syndrome, *Curr. Ther. Res.,* **9**:514-516, 1967.
164. Simeon, J., Fuchs, M., Nikolovski, O., and Bucci, L.: Ketipramine in the therapy of depression in outpatients, *Psychosomatics,* **2**:342-346, 1970.
165. Siwers, B., Freyschuss, U., Hamberger, B., Tuck, D., Malmfors, T., and Sjoqvist, F.: A quantitative approach to the initial clinical trial of tricyclic antidepressants: a comparison of Leo 640 and nortriptyline, *Eur. J. Clin. Pharmacol.,* **3**:12-17, 1970.
166. Squires, R.: Antagonism of p-chloroamphetamine (PCA) induced depletion of 5-HT from rat brain by some thymoleptics and other psychotropic drugs, *Acta Pharmacol. Toxicol.,* **31**, Suppl. 1, 35, 1972.
167. Sterling-Winthrop, Belgian Patent 714,439 (U.S. Priority 10-8-67).
168. Suchowsky, G. K. and Pegrassi, L.: The pharmacology of 4H-3-methylcarboxyamide-1,3-benzoxazine-2-one (F. I. 6654), a compound acting on the central nervous system, *Arzneim. Forsch.,* **19**:643-648, 1969.
169. Suchowsky, G. K., Pegrassi, L., Bonsignori, A., Bertazzoli, C., and Chielie, T.: Some pharmacological properties of 4H-3-methylcarboxamide 1,3-benzoxazine-2-one (FI 6654), *Eur. J. Pharmacol.,* **6**327-332, 1969.
170. Suchowsky, G. K., Pegrassi, L., Moretti, A., and Bonsignori, A.: The effect of 4H-3-methylcarboxamide-1,3-benzoxazine-2-one (FI 6654) on monoaminoxidase and cerebral 5-HT, *Arch. Int. Pharmacodyn.,* **182**:332-340, 1969.
171. Sugerman, A. A. and Med., M. B.: A pilot study of MK-741 in chronic schizophrenics, *Curr. Ther. Res.,* **8**:479-482, 1966.
172. Taber, R. I., Barnett, A., and Roth, F. E.: The pharmacology of SCH 12650, a potential antidepressant agent, *The Pharmacologist,* **11**::247, 1969.
173. Theobald, W., Buch, O., Kunz, H. A., and Morpurgo, C.: Zur pharmakologie des antidepressivums 3-chlor-5-(3-dimethylamino-propyl)-10,11-dihydro-5H-dibenz[b,f] azepin HCl, *Arzneim. Forsch.,* **17**:561-564, 1967.
174. Theobald, W., Buch, O., Kunz, H. A., Morpurgo, C., Stenger, E. G., and Wilhelmi, G.: Vergleichende pharmakologische untersuchungen mit tofranil® pertofran® und insidon®, *Arch. Int. Pharmacodyn.,* **148**:560-596, 1964.
175. Trepanier, D. L. and Sunder, S.: 3,4-dihydroisocarbostyril and 1,2,3,4-tetrahydroisoquinoline derivatives of ephedrine, *J. Med. Chem.,* **16**:342-347, 1973.
176. Tuck, J. R., Kahan, E., and Siwers, B.: Biological and pharmacokinetic evidence for generic equivalence of three imipramine prepara-

tions: comparison with a new imipramine analogue, *Acta Pharmacol. Toxicol.,* **32**:304-313, 1973.
177. Tuomisto, J. and Mannisto, P.: Amine uptake and thyrotropin-releasing hormone, *Lancet,* **1**:836, 1973.
178. Ursillo, R. C. and McCulloch, J. A.: The effect of elantrine, a new anti-parkinsonism agent, on drug-induced tremor in mice, *Arch. Int. Pharmacodyn.,* **197**:132-140, 1972.
179. Vagne, A., Manier, M., Brunet, M. A., and Boucherle, A.: Activités pharmacologiques de la NN' dimethyl-diphénoxy 2-2 éthylamine *Therapie,* **26**:553-561, 1971.
180. Van Der Burg, W. J., Bonta, I. L., Delobelle, J., Ramon, C., and Vargaftig, B.: A novel type of substituted piperazine with high antiserotonin potency, *J. Med. Chem.,* **13**:35-39, 1970.
181. Van Der Vis-Melsen, M. J. E., and Wiener, J. B.: Improvement in mental depression with decreased thyrotropin response after administration of thyrotropin-releasing hormone, *The Lancet,* **II**:1415, 1972.
182. Van Praag, H. M. and Korf, J.: 4-chloramphetamines. chance and trend in the development of new antidepressants, *J. Clin. Pharmacol.,* **13**:3-14, 1973.
183. Van Praag, H. M., Korf, J., van Woudenberg, F., and Kits, T. P.: Influencing the human indoleamine metabolism by means of a chlorinated amphetamine derivative with antidepressive action (p-Chloro-N-methylamphetamine), *Psychopharmacologia,* **13**:145-160, 1968.
184. Vargaftig, B. B., Coignet, J. L., de Vos, C. J., Grijsen, H., and Bonta, I. L.: Mianserin hydrochloride: peripheral and central effects in relation to antagonism against 5-hydroxytryptamine and tryptamine, *Eur. J. Pharmacol.,* **16**:336-346, 1971.
185. Villani, F. J. and Mann, T. A.: 5-(dimethylaminopropyl)-10, 11-dihydro-5H-benzo[2,3]pyrido[6,7-b]azepine, *J. Med. Chem.,* **11**:894-895, 1968.
186. Villani, F. J., Tavares, R. F., and Ellis, C. A.: Oximino ethers: dialkylaminoalkyl derivatives, *J. Pharm. Sci.,* **58**:138-140, 1969.
187. Voith, K. and Herr, F.: Psychopharmacological evaluation of a new antidepressant, butriptyline, *Arch. int. Pharmacodyn.,* **183**:318-331, 1969.
188. Walker, G. N. and Engle, A. R.: Synthesis of 10,11-dihydro-5,10-ethano-5H-dibenzo[a,d]cycloheptenes with various side chains at postion 12, *J. Org. Chem.,* **37**:4294-4302, 1972.
189. Wheatley, D.: Comparative trial of a new mono-amine oxidase inhibitor in depression, *Br. J. Psychiat.,* **117**:573-574, 1970.
190. Wheatley, D.: Clinical evaluation of a new chemical compound with antidepressant properties, *Br. J. Psychiat.,* **121**:621-622, 1972.
191. Wilhelm, M.: The chemistry of polycyclic psycho-active drugs—serendipity or systematic investigation? *in* Kielholz, P., editor: *Depressive illness,* Hans Huber, Vienna, 1972, pp. 129-137.
192. Wolpert, A., White, L., Dana, L., Sugerman, A. A., Arengo, A. D., Simpson, G. M., Bishop, M. P., and Gallant, D. M.: Clinical pharmacological trial of loxapine succinate, *J. Clin. Pharmacology,* **10**:175-181, 1970.

193. Zimmerman, R. L., Vestre, N. D., Schiele, B. C., and Curran, J.: A controlled study of the effects of gamfexine in phenothiazine-treated patients, *Curr. Ther. Res.*, **12**:230-233, 1970.

2

Antidepressants—Psychoneuropharmacology

JOHN H. GOGERTY, PH.D.

I. PRELIMINARY SCREENING TECHNIQUES USED IN IDENTIFYING ANTIDEPRESSANT ACTIVITY

A. Behavioral Techniques

As a result of the clinical findings that certain tricyclic substances, such as imipramine, and the mono-amine oxidase inhibitors, such as iproniazid, were effective in treating depressive symptomatology, a number of investigators undertook the task of developing relatively simple procedures that would allow, over a short period of time, the screening of a large number of compounds for their antidepressant potential. Some investigators leaned toward the development of behavioral techniques since depression is represented by a behavioral change in humans. Irwin (21), operating on the hypothesis that psychotropic agents affect behavior, developed a battery of tests in rodents that allowed the rapid analysis of a compound's effects on a variety of physiological and behavioral parameters. A point made by Irwin in favor of his behavioral techniques as opposed to the more commonly used drug interaction studies (e.g., reversal of reserpine- or tetrabenazine-induced phenomena, potentiation of amphetamine-induced behavioral changes) was that one complicates the study by investigating the interaction of an unknown drug with a substance (e.g., reserpine) whose site(s) and mechanism of action are not completely understood. Irwin placed great emphasis on the understanding of the physiological mechanisms which underlie motor and sensory behavior and the interrelationships between these that result in the totality of behavior (21, 22). However, it remains a moot point whether these procedures are useful in identifying antidepressant activity since most, if not all, of the data generated by Irwin related to the clinically proven antidepressants and comparisons of unknown substances with the "profile" of behavioral effects provided by these clinically accepted agents. Because the clinical entity of depression represents the result of possible genetic, social, and/or neurochemical interactions (1), it would appear that using "normal" animals in simplified screening procedures, whether they be rodents or not, would not result in identifying compounds having a profile of activity that is much different than that of the available clinically accepted substances.

In attempts to find a species that is superior to rodents in evaluating the behavioral effects of drugs, several investigators have discussed the use of cats (30, 31, 22, 25). Recognizing that the cat responds differently than other species to such centrally-acting substances as morphine and the benzodiazepines, it was the opinion of these investigators that the cat offers a behavioral syndrome which allows for more concise interpretation of inter- and intra-species social interaction and for more objective analyses of innate behavior (e.g., grooming, anxiety, hostility, depressive syndrome, etc.). The factors used by Kinnard et al. (25) to evaluate drug action on cat behavior are shown in Table I. Although the authors point out that the behavioral measurements used allow one to separate such distinctly different substances as pentobarbital, chlorpromazine, imipramine, and d-amphetamine, it must be remembered that many of the measures involve anthropomorphic interpretation of behavioral responses. This fact invites questioning of the true objectivity of the test. In addition, no attempt was made to identify the potential clinical significance of a profile of activity presented; for example, by imipramine as compared to that presented by chlorpromazine.

Insofar as measurements of drug effects on overt behavior are concerned, the use of nonhuman primates would appear to be the best species for reproducing the clinical disease state (i.e., depression) in animals and, therefore, the most useful model for predicting drug responses in man. It must be recognized, however, that monkeys are not the most available species and that the techniques required for reproduction of these disease states are often time-consuming and expensive. Although primates have been used as far back as the late 1950's in attempts to reproduce the clinical entity of depression (36, 24), the use of these models for the testing of potential antidepressants has not evolved. One of the more attractive techniques has been devised by Harlow (43), in which infant monkeys are separated from their mothers and the behavior of the infants is followed for a 4-week period. These investigators further showed that the age at which separation takes place and prior experience with separation are important in determining the reactions to separation in later life (43).

TABLE I
Factors used to evaluate drug action on cat behavior

Factor	Title	Major Positive Signs	Major Negative Signs
1	Social interaction	approaching pouncing pawing chasing fighting aggression	
2	Reaction with observer	purring contentment	indifference
3	General activity	amount of activity speed of movement exploring playing with objects catnip response	
4	Depressive syndrome	ataxia relaxation of nictitating membrane crying indifference[1]	grooming
5	Agitation	pacing thrashing tail pupil size	
6	Sleep	asleep	inactive but awake
7	Self-care	grooming object scratching crying	
8	Anxiety	piloerection hyperpnea	grooming
9	Hostility	hostility to observer hostility to second cat	crying

[1]minor positive sign.
Table obtained from Kinnard et al. (ref. 25)

Another behavioral technique considered by some as useful in identifying antidepressant activity is the one defined by Horowitz (20) in which the "muricide" (mouse-killing) behavior of rats is utilized as a behavioral parameter which can be predictably altered by known antidepressants. Horowitz has also used this procedure to identify the site in the brain through which antidepressants exert their primary effects (19). However, other workers (4) have presented data showing that this test is much more sensitive to CNS stimulants and appetite suppressants than it is to antidepressants.

B. Interaction with Autonomic Nervous System Functions

With the discovery of imipramine as a clinically useful antidepressant by Kuhn (26), preclinical reports relating to its pharmacological activities began to appear. Most notable among these reports was the one by Sigg (38), in which it was shown that imipramine, as distinguished from other "tricyclic" substances known at that time, produced a profound potentiation of the cardiovascular effects of exogenously administered catecholamines in animals. Because it was recognized that imipramine had little, if any, effect on the enzymes then assumed to be responsible for metabolism of catecholamines (i.e., mono-amine oxidase and catechol-o-methyl transferase), one had to assume that these results identified an interaction of potential antidepressants with the sympathetic nervous system that was clearly different than that heretofore known. When one then recalls Hess' original proposals regarding the interrelationships of the ergotropic (sympathetic) and trophotropic (parasympathetic) systems of the diencephalon (17) and the emphasis that was placed on the role of the sympathetic nervous system in controlling depression (as a result of the previous discovery that iproniazid, a mono-amine oxidase inhibitor, could effectively treat depression), it becomes clear why a simple cardiovascular autonomic interaction test, such as identified by Sigg, could become important as a primary screen to detect new antidepressant substances. However, as Stone (41) has shown, the established antidepressants are not the only drugs capable of potentiating the cardiovascular effects of catecholamines. Stone realized that the mechanisms accounting for potentiation of catecholamine responses in peripheral cardiovascular tissue probably cannot be related to similar mechanisms in a tissue such as the brain which requires a much more complex series of neuronal interactions for functional activity.

As a follow-up to this, Sigg presented a novel, but more complex, procedure that would allow the identification of a drug's effects on either peripheral or central adrenergic systems (37). However, because of the complexities of the procedures involved and because no attempt was made to show that known antidepressant substances would influence central adrenergic function to a greater degree than peripheral activity, one questions whether this technique would serve any useful purpose in the identification of potential antidepressants.

C. Interaction with Drugs Affecting Central Biogenic Amines

With the advent of imipramine and iproniazid as effective antidepressants, a certain number of investigators attempted to define new pharmacological testing procedures for identifying novel antidepressants through the interaction of new drugs with agents that were known to have their primary effects on systems affecting central biogenic amines. Because imipramine was introduced at a time when the roles of norepinephrine, 5-hydroxytryptamine, and acetylcholine in the central nervous system were considered to be important but unknown (primarily because these substances would not penetrate the blood-brain barrier when injected), investigators attempted to use certain agents that would substitute for, deplete, or antagonize these neurohumoral agents.

For instance, Everett (13) showed that the precursor of dopamine and norepinephrine synthesis, dihydroxyphenylalanine (DOPA), when injected into mice, produces a reproducible and measureable behavioral stimulation that is potentiated by substances such as mono-amine oxidase inhibitors and by imipramine. That this became one of the more established preliminary tests for antidepressants was because of its simplicity and reproducibility. Unfortunately, it is now recognized that many "false positives" (i.e., substances active in this test but subsequently shown to be not active in other testing procedures or in the clinic as antidepressants) can be obtained with this procedure. That DOPA can be converted to dopamine, which acts as a neurohumor in one neurophysiologic system, or to norepinephrine, which acts as a neurohumor in a different neurophysiologic system, may account for the unexpected results.

Other test procedures that interact an unknown substance with an agent known to alter biogenic amine metabolism are the tetrabenazine ptosis/catalepsy test (15) and the reserpine hypothermia test (14, 39). That tetrabenazine and reserpine are chemically related (both induce a depletion of brain catecholamines) and that reserpine has been shown clinically to produce depression in humans (11) provide additional arguments in favor of the use of these tests for defining antidepressant agents. However, the facts that both tetrabenazine and reserpine alter the brain levels of many amines in addition to norepinephrine and that a complete understanding of the biochemical, physiological, and behavioral mechanisms surrounding depressive illnesses is not available, have shown that these tests are again not as predictive as one might wish.

On the other hand, certain investigators (6, 7) have adopted the approach that at least part of the beneficial effects obtained with antidepressants are due to their anticholinergic properties. To this end, these individuals and others (see Spencer, 39) have developed procedures to either measure the hypothermia in mice produced by agents such as oxotremorine, or measure the electroencephalographic arousal produced in rabbits by agents such as nicotine or physostigmine. That certain anticholinergic agents presently available do not possess significant antidepressant activity makes one question the validity of this approach. However, it is argued that the primary reason for the ineffectiveness of substances such as atropine, benzotropine, or trihexyphenidyl is due to their peripheral effects and the lack of specific central anticholinergic activity. Blackwell et al (7) have stated that the anticholinergic activity of presently available antidepressants is probably not responsible for the antidepressant activity, but may account for the sedative action observed with these drugs.

Finally, it would be incomplete to discuss drug interaction techniques in developing new antidepressant substances without citing the use of amphetamine interactions as a means of preliminary testing for antidepressants. These procedures have utilized such simple techniques as the ability of amphetamine to increase locomotor activity of small animals, as measured in activity cages, to the more sophisticated tests used particularly by Stein and coworkers (40) wherein the self-stimulation technique of Olds (32) is employed to measure the effects of amphetamine and interaction of same with unknown drugs on self-stimulation behavior in rats having electrodes implanted in specific brain areas (i.e., the ascending adrenergic pathway for reward). Again, the more simple test procedures that measure the general CNS stimulant activity of amphetamines can lead to "false positives" (e.g., barbiturates, benzodiazepines), whereas the self-stimulation procedure allows a more definitive localization of amphetamine in a neural network presumed to be related to "drive" behavior. In the latter test, the only substance (other than psychostimulants and the standard antidepressants) shown to produce a potentiation of amphetamine is iprindole, a drug known to inhibit the metabolism of amphetamine (27). Interestingly, iprindole is not active in the other "standard" testing procedures which are used to define potential antidepressant activity. Iprindole is also not active in another test procedure, to be discussed presently, that is considered by some (present author included) as a much more reliable predictor of antidepressant activity (i.e., potentiation of 5-hydroxytryptophane-induced facilitation of monosynaptic potentials in the cat DR-VR preparation).

In referring to the cat dorsal-ventral root (DR-VR) preparation and the effects of 5-hydroxytryptophane (5-HTP) and antidepressants on this preparation, one is reminded of the original studies by Sigg (38) in which he showed that imipramine not only potentiated the cardiovascular response to catecholamines but also potentiated the effects obtained with 5-hydroxytryptamine (5-HT, serotonin). This highly technical and sophisticated preparation, as originally described by Lloyd (28), was used by Anderson and coworkers (3) in an attempt to define the role of 5-HT in modulating neuronal activity in the spinal cord. In considering the results presented by Anderson, and the previous data of Sigg, on the interaction of antidepressants with 5-HT, the DR-VR preparation seemed to be a natural, albeit quite difficult, procedure to use in order to study the effects of antidepressants on 5-HT function in a specific neuronal system. Indeed, investigations over the past several years in the present author's laboratory and in other laboratories around the world (10, 29) have shown that the ability of a substance to potentiate 5-HTP-induced facilitation of monosynaptic spikes in the cat or rat DR-VR preparation is restricted to the presently marketed and proven antidepressant substances (see Fig. 1). The relevance of these data regarding pre-

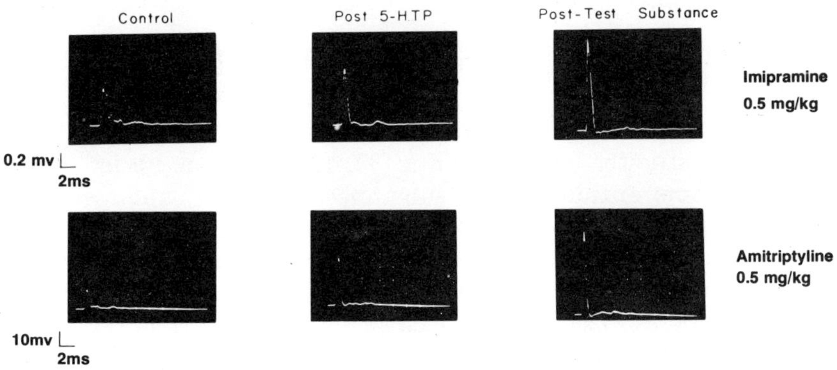

FIGURE 1 Effects of 5-hydroxytryptophane and antidepressants on mono- and polysynaptic spikes obtained in the dorsal-ventral root preparation of the cat. The left hand part of the graph shows the spike potentials obtained under control conditions with the middle portion demonstrating the effect of 5-hydroxytryptophane (75 mg/kg i.v.) on the spike phenomena approximately 80 minutes after the administration of 5-hydroxytryptophane. The right hand portion shows the effect of standard antidepressants on the 5-hydroxytryptophane facilitated monosynaptic spikes. The antidepressants have no effect *per se* in the dorsal-ventral root preparation.

dictability of antidepressant activity as compared to the self-stimulation procedure of Stein (40) should receive a stern test over the coming year inasmuch as iprindole, as mentioned previously, is not active in the DR-VR preparation whereas two new potential antidepressants (one from Ayerst and one from Sandoz) have shown activity in this preparation and are presently undergoing early clinical trials. Of possible relevance to the total picture is the finding of Carlsson and coworkers (9) who showed that the amine pump of central 5-HT neurons was more sensitive than that of central noradrenaline (NA) neurons to imipramine, chlorimipramine, and amitriptyline. Interestingly, one substance (a compound by the name of quipazine) was found in the DR-VR preparation to mimic the effects of 5-HTP. However, when this agent was taken into the clinics as a potential antidepressant, it was shown to produce significant nausea and vomiting and could not be pursued further.

Obviously, the one ideal preliminary screening technique for reliably predicting antidepressant activity has not as yet been identified. To this end, data are presented (Table II and Fig. 2) which show the effects of two "antidepressant" substances in a variety of preliminary testing procedures as carried out in the author's laboratories.

II. ELECTROPHYSIOLOGICAL EFFECTS OF ANTIDEPRESSANTS

A. Effects on Spontaneous Electroencephalographic (EEG) Activity

Very little work, apart from that presented by some of the original investigators of imipramine (38, 42), has been carried out on the effects of antidepressant substances on the resting awake EEG of animals. To the extent that studies have been completed, it has been found that antidepressants such as imipramine and amitriptyline, in contrast to the mono-amine oxidase inhibitors, produce a synchronized sleep-like pattern with impairment of the EEG alerting response obtained following sensory stimulation. However, this EEG alteration does not correlate, in time or intensity, with behavioral changes and thus might be more directly related to the central anticholinergic properties of these agents. Bradley and Key (8) have shown a similar dissociation between EEG and behavioral changes with substances such as atropine. It is thus concluded that studies on the effects of potential antidepressants on the EEG of normal resting awake animals would have little relevance in determining the overall profile of a compound. It should be mentioned, however, that Itil and coworkers

TABLE II
Comparison of the pharmacological profiles of amitriptyline and imipramine.

Test	Central Nervous System Effects of Marketed Antidepressants (ED_{50} mg /kg) Amitriptyline	Imipramine
Acute Mouse Toxicity (mg/kg i.p.)[1]	63.0± 4.8	87.5±11.0
Acute Mouse Toxicity (mg/kg p.o.)[1]	159.8±20.6	206.7±29.0
Acute Rat Toxicity (mg/kg p.o.)[1]	186.5±27.5	182.0±18.0
Mice Clonic Conv. (mg/kg i.p.)[2]	31.9± 2.4	N.A. @87.5
Mice Docility (mg/kg i.p.)[2]	N.A.*@22.2	83.4±11.7
Mice 41-178 Ext. Antag. (mg/kg i.p.)[3]	11.9± 1.6	35.5±22.2
Mice 41-178 Death Antag. (mg/kg i.p.)[3]	>22.2	>88.8
Mice Hxb. Reind. (mg/kg i.p.)[4]	19.0± 5.5	>44.4
Aggressive Mice Antag. (mg/kg i.p.)[5]	13.4± 2.8	21.3± 9.7
Mice RSP Hypotherm. Rev. (mg/kg i.p.)[6]	see accompanying graph	
Rat Anti-"Muricide" Activity (mg/kg p.o.)[7]	>100.0	55.0
Oxotremorine Antag. (mg/kg i.p.)[8]	> 26.6	> 26.6
Oxotremorine Antag. (mg/kg p.o.)[8]	> 88.8	>177.6
5-HTP Potent (DR-VR) (mg/kg i.v.)[9]	82% @ 0.5	95% @ 0.5
	see accompanying graph	

*N.A. = not active

[1] Determined by the method of Litchfield and Wilcoxon using 10 animals per dose (*J. Pharmacol. Exp. Ther.*, **96**:99, 1949).
[2] Anal. of behavior used modification of method of S. Irwin (see ref. 22)
[3] 41-178 = N-sulfamoylazepine, a substance producing pentylenetetrazole-like convulsions (see Iorio, L. C., Ryan, E. A., Kerestan, S. P. and Gogerty, J. H.: Analeptic effects of N-Sulfamoyl-Hexahydro-Azepine, SaH 41-178, *Arch. Int. Pharmacodyn.*, **200:**255-265, 1972)
[4] Modified method of C. F. Winter: *J. Pharmacol. Exp. Ther.*, **94**:7 (1948), was used in which animals were administered compd. immediately following recovery from hexobarbital anesthesia (70 mg/kg i.v.) and reinduction of "anesthesia" (loss of righting) was measured from that time.
[5] Modification of method of R. E. Tedeschi, et al.: *J. Pharmacol. Exp. Ther.*, **125**:28 (1959)
[6] Modification of the method presented by P. S. J. Spencer (see ref. 39)
[7] Modification of the method of Z. P. Horowitz (see ref. 19)
[8] Modification of the method of Everett: *Science,* **124**:79, 1956.
[9] Modification of the method of Anderson, E. G. (see ref. 3)

(23) have recently proposed that mianserin (GB-94) has antidepressant properties, based solely on results obtained from EEG studies in normal human volunteers. Because this compound provided no pharmacological activity suggestive of antidepressant activity, we shall watch with interest its development, with par-

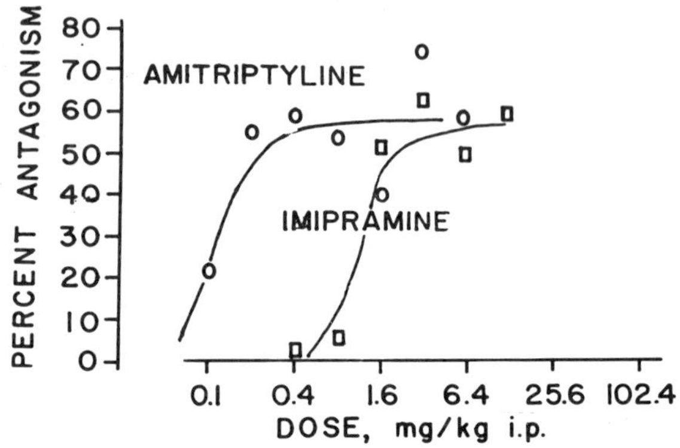

FIGURE 2 Comparison of the effects of amitriptyline (O) and imipramine (□) on reserpine-induced hypothermia in mice. The ordinate shows the percent antagonism of reserpine-induced hypothermia obtained when the antidepressants are administered at selected doses (listed on the abcissa) intraperitoneally two hours following the administration of an intraperitoneal dose of 5 mg/kg of reserpine to mice.

ticular regard to future consideration of the computerized methodology utilized by these investigators. It is also of interest that lithium has been proposed to have "antidepressant" activity and, following chronic administration to cats, produces a significant slowing of EEG activity recorded from cortical and subcortical loci (5). Accompanying this EEG change was a change in the spontaneous behavior of the animals; they did not like to be handled and developed a "withdrawing" behavior. When one compares this behavioral effect to that described by Kinnard (25) for imipramine, one would have to question the interpretation placed upon both the EEG effects and the relevance of the behavioral changes produced by either lithium or imipramine to their clinical potential as antidepressants. Indeed, it may be that lithium acts as an "antidepressant" by the fact that it reduces manic behavior and thereby breaks the manic-depressive cycle.

Although the study of antidepressant effects on the resting awake spontaneous EEG has proven to be unrewarding, the analysis of effects of these substances on the EEG pattern of sleeping animals might provide more fruitful results. It is well recognized that the clinical state of depression is accompanied by significant changes in sleep patterns (44, 16). Hishikawa and coworkers (18) compared the effects of imipramine, desmethylimipramine, and chlorpromazine on the sleep-wakefulness cycle of normal cats and found that antidepressants prolonged the time spent in sleep, decreased the number of awakenings, decreased the number of REM episodes, and decreased the total time spent in REM sleep. The effect of antidepressants on total sleep would appear to relate positively to the clinical situation since depressed patients show frequent awakenings and decreased sleep time. However, the effect on REM episodes would be considered negative since depressed patients also show a decrease in REM time. One of the problems that obviously exists with this type of correlation is again the fact that the animal model does not correlate with the clinical condition (unless cats are considered to be genetically predisposed to "depressive" illnesses).

B. Effects on Evoked Electrical Activity in Various Central Neural Systems

Attempts to define the site and neurophysiological mechanism of action of antidepressants have brought forth a number of provocative hypotheses regarding brain function, in addition to providing specific neuropharmacological data regarding the possible site(s) of action of the ideal antidepressants. Since the original findings of Bradley and Key (8) on the depressant effects of imipramine EEG arousal, which is induced by electrical stimulation of nuclei within the reticular formation, numerous investigators have studied the effects of antidepressants on those neuronal circuits considered to be more closely associated with the control of emotions than is the reticular formation. In this regard, the late Hernandez-Peon and coworkers (34) showed that imipramine would enhance "arousal discharges" elicited in the ol-factory bulb by presentation of unfamiliar visual or auditory stimuli whereas at the same time cortical electrical activity was slowed. In an additional study, these investigators (33) showed that the threshold for rage behavioral response induced by hypothalamic stimulation is reduced by low doses of imipramine whereas higher doses produce depression of excitability within both hypothalamic and amygdaloid nuclei. These data were essentially duplicated by Dubinsky and Goldberg (12). In addition, Allikmets and Delgado (2) showed that imipramine injected directly into the amygdaloid nuclei of restrained rhesus monkeys would raise the threshold required to obtain behavioral "attention" or electrical seizure elicited from electrodes placed in the amygdala. These results and those of Schmitt (35) point to the fact that "low doses" of imipramine enhance the electrical activity within various rhinencephalic and midbrain nuclei known to be associated with increased arousal (or alertness), whereas higher doses produce depression of neurophysiologic activity in these same areas. With these facts in mind, it should be recalled that imipramine produces a potentiation of catecholamine and/or 5-hydroxytryptamine-induced activities at relatively low doses whereas depressant activities are obtained at higher doses. Which one, or all, of these effects are responsible for the antidepressant effects provided by compounds such as imipramine is still to be determined, but it seems encouraging to note that an area of the central nervous system that contains a relatively high concentration of 5-hydroxytryptamine (i.e., the amygdala) demonstrates a similar responsiveness to low doses of antidepressants, such as imipramine, as does the 5-HTP-induced potentiation of DR-VR monosynaptic spikes.

ACKNOWLEDGEMENTS

I would like to express my personal appreciation to Mrs. Elizabeth Pfister for the typing of this manuscript.

REFERENCES

1. Akiskal, H. S. and McKinney, W. T. Jr.: Depressive disorders: Toward a unified hypothesis, *Science,* **182**:20-29, 1973.
2. Allikmets, L. and Delgado, J. M. R.: Injection of antidepressants in the amygdala of awake monkeys, *Arch. Int. Pharmacodyn.,* **175**:170-178, 1968.
3. Anderson, E. G. and Shibuya, T.: The effects of 5-Hydroxytryptophan and 1-Tryptophan on spinal synaptic activity, *J. Pharm. & Exp. Therap.,* **153**:352-360, 1966.
4. Barnes, H. W., Cunningham, B. L., Penberthy, C., and Gogerty, J. H.: Effects of various CNS-active substances and CNS-modifying influences on mouse-killing behavior of rats, *The Pharmacologist,* **9**:200, 1967.
5. Barratt, E. S., Creson, D. L., and Russell, G.: The effects of lithium salts on brain activity in the cat, *Amer. J. Psychiat.,* **125**:122-128, 1968.
6. Benesova, O. and Nahunek, K.: Correlation between the experimental data from animal studies and therapeutical effects of antidepressant drugs, *Psychopharmacologia* (Berl.), **20**:337-347, 1971.
7. Blackwell, B., Lipkin, J. O., Meyer, J. H., Kuzma, R., and Boulter, W. V.: Dose responses and relationships between anticholinergic activity and mood with tricyclic antidepressants, *Psychopharmacologia* (Berl.), **25**:205-217, 1972.
8. Bradley, P. B. and Key, B. J.: A comparative study of the effects of drugs on the arousal system of the brain, *Brit. J. Pharmacol.,* **14**:340-349, 1959.
9. Carlsson, A., Jonason, J., Lindqvist, M., and Fuxe, K.: Demonstration of extraneuronal 5-Hydroxytryptamine accumulation in brain following membrane-pump blockade by chlorimipramine, *Brain Research,* **12**:456-460, 1969.
10. Clineschmidt, B. V., Pierce, J. E., and Sjoerdsma, A.: Interactions of tricyclic antidepressants and 5-Hydroxyindolealkylamine precursors on spinal monosynaptic reflex transmission, *J. Pharm. & Exp. Therap.,* **179**:321-323, 1971.
11. Davies, E. B.: *Depression,* Cambridge Univ. Press, New York, 1964.
12. Dubinsky, B. and Goldberg, M. E.: The effect of imipramine and

selected drugs on attack elicited by hypothalamic stimulation in the cat, *Neuropharmacology,* **10**:537-545, 1971.
13. Everett, G. M. and Wiegand, R. G.: Central amines and behavioral states: A critique and new data, *in* Paton, W. D. M., editor: *First International Pharmacological Meeting,* Stockholm, 1961, Vol. 8, The MacMillan Company, New York, 1962, pp. 85-92.
14. Garattini, S., Giachetti, A., Jori, A., Pieri, L., and Valzelli, L.: Effect of imipramine, amitriptyline and their monomethylderivatives in reserpine activity, *J. Pharm. Pharmacol.,* **14**:509-514, 1962.
15. Giurgea, M., Dauby, J., Levis, S., and Giurgea, C.: Un test modifié pour le screening des produits antidépressifs, *Med. Exp.* (Basel), **9**:249-262, 1963.
16. Hartman, E.: Mania, depression, and sleep, *in* Kales, A., editor: *Sleep, Physiology and Pathology, A Symposium,* J. B. Lippincott, Philadelphia, 1969, pp. 183-191.
17. Hess, W. R.: *Diencephalon, Autonomic and Extrapyramidal Functions,* Grune & Stratton, New York, 1954.
18. Hishikawa, Y., Nakai, K., Ida, H., and Kaneko, Z.: The effect of imipramine, desmethylimipramine and chlorpromazine on the sleep-wakefulness cycle of the cat, *EEG & Clin. Neurophys.,* **19**:518-521, 1965.
19. Horowitz, Z. P., Piala, J. J., High, J. P., Burke, J. C., and Leaf, R. C.: Effects of drugs on the mouse-killing (muricide) test and its relationship to amygdaloid function, *Int. J. Neuropharmacol.,* **5**:405-411, 1965.
20. Horowitz, Z. P.: Psychoactive drugs and limbic system of the brain, *Psychosomatics,* **6**:281-286, 1965.
21. Irwin, S.: Drug screening and evaluative procedures, *Science,* **136**:123-128, 1962.
22. Irwin, S.: Drug screening and evaluation of new compounds in animals, *in* Nodine, J. H. and Siegler, P. E., editors: *Animal and Clinical Pharmacologic Techniques in Drug Evaluation,* Year Book Medical Publishers, Inc., Chicago, 1964, pp. 36-54.
23. Itil, T. M., Polvan, N., and Hsu, W.: Clinical and EEG effects of GB-94, a "tetracyclic" antidepressant (EEG model in discovery of a new psychotropic drug), *Current Therap. Research,* **14**:395-413, 1972.
24. Kaufman, I. C. and Rosenblum, L. A.: Depression in infant monkeys separated from their mothers, *Science,* **155**:1030-1031, 1967.
25. Kinnard, W. J., Barry, H. III., Watzman, N., and Buckley, J. P.: Methods of evaluation of antidepressant activity, *in* Garattini, S. and Dukes, M. N. G., editors: *Antidepressant Drugs,* Excerpta Medica Foundation, Amsterdam, 1967, pp. 89-98.
26. Kuhn, R.: The treatment of depressive states with G22355 (imipramine hydrochloride), *Am. J. Psychiatry,* **115**:459-464, 1958.
27. Lemberger, L., Sernatinger, E., and Kuntzman, R.: Effect of desmethylimipramine, iprindole and DL-erythro-α-(3,4-dichlorophenyl)-β-(t-butyl amino) propanol HCl on the metabolism of amphetamine, *Biochemical Pharmacology,* **19**:3021-3028, 1970.
28. Lloyd, D. P. C.: Functional organization of the spinal cord, *Physiological Reviews,* **24**:1-17, 1944.
29. Meek, J., Fuxe, K., and Andén, N. E.: Effects of antidepressant drugs

of the imipramine type on central 5-Hydroxytryptamine neurotransmission, *Eur. J. Pharmacol.,* **9**:325-332, 1970.
30. Norton, S. and DeBeer, E. J.: Effects of drugs on the behavioral patterns of cats, *Ann. N. Y. Acad. Sci.,* **65**:249-257, 1956.
31. Norton, S.: Behavioral patterns as a technique for studying psychotropic drugs, *in* Garattini, S. and Ghetti, V., editors: *Psychotropic Drugs,* Elsevier, Amsterdam, 1957, pp. 73-82.
32. Olds, J.: A preliminary mapping of electrical reinforcing effects in rat brain, *J. Comp. Physiol. Psychol.,* **49**:281-285, 1956.
33. Penaloza-Rojas, J. H., Bach-Y-Rita, G., Rubio-Chevannier, H. F., and Hernandez-Peon, R.: Effects of imipramine upon hypothalamic and amygdaloid excitability, *Exp. Neurology,* **4**:205-213, 1961.
34. Rubio-Chevannier, H., Bach-Y-Rita, G., Penaloza-Rojas, J., and Hernandez-Peon, R.: Potentiating action of imipramine upon "reticular arousal", *Exp. Neurology,* **4**:214-220, 1961.
35. Schmitt, H.: Selective action of antidepressant drugs on some rhinencephalic and related structures, *in* Garattini, S. and Dukes, M. N. G., editors: *Antidepressant Drugs,* Excerpta Medica Foundation, Amsterdam, 1967, pp. 104-115.
36. Seay, W. and Harlow, H.: Maternal separation in the rhesus monkey, *J. Nerv. Ment. Dis.,* **140**:434-441, 1965.
37. Sigg, E. B. and Sigg, T. D.: Adrenergic modulation of central function, *in* Garattini, S. and Dukes, M. N. G., editors: *Antidepressant Drugs,* Excerpta Medica Foundation, Amsterdam, 1967, pp. 172-178.
38. Sigg, E. B.: Pharmacological studies with Tofranil, *Can. Psych. Ass. J.,* **4**:S75-S85, 1959.
39. Spencer, P. S. J.: Antagonism of hypothermia in the mouse by antidepressants, *in* Garattini, S. and Dukes, M. N. G., editors: *Antidepressant Drugs,* Excerpta Medica Foundation, Amsterdam, 1967, pp. 194-204.
40. Stein, L.: Psychopharmacological substrates of mental depression, *in* Garattini, S., and Dukes, M. N. G., editors: *Antidepressant Drugs,* Excerpta Medica Foundation, Amsterdam, 1967, pp. 130-140.
41. Stone, C. A.: Relationship of some autonomic actions to potential antidepressant activity among antidepressant drugs, *in* Garattini, S. and Dukes, M. N. G., editors: *Antidepressant Drugs,* Excerpta Medica Foundation, Amsterdam, 1967, pp. 158-163.
42. Van Meter, W. G., Owens, H. F., and Himwich, H. E.: Effects of tofranil, an antidepressant drug, on electrical potentials of rabbit brain, *Can. Psych. Ass. J.,* **4**:S113-S119, 1959.
43. Young, L., Suomi, S., Harlow, H., and McKinney, W.: Early stress and later response to separation in rhesus monkeys, *Am. J. Psychiatry,* **130**:400-405, 1973.
44. Zung, W. K.: The pharmacology of disordered sleep, JAMA, **211**:1532-1534, 1970.

3

Antagonism of Reserpine-Like Activity

CARLOS J. E. NIEMEGEERS, D.SC.

I. INTRODUCTION

The clinical use of reserpine in humans has been associated with the occurrence of severe depressive reactions (11, 16, 51, 60), and since reserpine-induced symptoms in animals were found to be antagonized by imipramine-like drugs, the antagonism or reversal of reserpine-like activity has been introduced as a pharmacological test to detect drugs with potential "antidepressant" activity.

In earlier described methods (Table I), antagonism or reversal of palpebral ptosis, hypothermia, and sedation were the criteria used for evaluating antidepressant activity. The challenging drugs currently used for inducing these symptoms are reserpine, tetrabenazine, or the benzoquinolizine derivative, Ro-4-1284.

In this chapter we describe a modified anti Ro-4-1284 test in mice (14), and report on the results obtained in this test with 67 different drugs belonging to several pharmacological classes (cfr addendum). A comparison of antidepressants with drugs of other pharmacological classes provides necessary perspectives on the potentials of this test in preclinical screening.

II. TEST PROTOCOL

The experimental animals are male inbred albino mice (Swiss substrain) from our own breeding, fasted overnight and weighing 22 ±3 g. Thirty minutes prior to testing drinking water is removed from the cages, whereafter the mice are individually marked and placed in groups of 3 in a makrolon observation cage (11 ×12 ×17 cm). The experiments are carried out in an air conditioned room (21±1° C; R. H. 65±5%) by unbiased trained technicians, using coded solutions of freshly prepared test drugs. Aqueous solutions of the compounds to be investigated are injected subcutaneously (0.1 ml/10 g body weight). Insoluble compounds are administered orally as freshly prepared aqueous suspensions, containing 1%

TABLE I
Experimental studies concerned with the antagonism of reserpine-like symptoms in different animal species

Symptoms studied	Challenging drugs	Animal species	References
Palpebral opening	Reserpine	Mice	(1, 8, 9, 13, 20, 23, 25, 46, 47, 49, 56, 77)
		Rats	(18, 44)
		Rabbits	(28, 45)
	Tetrabenazine	Mice	(3, 29, 68)
		Rats	(27, 48)
Temperature	Reserpine	Mice	(2, 3, 8, 9, 15, 22, 25, 26, 27, 29, 30, 46, 47, 50, 55, 67, 74, 75, 76)
		Rats	(3, 4, 5, 21, 22, 40)
	Tetrabenazine	Mice	(22)
		Rats	(22)
Sedation	Reserpine	Mice	(27, 56, 63, 66)
		Rats	(7)
	Tetrabenazine	Mice	(38)
		Rats	(43, 59)
	Ro-4-1284	Rats	(6, 7)
Palpebral opening + Temperature	Reserpine	Mice	(8, 9)
		Rats	(17)
Palpebral opening + Sedation	Reserpine	Mice	(12, 30, 58, 61)
		Rats	(39, 70*, 72)
	Tetrabenazine	Mice	(43, 61, 75, 76)
		Rats	(24, 69)
	Ro-4-1284	Rats	(10, 70*, 72)
Palpebral opening + Temperature + Sedation	Reserpine	Mice	(41, 42, 43, 68)
		Rats	(71)
	Tetrabenazine	Rats	(71)
	Ro-4-1284	Rats	(71)

*Pupil diameter mentioned but not studied.

polysorbate 80 and homogenized by means of ultrasonic sterring. The successive dose levels are selected from the following geometrical series .01, .02, .04, ... 80.0, 160, 320 mg/kg body weight. In a single experiment, one group of 3 mice receives saline, whereas the other groups are treated with one dose each of the test drugs. The same doses of these compounds are tested a second time during another experiment so that each dose level is given to 6 mice in 2 different experiments on separate days.

Fifteen minutes after administration of the drugs all mice are subcutaneously injected with 10 mg/kg Ro-4-1284 (0.1 ml/10 g body weight). Fifteen, 30, and 60 minutes after Ro-4-1284, palpebral opening and spontaneous locomotor activity are observed and scored in all mice individually, without disturbing them in any way. The score system for palpebral opening (57) is as follows:

0: eyelids completely closed
1: eyelids opened for 1/4
2: eyelids opened for 2/4
3: eyelids opened for 3/4
4: eyelids opened for 4/4
5: Exophthalmia

Spontaneous locomotor activity is scored
-1: for prostration
0: for sedation
1: for slight irregular motility
2: for pronounced, more regular motility
3: for continuous hypermotility

Immediately following the last behavioral scoring (60 minutes after Ro-4-1284), the pupil diameter is measured using a graduated microscope, (53, 54) and expressed in 1/25 mm units, and the oesophageal temperature is determined ($\pm$.01°C) with a thermistor (Ellab), of which the thermosensitive probe (1.0 mm diameter) is inserted orally to a constant depth of 4 cm. Statistical significance ($P \leq .05$) of the results is calculated according to the Kolmogorov-Smirnov two-sample test (62).

III. ACTIVITY OF TEST DRUGS

A. Effects of Ro-4-1284

Table II summarizes control data from 1,000 mice pretreated with saline, obtained over a period of approximately five years. Within 5 to 10 minutes following the Ro-4-1284 challenge, all controls assume a definite ptosis (palpebral opening score 0 or 1) accompanied by very marked sedation (locomotor activity score 0). Sixty minutes after Ro-4-1284 hypothermia (i.e. temperature less than 35.9°C; median 32.0-32.9°C) and miosis (i.e. pupil diameter ranging from 0 to 6 units; median 3 to 4 units) are seen in all controls. Short bursts of activity are sometimes noted in a very small number of the control mice. As the animals are in no way

TABLE II
Occurrence of symptoms in 1,000 control mice pretreated with saline and challenged with 10 mg/kg S. C. Ro-4-1284 (percent of mice showing the symptoms).

Parameter	Time in min after Ro-4-1284	Scores and intervals			
		0	1	2	3
Palpebral opening (scores)	15	59.1	35.9	5.0	0
	30	88.6	11.1	0.3	0
	60	97.3	2.7	0.	0
Locomotor activity (scores)	15	98.7	1.3	0	0
	30	99.8	0.2	0	0
	60	110.	0.	0	0
		≤35.9	36-36.9	37-37.9	38-38.9
Temperature (° C)	60	97.7	1.9	0.4	0
		0-6	7-12	13-18	19-24
Pupil diameter (1/25 mm)	60	98.2	1.8	0	0

disturbed throughout the experimental session, their behavior remains essentially unchanged until temperature and pupil diameter are determined at the end of the experiment.

B. Interaction with test drugs

The results obtained with a number of compounds that belong to different chemical and pharmacological classes, are illustrated in Figures 1-7 as synoptic Anti-Ro-4-1284-Profiles. In these profiles, six consecutive dose levels are ranked by numbers. Dose (#1), is the highest inactive dose on the parameter that is most selectively affected by the compounds studied. The subsequent doses are numbered 2 to 6. For the six doses, the median value of each parameter at different time intervals is derived from pooling the data of all drugs tested in that class. These medians are represented by a solid bar if the Ro-4-1284 effect is significantly ($p<.05$) antagonized, and by a shaded bar if the Ro-4-1284 effect is significantly potentiated. Thus, for palpebral opening median scores at 3 time intervals (3 blocks: 15, 30, and 60 minutes) range from 0 to 5. The median scores of locomotor activity vary from 0 to 3; shaded bars indicating prostration with a maximum median value of 1. With regard to body temperature and pupil diameter, solid bars indicate median degrees centigrade and median units respectively significantly higher than controls; shaded bars indicate that results are significantly inferior to control values without any further quantitative precision. The synoptic Anti-Ro-4-1284 Profiles thus provide easily accessible information on the lowest effective dose for each parameter, on the extent of the drug effects, on the dose-response relationship, and on the relationship of drug effects on different parameters, typical for that class of drugs.

The following terms are adopted in the description of drug effects:

Counteraction: indicates the antagonizing effect of a compound on Ro-4-1284-induced symptoms, up to a value or score that does not essentially differ from values and scores found in normal, untreated mice.

Reversal: pertains to an antagonizing effect up to an extent that largely exceeds normality. Thus, reversal of all symptoms studied is characterized by exophthalmia (score 5), hyperthermia (>38.0°C), excitation (score 3), and mydriasis (≥19-24 units).

Consistent: refers to the dose-response relationship. Thus, "inconsistent antagonism" means that the extent of the antagonism does not regularly increase with increasing doses.

Potentiation: means that the Ro-4-1284-induced symptoms are significantly increased by the test drug.

1. *Anticholinergics*

Five anticholinergics were studied at the following 6 dose levels:

atropine: 0.01 to 0.31 mg/kg S. C.
dexetimide: 0.01 to 0.31 mg/kg S. C.
isopropamide: 0.01 to 0.31 mg/kg S. C.
benztropine: 0.08 to 2.50 mg/kg S. C.
benactyzine: 1.25 to 40.0 mg/kg S. C.

Atropine, dexetimide (33, 36), benztropine, and benactyzine are central, and isopropamide (19, 73) is a peripheral anticholinergic.

The synoptic anti-Ro-4-1284 profile derived from the results obtained with these 5 compounds is shown in Figure 1.

The activity of all five anticholinergics consists of counteracting and reversing Ro-4-1284-induced miosis, without significantly affecting the other parameters studied. The low doses required to produce mydriasis and the lack of any other effect in this test indicate that the miosis-reversing activity of the anticholinergics is a highly selective and specific property of this class of drugs.

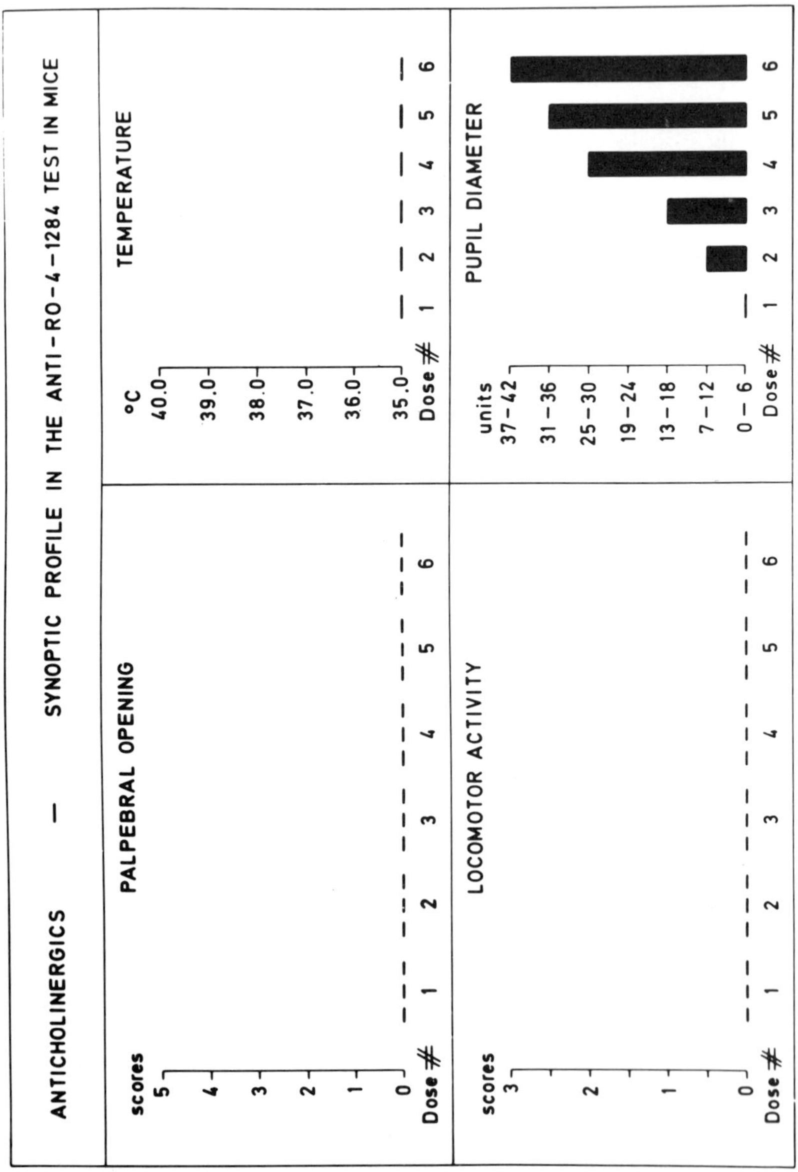
ANTICHOLINERGICS — SYNOPTIC PROFILE IN THE ANTI-RO-4-1284 TEST IN MICE
PALPEBRAL OPENING
scores
5
4
3
2
1
0
Dose #
1
2
3
4
5
6
TEMPERATURE
°C
40.0
39.0
38.0
37.0
36.0
35.0
Dose #
1
2
3
4
5
6
LOCOMOTOR ACTIVITY
scores
3
2
1
0
Dose #
1
2
3
4
5
6
PUPIL DIAMETER
units
37-42
31-36
25-30
19-24
13-18
7-12
0-6
Dose #
1
2
3
4
5
6

FIGURE 1

2. Monoamine oxidase inhibitors

Five monoamine oxidase (MAO) inhibitors were studied at the following 6 dose levels:

tranylcypromine: 0.31 to 10.0 mg/kg S. C.
pheniprazine: 0.63 to 20.0 mg/kg S. C.
modaline: 1.25 to 40.0 mg/kg S. C.
pargyline: 10.0 to 320 mg/kg S. C.
iproniazid: 10.0 to 320 mg/kg S. C. given 16 hours before Ro-4-1284.

The synoptic anti-Ro-4-1284 profile derived from the results obtained with these 5 compounds is shown in Figure 2. The common anti-Ro-4-1284 actions shared by all MAO inhibitors tested are reversal of palpebral ptosis, reversal of hypothermia, and reversal of sedation. The effect on miosis ranged from counteraction to reversal. The MAO inhibitors are found to possess the most pronounced antagonism of Ro-4-1284-induced symptoms of all drugs tested.

3. Sympathomimetics

a) Direct acting

Five compounds of this class were tested at the following dose levels:

oxymetazoline: 0.005 to 0.16 mg/kg S. C.
xylometazoline: 0.04 to 1.25 mg/kg S. C.
naphazoline: 0.04 to 1.25 mg/kg S. C.
tramazoline: 0.08 to 2.50 mg/kg S. C.
tetrahydrozoline: 0.63 to 20.0 mg/kg S. C.

The synoptic anti-Ro-4-1284 profile derived from the results obtained with these 5 compounds is shown in Figure 3. All direct sympathomimetics tested reverse Ro-4-1284-induced palpebral ptosis and produce no effects on locomotor activity. Effects on hypothermia are slight and erratic. Miosis is only counteracted to some extent at doses exceeding those reported.

b) Indirect acting

Five compounds of this class were tested at the following dose levels:

amphetamine: 0.08 to 2.50 mg/kg S. C.
methylamphetamine: 0.08 to 2.50 mg/kg S. C.
hydroxyamphetamine: 0.16 to 5.00 mg/kg S. C.
ephedrine: 0.63 to 20.0 mg/kg S. C.
tyramine: 20.0 to 640 mg/kg S. C.

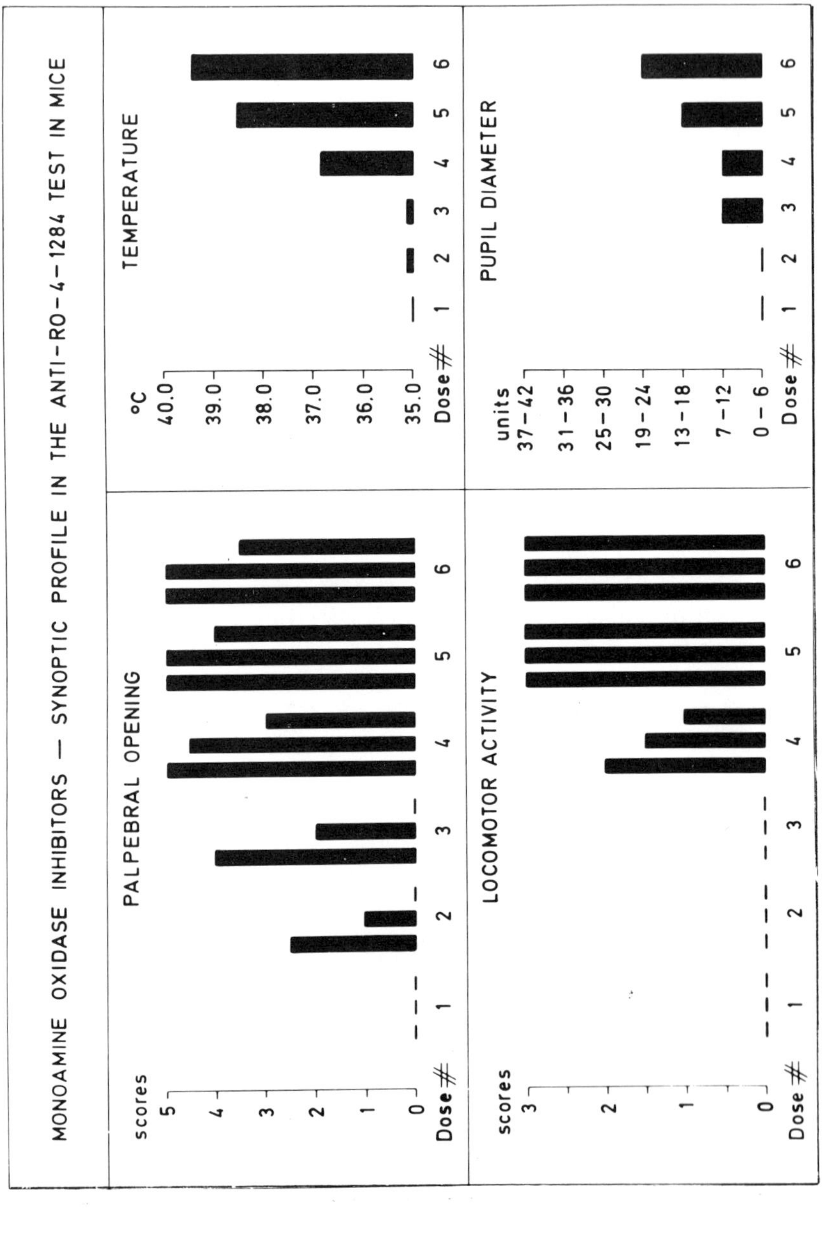
MONOAMINE OXIDASE INHIBITORS — SYNOPTIC PROFILE IN THE ANTI-RO-4-1284 TEST IN MICE
PALPEBRAL OPENING
scores
5
4
3
2
1
0
Dose #
1 2 3 4 5 6
TEMPERATURE
°C
40.0
39.0
38.0
37.0
36.0
35.0
Dose #
1 2 3 4 5 6
LOCOMOTOR ACTIVITY
scores
3
2
1
0
Dose #
1 2 3 4 5 6
PUPIL DIAMETER
units
37−42
31−36
25−30
19−24
13−18
7−12
0−6
Dose #
1 2 3 4 5 6

FIGURE 2

The synoptic anti-Ro-4-1284 profile derived from the results obtained with these 5 compounds is shown in Figure 4. All these compounds consistently antagonize and reverse Ro-4-1284-induced ptosis. Ro-4-1284-induced sedation is reversed with amphetamine and methylamphetamine at relatively low doses and with hydroxyamphetamine and ephedrine at doses higher than those reported (i.e. 80.0 and 160 mg/kg). Tyramine has no effect in this respect. Ro-4-1284-induced hypothermia is counteracted by all five drugs, most pronounced however with ephedrine and much less with tyramine. Ro-4-1284-induced miosis is counteracted by all these drugs, but with hydroxyamphetamine only at 80.0 mg/kg and above.

4. Antidepressants

Twenty-four so called "antidepressants" were studied at the following dose levels:

a) tricyclics:

desipramine: 0.02 to 0.63 mg/kg S. C.
protriptyline: 0.02 to 0.63 mg/kg S. C.
nortriptyline: 0.16 to 5.00 mg/kg S. C.
dibenzepine: 0.31 to 10.0 mg/kg S. C.
imipramine: 0.31 to 10.0 mg/kg S. C.
iopramine: 0.31 to 10.0 mg/kg P. O.
noxiptilin: 0.31 to 10.0 mg/kg S. C.
amitryptyline: 0.63 to 20.0 mg/kg S. C.
amoxapine: 0.63 to 20.0 mg/kg P. O.
doxepin: 0.63 to 20.0 mg/kg S. C.
melitracene: 0.63 to 20.0 mg/kg S. C.
maprotiline: 0.63 to 20.0 mg/kg S. C.
norpropazepine: 0.63 to 20.0 mg/kg S. C.
northiaden: 0.63 to 20.0 mg/kg S. C.
clomipramine: 1.25 to 40.0 mg/kg S. C.
pizotifen: 1.25 to 40.0 mg/kg S. C.
prothiaden: 1.25 to 40.0 mg/kg S. C.
butriptyline: 2.50 to 80.0 mg/kg S. C.
propazepine: 2.50 to 80.0 mg/kg S. C.
ketipramine: 5.00 to 160 mg/kg S. C.
opipramol: 5.00 to 160 mg/kg S. C.

b) others:

amedalin: 0.08 to 2.50 mg/kg S. C.
talopram: 0.08 to 2.50 mg/kg S. C.
talsupram: 0.08 to 2.50 mg/kg S. C.

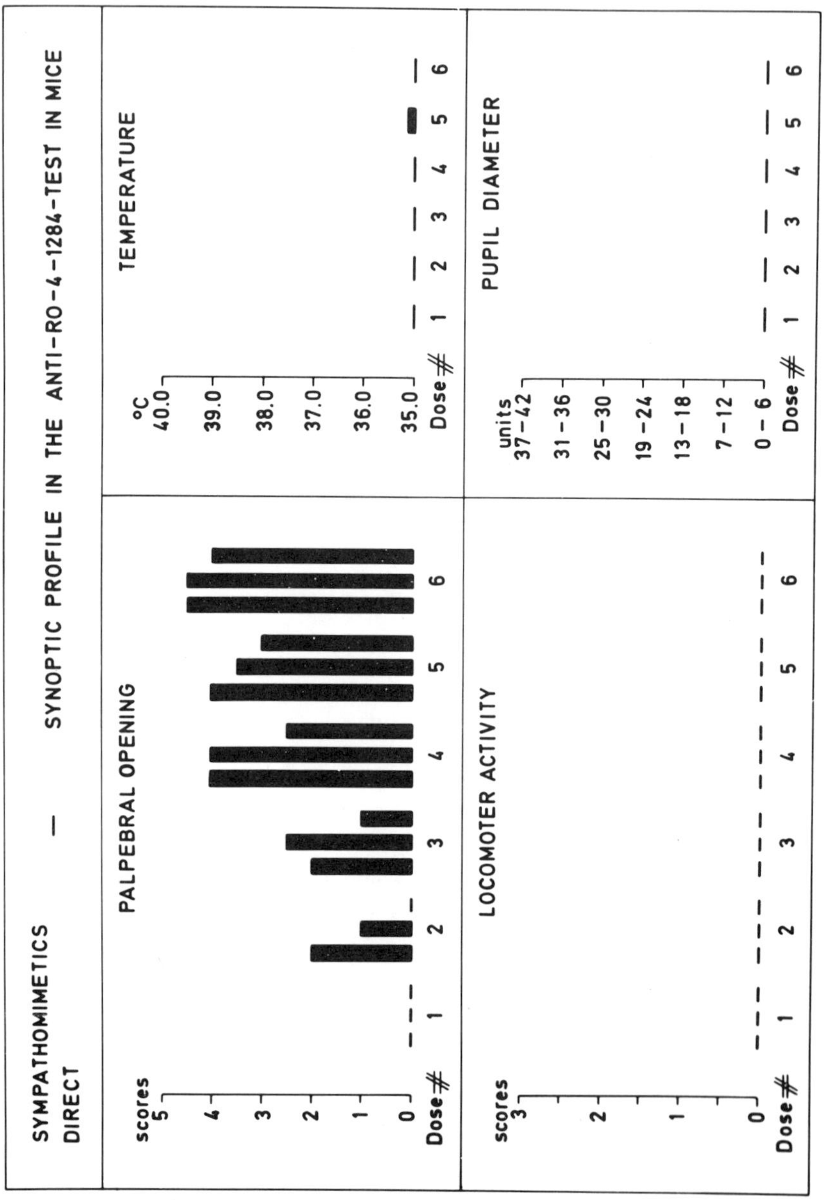
SYMPATHOMIMETICS — SYNOPTIC PROFILE IN THE ANTI-RO-4-1284-TEST IN MICE
DIRECT
PALPEBRAL OPENING
TEMPERATURE
LOCOMOTER ACTIVITY
PUPIL DIAMETER
scores
°C
units
Dose #

FIGURE 3

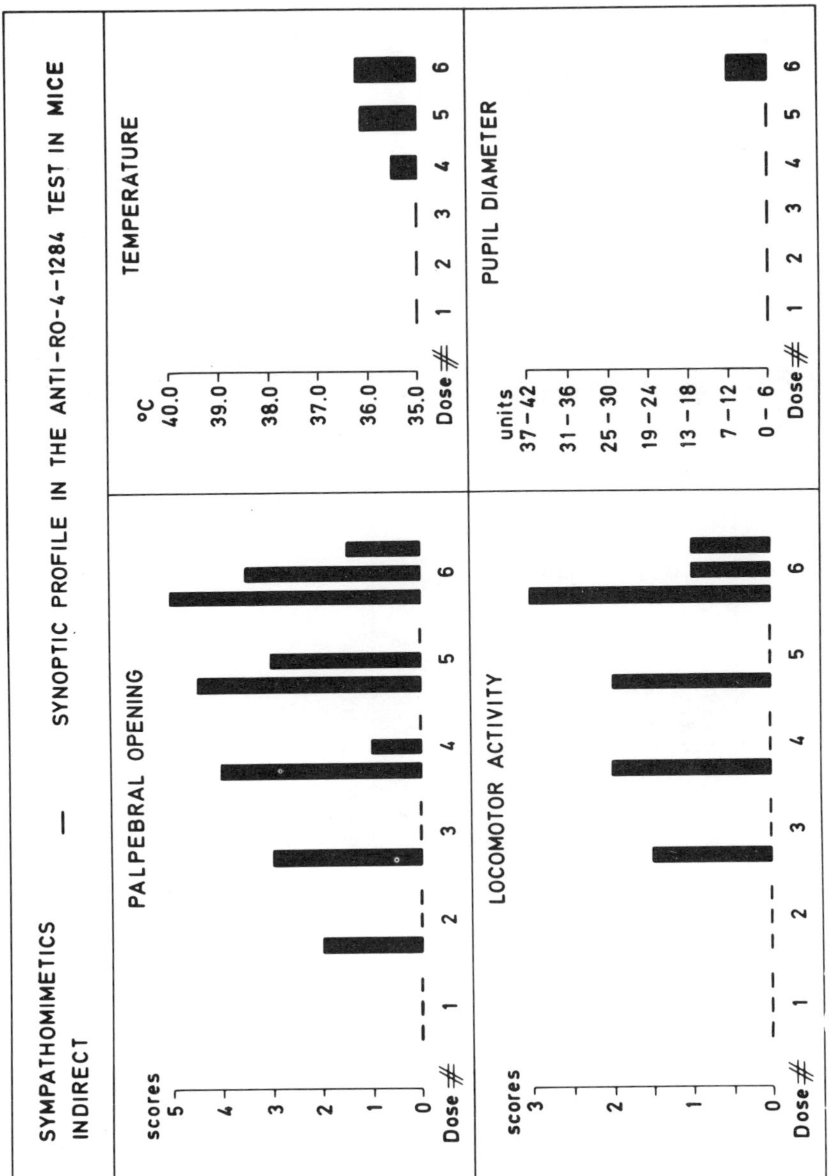

SYMPATHOMIMETICS — SYNOPTIC PROFILE IN THE ANTI-RO-4-1284 TEST IN MICE
INDIRECT
PALPEBRAL OPENING
scores
5
4
3
2
1
0
Dose #
1
2
3
4
5
6
TEMPERATURE
°C
40.0
39.0
38.0
37.0
36.0
35.0
LOCOMOTOR ACTIVITY
3
2
1
0
PUPIL DIAMETER
units
37 - 42
31 - 36
25 - 30
19 - 24
13 - 18
7 - 12
0 - 6

FIGURE 4

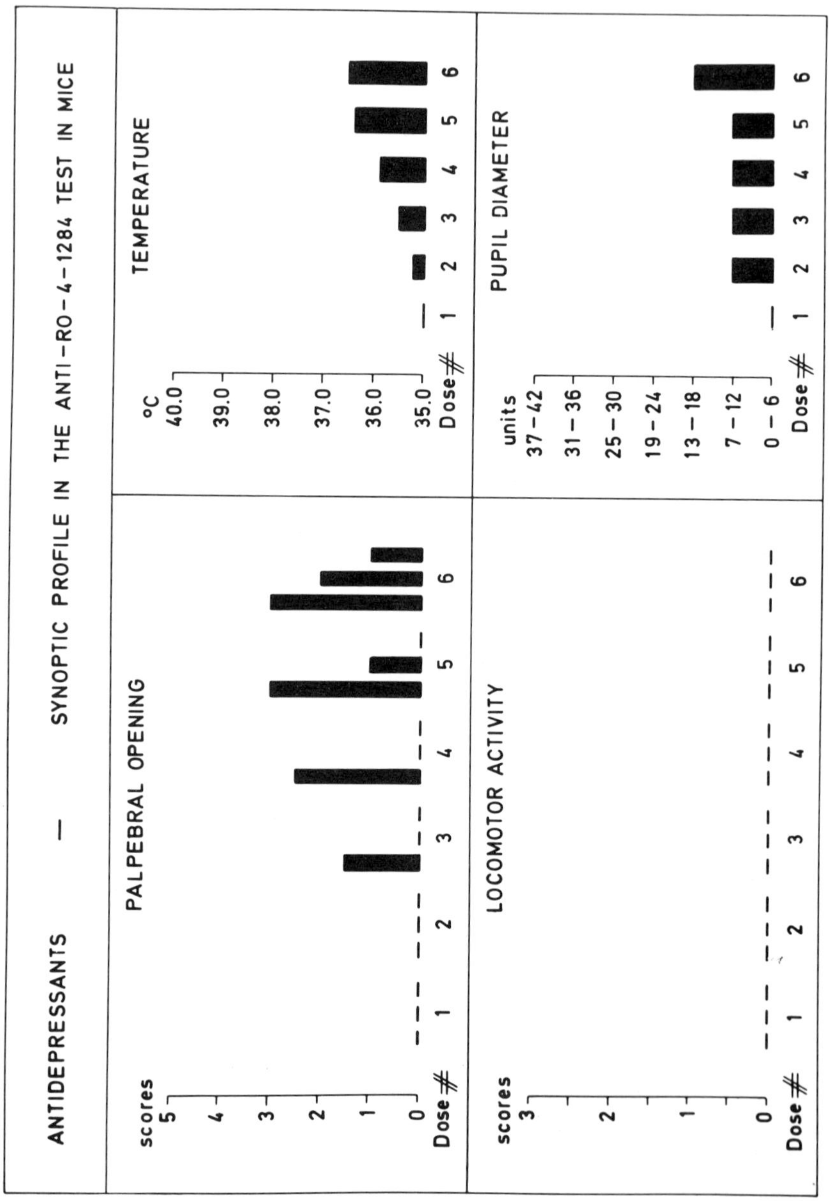
ANTIDEPRESSANTS — SYNOPTIC PROFILE IN THE ANTI-RO-4-1284 TEST IN MICE
PALPEBRAL OPENING
scores
5
4
3
2
1
0
Dose #
1 2 3 4 5 6
TEMPERATURE
°C
40.0
39.0
38.0
37.0
36.0
35.0
Dose #
1 2 3 4 5 6
LOCOMOTOR ACTIVITY
scores
3
2
1
0
Dose #
1 2 3 4 5 6
PUPIL DIAMETER
units
37 – 42
31 – 36
25 – 30
19 – 24
13 – 18
7 – 12
0 – 6
Dose #
1 2 3 4 5 6

FIGURE 5

The synoptic anti-Ro-4-1284 profile derived from the results obtained with these 24 compounds is shown in Figure 5. All compounds of this class counteract Ro-4-1284-induced ptosis. However, a reversing action within the dose range mentioned is not observed. At doses exceeding those reported reversal is occasionally seen and most pronounced with talopram, talsupram, and amedalin, 3 compounds not belonging to the tricyclic series.

Ro-4-1284-induced hypothermia is counteracted although not always consistently. Clomipramine and opipramol are two exceptions that do not affect body temperature even at doses up to 160 mg/kg. During the first observation, 15 minutes after Ro-4-1284, sedation is counteracted with 10 mg/kg of desipramine, and with 160 mg/kg of imipramine. However, amitryptyline, clomipramine, doxepin, opipramol, and prothiaden potentiate sedation at the highest dose reported and at higher doses potentiation also occurs with imipramine and propazepine.

All "antidepressants" counteract Ro-4-1284-induced miosis. Within the dose range described reversal is observed with amitryptyline, butriptyline, pizotifen, and prothiaden. At doses exceeding those reported mydriasis is also observed for doxepin (160 mg/kg), imipramine (160 mg/kg), melitracene (40.0 and 80.0 mg/kg), maprotiline (80.0 mg/kg), nortriptyline (40.0 mg/kg), noxiptiline (40.0 mg/kg), northiaden (80.0 mg/kg), protriptyline (5.00 and 10.0 mg/kg), talopram (20.0 and 40.0 mg/kg), and talsupram (20.0 and 40.0 mg/kg)

5. Analgesics

Six analgesics were tested at the following dose levels:

fentanyl: 0.02 to 0.63 mg/kg S. C. (34)
dextromoramide: 0.31 to 10.0 mg/kg S. C. (32)
cyclazocine: 0.31 to 10.0 mg/kg S. C.
piritramide: 1.25 to 40.0 mg/kg S. C. (31)
meperidine: 2.50 to 80.0 mg/kg S. C.
morphine: 5.00 to 160 mg/kg S. C.

The synoptic anti-Ro-4-1284 profile derived from the results obtained with these 6 compounds is shown in Figure 6.

Ro-4-1284-induced palpebral ptosis is counteracted consistently with cyclazocine and pethidine, inconsistently with the other compounds. No effect is noted on Ro-4-1284-induced sedation, except for a potentiation with cyclazocine at doses exceeding the mentioned range (40.0 and 80 mg/kg). Ro-4-1284-induced hypothermia and miosis are inconsistently counteracted and only at high dose levels.

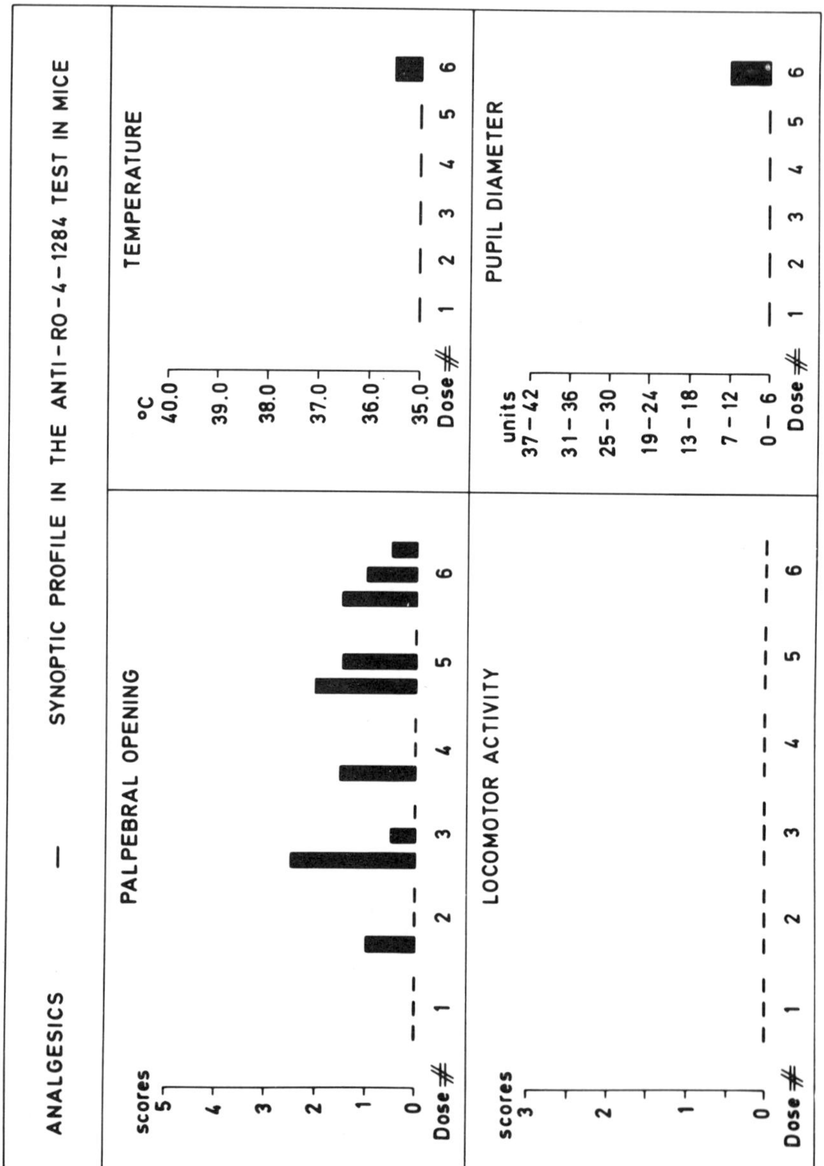
ANALGESICS — SYNOPTIC PROFILE IN THE ANTI-RO-4-1284 TEST IN MICE
PALPEBRAL OPENING
scores
5
4
3
2
1
0
Dose #
1 2 3 4 5 6
TEMPERATURE
°C
40.0
39.0
38.0
37.0
36.0
35.0
Dose #
1 2 3 4 5 6
LOCOMOTOR ACTIVITY
scores
3
2
1
0
Dose #
1 2 3 4 5 6
PUPIL DIAMETER
units
37 – 42
31 – 36
25 – 30
19 – 24
13 – 18
7 – 12
0 – 6
Dose #
1 2 3 4 5 6

FIGURE 6

6. Miscellaneous compounds

Several other compounds were found to antagonize the symptoms induced by Ro-4-1284. Table III shows the dose levels given and the results obtained with 12 of these compounds.

Cocaine, a compound with an amphetamine-like CNS profile (65) is found to produce anti-Ro-4-1284 effects comparable to those of amphetamine.

The antihistaminics, chlorpheniramine and diphenhydramine, counteract Ro-4-1284-induced palpebral ptosis, hypothermia, miosis, and to a smaller extent sedation. Mazindol reverses ptosis, and counteracts hypothermia and miosis, while locomotor activity is enhanced at 40.0 mg/kg.

Comparable but less pronounced effects are found with xylazine, a compound with various pharmacological properties (64).

Clonidine and guanethidine counteract and bretylium reverses Ro-4-1284-induced ptosis. Locomotor activity is unaffected by all three compounds. Hypothermia is slightly and inconsistently counteracted. Clonidine and guanethidine counteract miosis, while bretylium does not affect this parameter.

The main effects of pilocarpine and eserine are counteraction of Ro-4-1284-induced palpebral ptosis. Pilocarpine inconsistently potentiates hypothermia. Eserine potentiates sedation at the highest subtoxic dose level.

The anti-Ro-4-1284 profile of tolazoline is similar to that of the direct sympathomimetics.

Finally, apomorphine, whose neuro-psychopharmacological properties have been described recently by Puech et al (52), has a unique profile since it is the only compound reversing Ro-4-1284-induced sedation without affecting any of the other parameters studied.

7. Chlordiazepoxide and diazepam

The synoptic profile (Figure 7) is derived from chlordiazepoxide subcutaneously (5.00 to 160 mg/kg) and diazepam orally (0.63 to 40.0 mg/kg). Both muscle relaxants produce a significant counteraction of Ro-4-1284-induced ptosis and potentiate hypothermia. Chlordiazepoxide potentiates Ro-4-1284-induced sedation at 160 mg/kg; diazepam has a similar effect at 80 mg/kg.

8. Neuroleptics

Several neuroleptics (35, 37) were tested: haloperidol (0.16 to 5.00 mg/kg S. C.), pimozide (0.31 to 10.0 mg/kg S. C.), pipamperone and chlorpromazine (1.25 to 40.0 mg/kg S. C.).

TABLE III
Activity profiles of several drugs in the anti-Ro-4-1284 test

Drugs	Dose #	Effects[1] on Ro-4-1284 induced																							
		Palpebral ptosis						Sedation						Hypothermia						Miosis					
		1	2	3	4	5	6	1	2	3	4	5	6	1	2	3	4	5	6	1	2	3	4	5	6
cocaine (S. C.)	2.50 to 80.0	0	+	+	+	++	++	0	0	+	+	+	++	0	0	+	+	+	+	0	0	0	+	+	+
chlorpheniramine (S. C.)	2.50 to 80.0	0	+	+	+	++	+	0	0	0	0	0	+	0	0	0	+	+	+	0	+	+	+	+	+
diphenhydramine (S. C.)	1.25 to 40.0	0	0	0	+	+	+	0	0	0	0	0	+	0	0	+	+	+	+	0	0	0	+	+	++
mazindol (O. R.)	0.16 to 5.00	0	+	+	+	++	++	0	0	0	0	0	0	0	+	+	+	+	+	+	+	+	+	+	+
xylazine (S. C.)	0.31 to 2.50	0	+	+	+	+	+	0	0	0	0	0	0	0	+	+	+	+	+	0	0	0	+	+	+
clonidine (S. C.)	0.01 to 0.31	0	+	+	+	+	+	0	0	0	0	0	0	0	+	+	+	+	0	0	0	0	0	+	+
guanethidine (S. C.)	5.00 to 160	0	0	0	+	+	+	0	0	0	0	0	0	0	0	0	+	+	+	0	0	0	0	0	+
bretylium (S. C.)	0.31 to 10.0	0	+	+	+	++	++	0	0	0	0	0	0	0	0	0	+	+	+	0	0	0	0	0	0
pilocarpine (S. C.)	0.31 to 10.0	0	+	+	+	+	+	0	0	0	0	0	0	0	-	0	0	-	-	0	0	0	0	0	+
eserine (S. C.)	0.01 to 0.31	0	0	0	+	+	+	0	0	0	0	0	-	0	0	0	0	0	0	0	0	0	0	0	0
tolazoline (S. C.)	1.25 to 40.0	0	+	+	+	+	+	0	0	0	0	0	0	0	0	0	0	0	0	0	0	0	0	0	0
apomorphine (S. C.)	0.63 to 20.0	0	0	0	0	0	0	0	+	+	+	+	++	0	0	0	0	0	0	0	0	0	0	0	0

[1]0 no change; + counteraction; ++ reversal; - potentiation

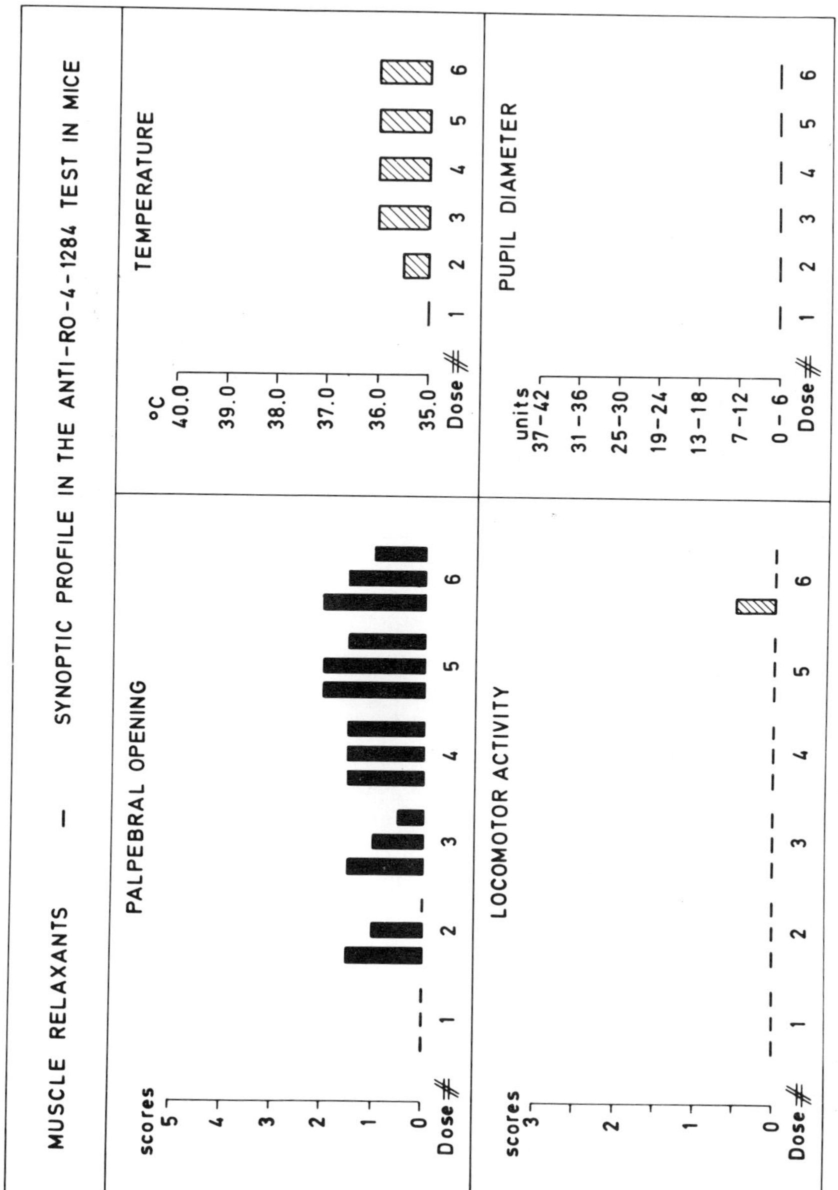
MUSCLE RELAXANTS — SYNOPTIC PROFILE IN THE ANTI-RO-4-1284 TEST IN MICE
PALPEBRAL OPENING
scores
5
4
3
2
1
0
Dose #
1
2
3
4
5
6
TEMPERATURE
°C
40.0
39.0
38.0
37.0
36.0
35.0
Dose #
1
2
3
4
5
6
LOCOMOTOR ACTIVITY
scores
3
2
1
0
Dose #
1
2
3
4
5
6
PUPIL DIAMETER
units
37–42
31–36
25–30
19–24
13–18
7–12
0–6
Dose #
1
2
3
4
5
6

FIGURE 7

These compounds do not affect Ro-4-1284-induced palpebral ptosis and sedation with the exception of chlorpromazine, which potentiates the sedative effects of Ro-4-1284 at 5.00 mg/kg and above. A slight inconsistent potentiation of hypothermia and miosis is further observed for all 4 drugs.

IV. PITFALLS AND USEFULNESS OF THE TEST

From the present study with 68 different compounds, it may be concluded that Ro-4-1284-induced symptoms in mice can be antagonized by many chemical agents, possessing a variety of pharmacological actions. This would indicate that the anti-Ro-4-1284 test in mice is by no means a selective test for antidepressant activity. However in the absence of more selective tests, the anti-Ro-4-1284 test may be used with caution to screen potential drugs with antidepressant activity. These cautions are discussed below.

As evidenced by their synoptic anti-Ro-4-1284 profile, the imipramine-like antidepressants studied, counteract Ro-4-1284-induced palpebral ptosis, hypothermia, and miosis, without affecting sedation. However, Ro-4-1284-induced palpebral ptosis is also counteracted by tranylcypromine, pheniprazine, modaline, pargyline and iproniazid, by oxymetazoline, xylometazoline, naphazoline, tramazoline, tetrahydrozoline, amphetamine, methylamphetamine, hydroxyamphetamine, ephedrine and tyramine, by fentanyl, dextromoramide, cyclazocine, piritramide, pethidine and morphine, by chlordiazepoxide and diazepam, and by a variety of compounds such as cocaine, chlorpheniramine, diphenhydramine, mazindol, xylazine, clonidine, guanethidine, bretylium, pilocarpine, eserine, and tolazoline. Hypothermia is counteracted by tranylcypromine, pheniprazine, modaline, pargyline, and iproniazid, by amphetamine, methylamphetamine, hydroxyamphetamine, ephedrine, and tyramine, and also by cocaine, chlorpheniramine, diphenhydramine, mazindol, xylazine, clonidine and bretylium. Miosis is counteracted by atropine, dexetimide, isopropamide, benztropine and benactyzine, by tranylcypromine, pheniprazine, modaline, pargyline and iproniazid, by amphetamine, methylamphetamine, hydroxyamphetamine, ephedrine and tyramine, by cocaine, chlorpheniramine, diphenhydramine, mazindol, xylazine, clonidine, guanethidine and pilocarpine, and at very high doses even by oxymetazoline, xylometazoline, naphazoline, tramazoline, and xylometazoline.

Nevertheless all the classical antidepressants counteract the three above mentioned symptoms within the same dose range and in a rather characteristic manner, allowing the construction of a

ADDENDUM 1

I ANTICHOLINERGICS		**III a SYMPATHOMIMETICS – DIRECT**	
ATROPINE	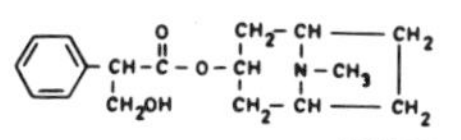 1/2 H_2SO_4	OXYMETAZOLINE	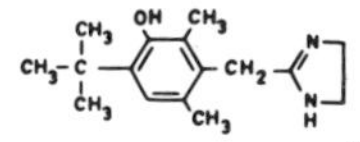 HCl
DEXETIMIDE	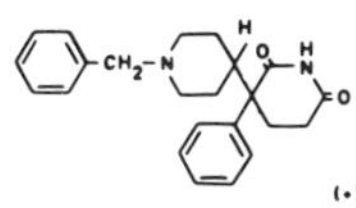 (+)-(S)-HCl	XYLOMETAZOLINE	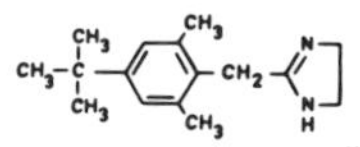 HCl
ISOPROPAMIDE	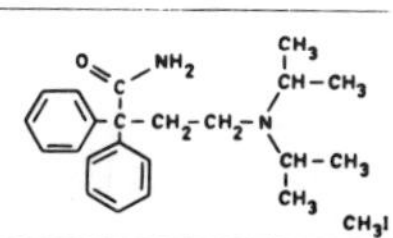 CH_3I	NAPHAZOLINE	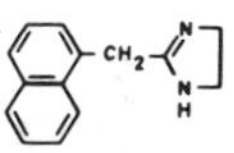 HCl
BENZTROPINE	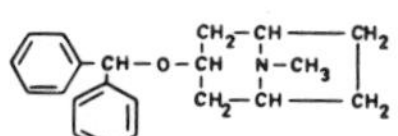 CH_3SO_3H	TRAMAZOLINE	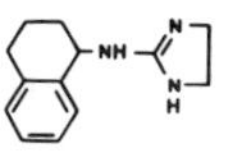 HCl
BENACTYZINE	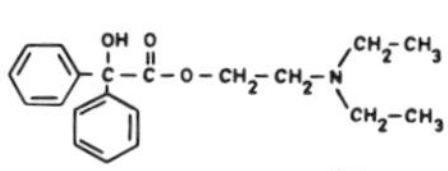 HCl	TETRAHYDROZOLINE	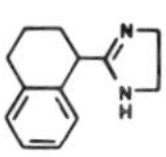 HC:
II MONOAMINE OXIDASE INHIBITORS		**III b SYMPATHOMIMETICS – INDIRECT**	
TRANYLCYPROMINE	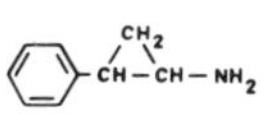 1/2 H_2SO_4	AMPHETAMINE	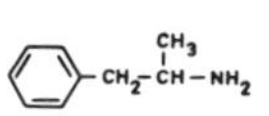 1/2 H_2SO_4
PHENIPRAZINE	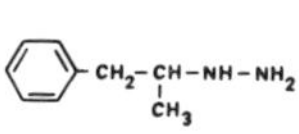 HCl	METHYLAMPHETAMINE	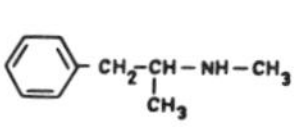 (+)-HCl
MODALINE	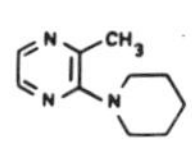 H_2SO_4	HYDROXYAMPHETAMINE	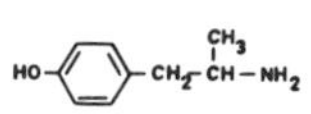 HBr
PARGYLINE	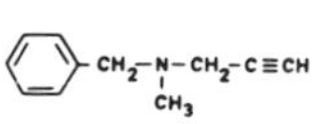 HCl	EPHEDRINE	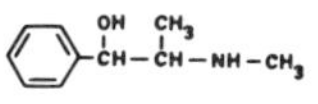 (-)-HCl
IPRONIAZID	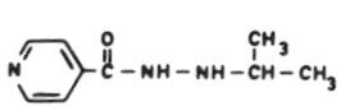	TYRAMINE	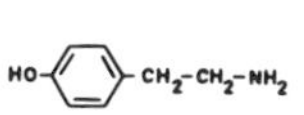 HCl

Antidepressants

ADDENDUM 2

IV ANTIDEPRESSANTS			
MELITRACENE	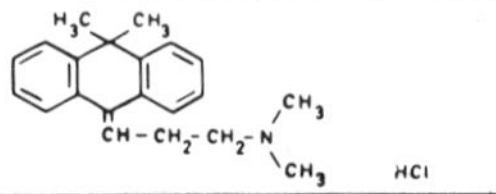	OPIPRAMOL	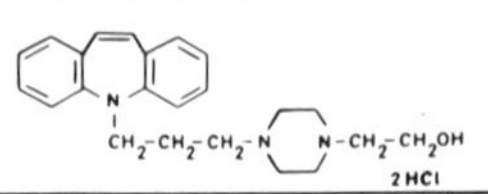
BUTRIPTYLINE	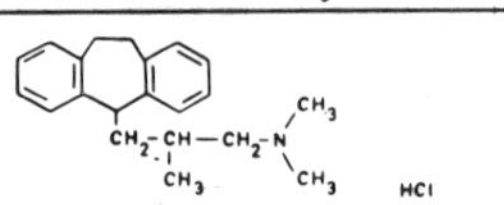	NORPROPAZEPINE	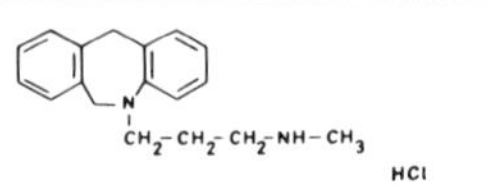
PROTRIPTYLINE	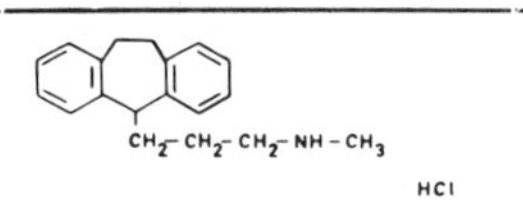	PROPAZEPINE	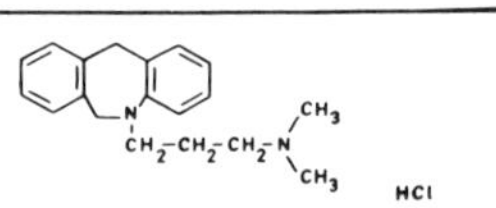
NORTRIPTYLINE	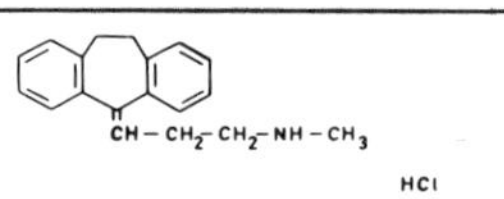	KETIPRAMINE	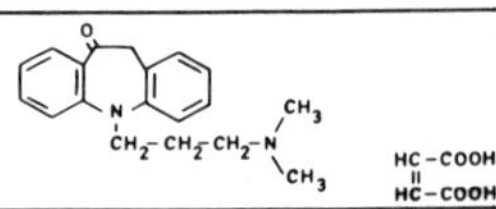
AMITRYPTYLINE	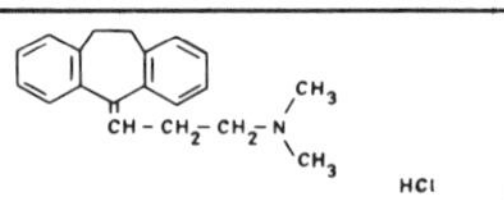	DOXEPIN	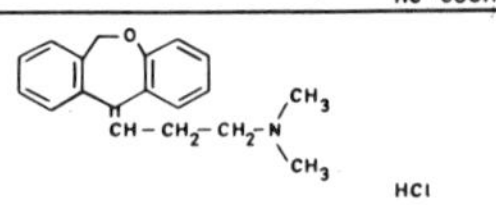
PIZOTIFEN	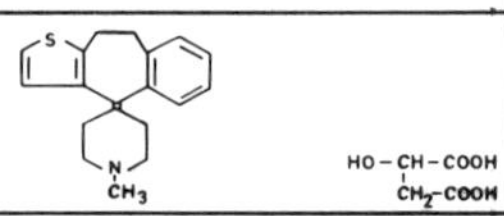	NORTHIADEN	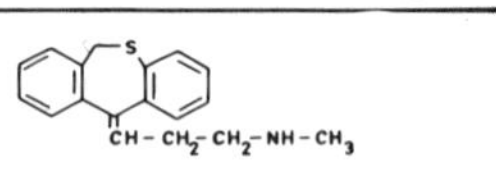
NOXIPTILIN	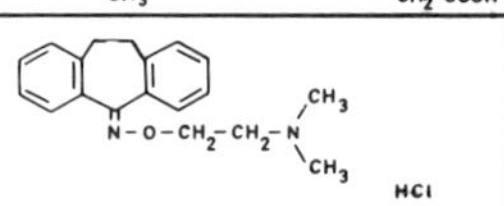	PROTHIADEN	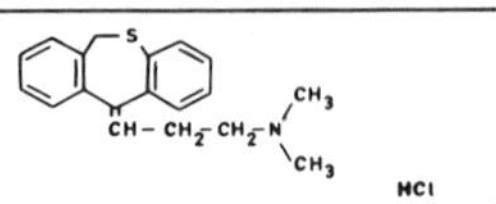
MAPROTILINE	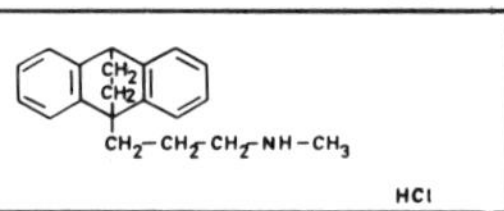	DIBENZEPINE	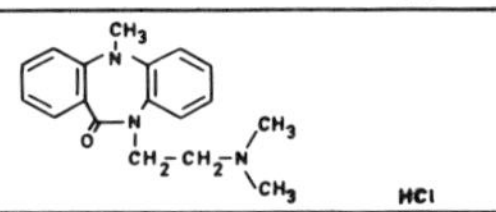
DESIPRAMINE	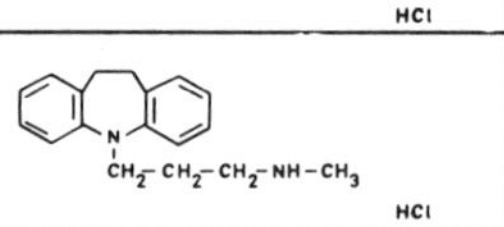	AMOXAPINE	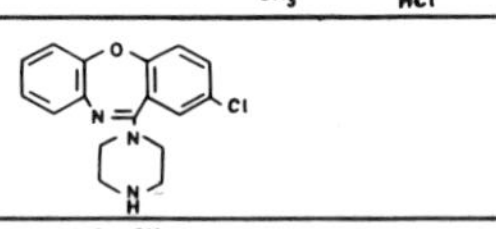
IMIPRAMINE	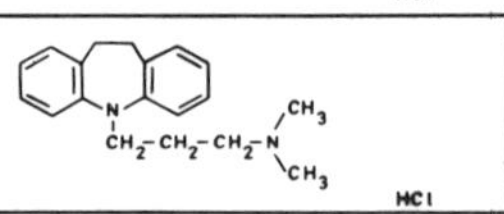	TALOPRAM	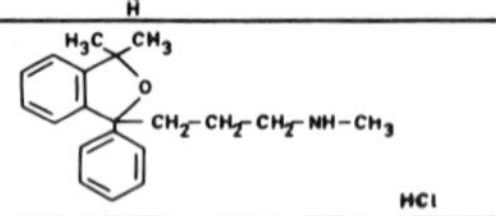
CLOMIPRAMINE	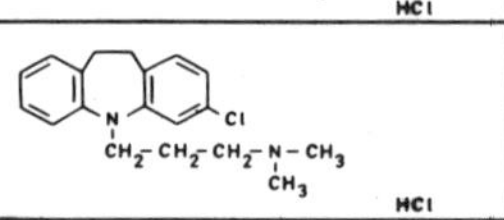	TALSUPRAM	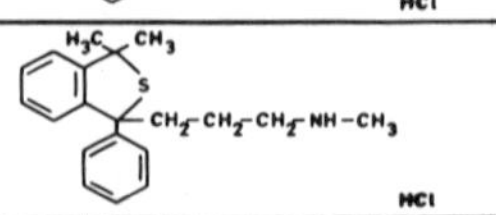
IOPRAMINE	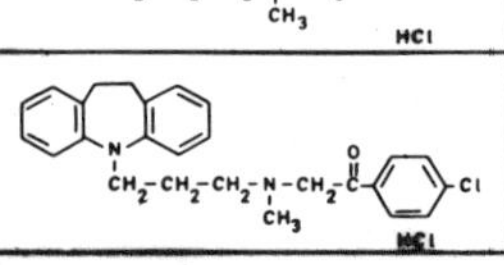	AMEDALIN	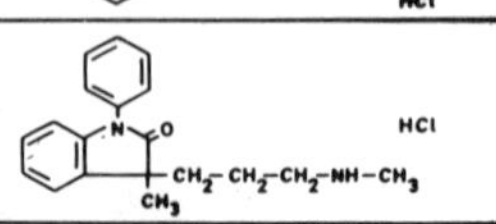

ADDENDUM 3

V	ANALGESICS
FENTANYL	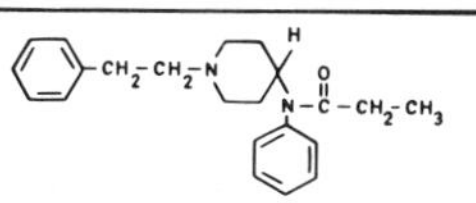
CYCLAZOCINE	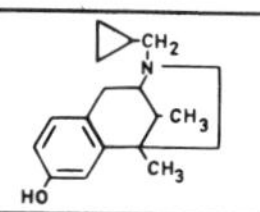
PIRITRAMIDE	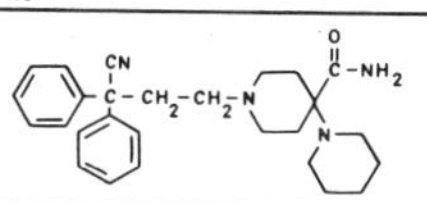
DEXTROMORAMIDE	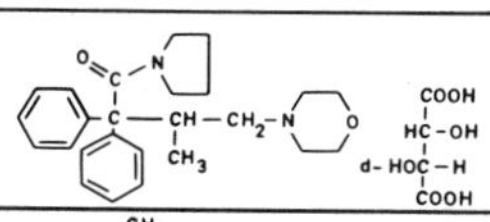
MORPHINE	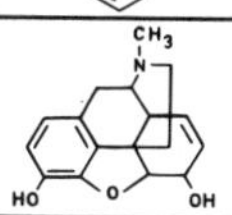 HCl

VII	MUSCLE RELAXANTS
CHLORDIAZEPOXIDE	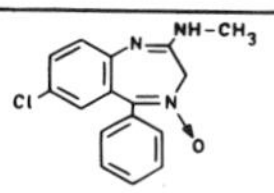 HCl
DIAZEPAM	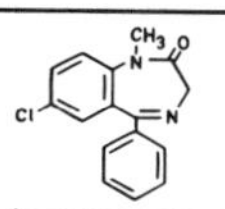

VIII	NEUROLEPTICS
HALOPERIDOL	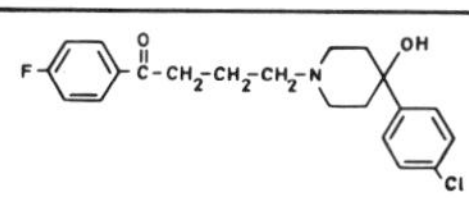
PIMOZIDE	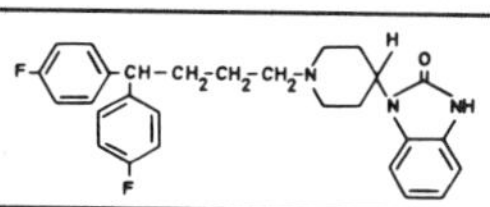
PIPAMPERONE	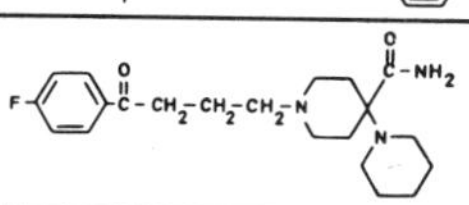
CHLORPROMAZINE	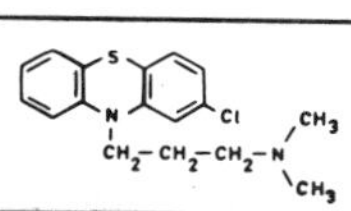

VI	MISCELLANEOUS
COCAINE	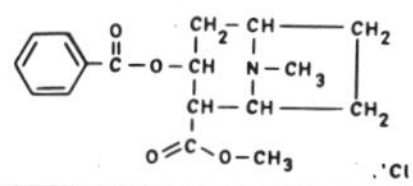
CHLORPHENIRAMINE	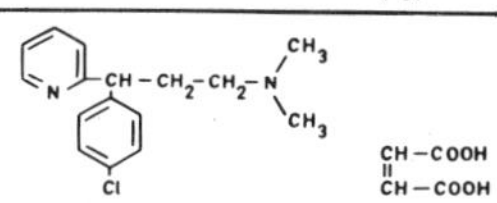
DIPHENHYDRAMINE	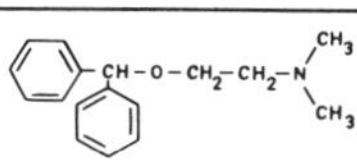 HCl
MAZINDOL	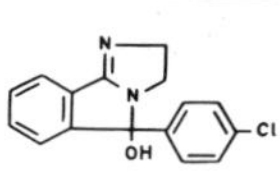
XYLAZINE	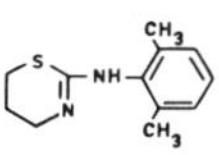
CLONIDINE	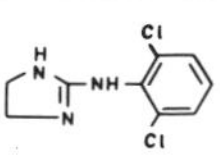
GUANETHIDINE	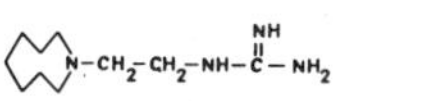 1/2 H_2SO_4
BRETYLIUM	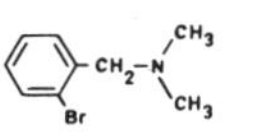 C_2H_5Br
PILOCARPINE	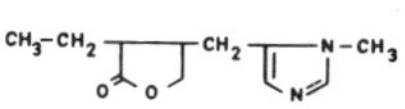 HCl
ESERINE	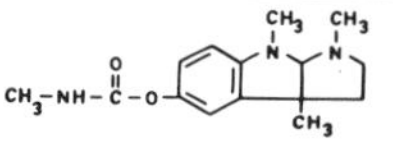 1/2 H_2SO_4
TOLAZOLINE	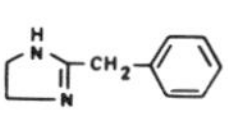
APOMORPHINE	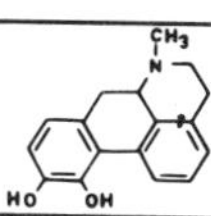 HCl

profile different from that of other compounds having similar qualitative properties.

Therefore, a standardized anti-Ro-4-1284 test in mice, as described, may be a useful tool for detecting and describing drugs with potential antidepressant activity, provided that quantitative and qualitative information on various aspects of the anti-Ro-4-1284 activity is taken into account.

REFERENCES

1. Aceto, M. D. and Harris, L. S.: Effect of various agents on reserpine-induced blepharoptosis, *Toxicol. Appl. Pharmacol.,* **7**:329-336, 1965.
2. Askew, B. M.: A simple screening procedure for imipramine-like antidepressant agents, *Life Sciences,* **10**:725-730, 1963.
3. Barnett, A., Taber, R. I., and Roth, F. E.: Activity of antihistamines in laboratory antidepressant test, *Int. J. Neuropharmac.,* **8**:73-79, 1969.
4. Bernardi, D., Jori, A., Morselli, P., Valzelli, L., and Garattini, S.: Further effects of imipramine and its desmethyl derivative on the hypothermia-induced by reserpine, *J. Pharm. Pharmacol.,* **18**:278-282, 1966.
5. Bernardi, D., Paglialunga, S., and Jori, A.: Peripheral and central components in the hyperthermic effect of desipramine in reserpinized rats, *J. Pharm. Pharmac.,* **20**:204-209, 1968.
6. Bickel, M. H. and Brodie, B. B.: Structure and antidepressant activity of imipramine analogues, *Int. J. Neuropharmacol.,* **3**:611-621, 1964.
7. Bickel, M. H., Sulser, F., and Brodie, B. B.: Monomethylanalogues of phenothiazines which exert a potent desmethylimipramine-like antidepressant action in rats, *Pharmacologist,* **4**:159, 1962.
8. Boissier, J. R., Simon, P., Fichelle-Pagny, J., and Lwoff, J. M.: La dibenzéprine (Noveril): quelques aspects de pharmacologie prévisonnelle, *Thérapie,* **21**:773-780, 1966a.
9. Boissier, J. R., Fichelle-Pagny, J., and Simon, P.: Activité anti-réserpine chez la souris de l'imipramine, de l'amitriptyline et de leurs dérivés monodesméthylés, *Thérapie,* 21:109-117, 1966 b.
10. Brodie, B. B., Bickel, M. H., and Sulser, F.: Desmethylimipramine, a new type of antidepressant drug, *Med. Exp.,* **5**:454-458, 1961.
11. Bunney, W. E. and Davis, J. M.: Norepinephrine in depressive reactions, *Arch. Gen. Psychiat.,* **13**:483-494, 1965.
12. Carlsson, A., Lindqvist, M., and Magnusson, T.: 3,4-dihydroxyphenylalanine and 5-hydroxytryptophan as reserpine antagonists, *Nature,* **180**:1200, 1957.
13. Chen, G. and Bohner, B.: The anti-reserpine effects of certain centrally-acting agents, *J. Pharmac. Exp. Ther.,* **131**:179-184, 1961.
14. Colpaert, F. C., Lenaerts, F. M., and Niemegeers, C. J. E. and Janssen, P. A. J.: A critical study of Ro-4-1284 antagonism in mice. *Arch. Int. Pharmacodyn,* **215**:189-239, 1975.
15. Cooper, F. and Schnieden, H.: Study of the mechanism of action of desipramine and chlorpromazine in reversing reserpine-induced hypothermia in mice, *Brit. J. Pharmac.,* **45**:162-163, 1972.
16. Coppen, A.: The biochemistry of affective disorders, *Brit. J. Psychiat.,* **113**:1237-1264, 1967.

17. Costa, E., Garattini, S., and Valzelli, L.: Interactions between reserpine, chlorpromazine and imipramine, *Experientia,* **16**:461-463, 1960.
18. Cotillo, P. and Bonaccorsi, A.: Observation on the interactions between desipramine and reserpine on adrenergic transmission in the rat, *J. Pharm. Pharmacol.,* **24**:103-107, 1972.
19. De Jongh, D. K., Van Proosdij-Hartzema, E. G., and Janssen, P. A. J.: Substituted phenylpropylamines. II. Pharmacological properties of basic butyrontriles and butyramides, *Arch. Int. Pharmacodyn.,* **103**:100-119, 1955.
20. Fielden, R. and Green, A. L.: Validity of ptosis as a measure of the central depressant action of reserpine, *J. Pharm. Pharmacol.,* **17**:185-187, 1965.
21. Garattini, S. and Jori, A.: Interactions between imipramine-like drugs and reserpine on body temperature, in Garattini S. and Dukes M. N. G.: *Antidepressant drugs, Exc. Med. Found.,* Amsterdam, N. Y. 1967, pp. 179-193.
22. Garattini, S., Giachetti, A., Jori, A., Pieri, L., and Valzelli, L.: Effect of imipramine, amitriptyline and their monomethyl derivatives on reserpine activity, *J. Pharm. Pharmacol.,* **14**:509-514, 1962.
23. Garattini, S., Giachetti, A., Pieri, L., and Re, R.: Antagonists of reserpine-induced eyelid ptosis, *Med. Exp.,* **3**:315-320, 1960.
24. Giurgea, M., Dauby, J., Levis, S., and Giurgea, C.: Un test antitétrabénazine modifié pour le screening des produits antidépressifs, *Med. Exp.,* **9**:249-262, 1963.
25. Gluckman, M. I. and Baum, T.: The pharmacology of iprindole, a new antidepressant, *Psychopharmacologia,* **15**:169-185, 1969.
26. Greenwood, D. T. and Sommerville, A. R.: The effect of immunosympathectomy on the responses of the mouse to reserpine and various antidepressant and stimulant drugs, *Psychopharmacologia,* **24**:231-237, 1972.
27. Gylys, J. A., Muccia, P. M. R., and Taylor, M. K.: Pharmacological and toxical properties of 2-methyl-3-piperidino-pyrazine, a new antidepressant, *Ann. N. Y. Acad. Sci.,* **107**:899-913, 1963.
28. Halliwell, G., Quinton, R. M., and Williams, F. E.: A comparison of imipramine, chlorpromazine and related drugs in various tests involving autonomic functions and antagonism of reserpine, *Brit. J. Pharmacol.,* **23**:330-350, 1964.
29. Herr, F., Voith, K., and Jaramillo, J.: The pharmacology of butriptyline, *J. Med.,* **2**:258-270, 1971.
30. Horovitz, Z. P., Furgiuele, A. R., High, J. P., and Burke, J. C.: Comparative activities of a substituted dibenzothiazepine of imipramine and of desipramine, *Arch. Int. Pharmacodyn.,* **151**:180-191, 1964.
31. Janssen, P. A. J.: Pirinitramide (R 3365), a potent analgesic with unusual chemical structure, *J. Pharm. Pharmacol.,* **13**:513-530, 1961.
32. Janssen, P. A. J. and Jageneau, A. H.: A new series of potent analgesics, dextro 2, 2-diphenyl-3-methyl-4-morpholino-butyryl-pyrrolidine and related basic amides, *J. Pharm. Pharmacol.,* **10**:14-21, 1958.
33. Janssen, P. A. J. and Niemegeers, C. J. E.: The peripheral and central anticholinergic properties of benzetimide (R 4929) and other atropine-like drugs as measured in a new anti-pilocarpine test in rats, *Psychopharmacologia,* **11**:231-254, 1967.
34. Janssen, P. A. J., Niemegeers, C. J. E., and Dony, J. G. H.: The

inhibitory effect of fentanyl and other morphine-like analgesics on the warm water induced tail withdrawal reflex in rats, *Arzneim.-Forsch.,* **13**:502-507, 1963.

35. Janssen, P. A. J., Niemegeers, C. J. E., and Schellekens, K. H. L.: Is it possible to predict the clinical effects of neuroleptic drugs (major tranquillizers) from animal data? Part I: 'Neuroleptic activity spectra' for rats, *Arzneim.-Forsch.,* **15**:104-117, 1965.
36. Janssen, P. A. J., Niemegeers, C. J. E., Schellekens, K. H. L., Demoen, P., Lenaerts, F. M., Van Nueten, J. M., Van Wijngaarden, F., and Brugmans, J.: Benzetimide and its optical isomers, *Arzneim.-Forsch.,* **21**:1365-1373, 1971.
37. Janssen, P. A. J., Niemegeers, C. J. E., Schellekens, K. H. L., Dresse, A., Lenaerts, F. M., Pinchard, A., Schaper, W. K. A., Van Nueten, J. M., and Verbruggen, F. J.: Pimozide, a chemically novel highly potent and orally long-acting neuroleptic drug, *Arzneim.-Forsch.,* **18**:261-279, 1968.
38. Jones, B. J., Tolman, B. D., and Roberts, D. J.: Studies on interactions involving antidepressive and other drugs with tetrabenazine and noradnamine on locomotor activity in mice, including details of the experimental design and statistical analysis, *Psychopharmacologia,* **18**:288-299, 1970.
39. Jori, A., Bonaccorsi, A., Valzelli, L., and Garattini, S.: New orally active monoamine oxidase (MAO)-inhibitors, *Life Sci.,* No.-**8**:611-617, 1963.
40. Jori, A., Carrara, M. C., Paglialunga, S., and Garattini, S.: Pharmacological studies on modaline sulphate (W 3207), *J. Pharm. Pharmacol.,* **17**:703-709, 1965.
41. Lapin, I. P.: Simple pharmacological procedures to differentiate antidepressants and cholinolytics in mice and rats, *Psychopharmacologia,* **11**:79-87, 1967 a.
42. Lapin, I. P.: Comparison of antireserpine and anticholinergic effects of antidepressants and of central and peripheral cholinolytics, *in* Garattini, S. and Duke, M. N. G.: *Antidepressant drugs,* Exc. Med. Found, Amsterdam, N. Y. 1967 b, pp. 266-278.
43. Lotti, V. J., Torchiana, M. L., and Porter, C. C.: Investigations on the action and mechanism of action of diphenylhydantion as an antagonist of tetrabenazine and reserpine, *Arch. Int. Pharmacodyn.,* **203**:107-116, 1973.
44. Lwoff, J. M., Larousse, C., Simon, P., and Boissier, J. R.: Profil psychopharmacologique d'un antidépresseur potentiel appartenant à la série pyridobenzodiazépine, *Thérapie,* **26**:451-457, 1971.
45. Maxwell, D. R. and Palmer, H. T.: Demonstration of antidepressant or stimulant properties of imipramine in experimental animals, *Nature,* **191**:84-85, 1961.
46. Metys, J. and Metysova, J.: Relationships between antireserpine and central cholinolytic effects of imipramine-like antidepressants, *in* Garattini, S. and Duke, M. N. G.: *Antidepressant drugs,* Exc. Med. Found., Amsterdam, N. Y. 1967, pp. 255-265.
47. Metysova, J. and Metys, J.: Pharmacological properties of the desmethyl derivatives of some antidepressants of imipramine type, *Int. J. Neuropharmacol.,* **4**:111-124, 1965.
48 Michaelis, W. and Stille, G.: Demethylation of imipramine and an-

titetrabenazine effect in the catalepsy and ptosis test, *Life Sci.,* **7**:99-106, 1968.
49. Møller-Nielsen, I., Nymark, M., Hougs, W. and Pedersen, V.: The pharmacological properties of Melitracen (N 7001) and Litracen (N 7049), *Arzneim.-Forsch.,* **16**:135-140, 1966.
50. Morpurgo, C. and Theobald, W.: Influence of imipramine-like compounds and chlorpromazine on the reserpine-hypothermia in mice and the amphetamine-hyperthermia in rats, *Med. Pharmacol. Exp.,* **12**:226-232, 1965.
51. Prange, A. J.: The pharmacology and biochemistry of depression, *Dis. Nerv. Syst.,* **25**:217-221, 1964.
52. Puech, A. J., Simon, P., Chermat, R., and Boissier, J. R.: Profile neuropsychopharmacologique de l'apomorphine, *J. Pharmacol. (Paris),* **5**:241-254, 1974.
53. Pulewka, P.: The eye of the white mouse as a pharmacological test object, *I. Arch. exp. Path. Pharmak.,* **168**:307-318, 1932.
54. Pulewka, P.: The eye of the white mouse as a pharmacological test object. II. The assay of therapeutic agents which contain atropine-like substances, *Arch. exp. Path. Pharmak.,* **180**:119-134, 1936.
55. Ribbentrop, A. and Schaumann, W.: Pharmakologische Untersuchungen mit Doxepin, einem Antidepressivum mit zentral anticholinerger und sedierender Wirkung, *Arzneim.-Forsch.,* **15**:863-868, 1965.
56. Rohte, O.: Observation of the grooming behaviour of reserpinized white mice as a method for investigating reserpine antagonism and synergism, *Psychopharmacologia,* **18**:154-161, 1970.
57. Rubin, B., Malone, M. H., Waugh, M. H., and Burke, J. C.: Bioassay of rauwolfia roots and alkaloids, *J. Pharm. Exp. Therap.,* **120**:125-136, 1957.
58. Saavedra, J. M. and Fischer, E.: Antagonism of β-phenyl-thylamine derivatives and serotonin blocking drugs upon serotonin, tryptamine and reserpine behavioral depression in mice, *Arzneim.-Forsch.,* **20**:952-957, 1970.
59. Scheel-Kruger, J. and Randrup, A.: Evidence for a cholinergic mechanism in brain involved in the tetrabenazine reversal by thymoleptic drugs, *J. Pharm. Pharmacol.,* **21**:403-406, 1969.
60. Schildkraut, J.: The catecholamine hypothesis of affective disorders: A review of supporting evidence, *Amer. J. Psychiat.,* **122**:509-522, 1965.
61. Segawa, T., Yajima, H., and Kawasaki, K.: Effects of 5-methoxytryptamine derivatives on reserpine-syndrome in mice, *Arch. Int. Pharmacodyn.,* **186**:129-132, 1970.
62. Siegel, S.: *Nonparametric statistics for the behavioral sciences,* McGraw-Hill, New York, 1956, p. 127.
63. Sigg, E. B., Gyermek, L., and Hill, R. T.: Antagonism to reserpine-induced depression by imipramine, related psychoactive drugs, and some autonomic agents, *Psychopharmacologia,* **7**:144-149, 1965.
64. Simon, P., Chermat, R., Puech, A. J., Goujet, M. A., and Boissier, J. R.: Profil psychopharmacologique d'un α-sympathomimétique central, la xylazine, analgésique et tranquillisant en médecine vétérinaire, *Thérapie,* **28**:735-751, 1973.
65. Simon, P., Sultan, Z., Chermat, R., and Boissier, J. R.: La cocaïne, une

substance amphétaminique? Un problème de psychopharmacologie expérimentale, *J. Pharmacol.,* **3**:129-142, 1972.
66. Smith, C. B. and Dews, P. B.: Antagonism of locomotor suppressant effects of reserpine in mice, *Psychopharmacologia,* **3**:55-59, 1962.
67. Spencer, P. S. J.: Antagonism of hypothermia in the mouse by antidepressants, *in* Garattini, S. and Dukes, M. N. G.: *Antidepressant drugs,* Exc. Med. Found., Amsterdam, N. Y. 1967, pp. 194-204.
68. Srinal, R. C., Singh, H. K., and Dhawan, B. N.: Experimental evidence for imipramine like activity of fenfluramine, *Arch. int. Pharmacodyn.,* **188**:320-331, 1970.
69. Stille, G., Lauener, H., and Eichenberger, E.: Ein pharmakologischer vergleich klinisch gebräuchlichen antidepressiva unter besonderer berücksichtigung von noveril, *Schweiz. Med. Woch.,* **95**:366-372, 1965.
70. Sulser, F., Bickel, M. H., and Brodie, B. B.: The action of desmethylimipramine in counteracting sedation and cholinergic effects of reserpine-like drugs, *J. Pharmacol. Exp. Ther.,* **144**:321-330, 1964.
71. Sulser, F. and Soroko, F.: On the role of rate of brain norepinephrine release in the antibenzoquinolizine action of desipramine, *Psychopharmacologia,* **8**:191-200, 1965.
72. Sulser, F., Watts, J., and Brodie, B. B.: On the mechanism of antidepressant action of imipramine-like drugs, *Ann. N. Y. Acad. Sci.,* **96**:279-286, 1962.
73. Van Proosdij-Hartzema, E. G., Janssen, P. A. J., and De Jongh, D. K.: Substituted phenylpropylamines. III. Anticholinergic activity of quaternary ammonium bases derived from R 55 (2, 2-diphenyl-4-diisopropylamino-butyramide), *Arch. int. Pharmacodyn.,* **103**:120-128, 1955.
74. Van Riezen, H. and Delver, A.: The effect of a number of drugs with different pharmacological properties upon reserpine-induced hypothermia in mice, *Arzneim.-Forsch.,* **10**:1562-1566, 1971.
75. Vernier, V. G., Alleva, F. R., Hanson, H. M., and Stone, C. A.: Pharmacological action of amitriptyline, noramitriptyline and imipramine, *Fed. Proc.,* **21**:419, 1962 a.
76. Vernier, V. G., Hanson, H. M., and Stone, C. A.: The pharmacodynamics of amitriptyline, *in* Nodine, J. H. and Moyer, J. H.: *Psychosomatic medicine,* Lea & Febiger, Philadelphia, 1962 b, pp. 683-690.
77. Wilson, S. P. and Tislow, R.: Differential antagonism of reserpine eyelid closure by imipramine and amphetamine, *Proc. Soc. Exp. Biol. Med.,* **109**:847-848, 1962.

4

Antidepressants and Mouse-Killing (Muricide) Behavior

JOHN R. VOGEL, PH.D.

I. INTRODUCTION

Widespread use of drugs in the treatment of depression began in the 1950's with the introduction of the monoamine oxidase inhibitor, iproniazid, and the dibenzazepine derivative, imipramine. It was subsequently found that monoamine oxidase inhibitors possess side effects and currently they are given only to patients who do not respond to other forms of treatment. On the other hand, imipramine and other dibenzazepine derivatives, commonly termed tricyclic antidepressants, with far less untoward reactions are reputed to have antidepressant activity.

One approach to the laboratory testing of new compounds for possible therapeutic activity is to measure their effectiveness in animal models of human disease states. At present there is no widely accepted animal model of human depression. Direct testing of new compounds for possible antidepressant activity has been largely impossible because most antidepressant drugs actually depress the behavior of laboratory animals (1). In this respect, the effect of these drugs may appear similar to that of tranquilizers. Therefore, several indirect approaches have been widely used. In general they are designed to measure: 1) antagonism of the behavioral depression produced by drugs such as tetrabenazine or 2) augmentation of the effects of psychostimulants such as amphetamine. These procedures are discussed in detail in chapters 3 and 2, and 6, respectively.

II. MOUSE-KILLING (MURICIDE) BY LABORATORY RATS

A novel approach to screening new compounds for possible antidepressant activity grew out of studies on the limbic system of the brain. Changes in behavior following stimulation or destruction of these structures indicated that the limbic system may play a major role in the control of affective reactions (2). Electrophysiological studies have indicated that functions of one of these structures, the amygdala, are selectively blocked by antidepressant drugs (3). For example, convulsive seizures elicited by electrical stimulation of the amygdala are inhibited by antidepressant drugs while those elicited by stimulation of the septum or hippocampus are not (4). Horovitz proposed that the amygdala might be the site of action of antidepressant drugs (5) and Horovitz, Ragozzino and Leaf (6) proposed that other behaviors controlled by the amygdala might also be inhibited by antidepressant drugs.

One behavior that appears to be controlled by the amygdala is mouse-killing by rats which was described by Karli (7). Some, but not all, laboratory rats spontaneously attack and kill mice. The attack-response patterns are relatively stereotyped. In general, rats strike at the cervical or upper thoracic portions of the mouse's spinal cord and kill by biting through the cord (see Fig. 1). Mouse-killing (which Horovitz termed muricide) is inhibited by lesions of the amygdala (7, 8), and by direct injection of imipramine, norepinephrine, or serotonin into the amygdala (9, 10, 11). In addition, muricide can be initiated in "non-killer" rats by implantation of crystalline eserine into the amygdala (11). This chapter will review the procedures that are used to measure the effects of drugs on muricide. Studies of the effects of drugs on muricide indicate that mouse-killing is markedly attenuated by drugs that have antidepressant activity in man.

III. PROCEDURES

A. Selection of Muricidal Rats

Rats are tested either directly upon receipt from the vendor or following a period of isolation and food deprivation. The effects of isolation on mouse-killing are unclear. Korn and Moyer (12) reported that isolation did not reliably increase mouse-killing behavior. However, Malick (personal communication) initiated muricide in some non-killer rats by isolating them for six weeks. Initial food deprivation does reliably increase the proportion of rats that kill mice (13). After several experiences with killing mice, deprivation may be discontinued and most rats will continue to kill mice. The rats are housed in individual cages which are separated from adjoining cages by metal partitions. An albino mouse, weighing approximately 20 g, is placed in each rat's cage. In the first test, mice are usually left in the cage for 30 to 120 minutes. Experienced "killers" have a short kill latency. Therefore, subsequent tests are gradually shortened to 5 minutes. Mice are removed from the cage shortly after they are killed in order to prevent the rats from eating them. Each rat is repeatedly tested with a mouse in order to determine that it reliably kills mice within 5 minutes. This selection procedure yields approximately 10 to 30 per cent "killers" in Sprague-Dawley derived and Long-Evans rats. Male and female rats do not differ with respect to incidence of mouse-killing.

B. Testing the Effects of Drugs on Muricide

Rats that reliably killed mice are tested with drugs. Each rat is pre-tested with a mouse prior to drug administration, and rats that fail to kill mice within 5 minutes are not tested with drugs. Drugs are typically administered intraperitoneally and the subjects are tested with mice at various intervals, usually 15, 30, 60, and 120 minutes after injection. The ED_{50}, i. e. that dose which inhibits killing in 50 per cent of the rats, is calculated according to the methods described by Litchfield and Wilcoxon (14) or Finney (15). A less precise estimation of the ED_{50} can be quickly obtained by graphical probit analysis as described by Miller and Tainter (16).

C. Rotarod Procedure

Inhibition of mouse-killing might simply reflect a general debilitation of the animal. Therefore, the subjects are also observed and the presence of ataxia is noted or they are tested for grip strength on a 60° inclined wire mesh screen (see Fig. 2). A more precise measure of neurological impairment can be obtained by testing the drugs in additional rats which are trained to walk on a slowly revolving rod (rotarod test (17). Ataxia, decreased grip, or an impairment of rotarod performance presumably reflects a general debilitation of the animal. The ratio of the ED_{50} for debilitation to the ED_{50} for inhibition of muricide is calculated. Ratios greater than 1.0 indicate that mouse-killing was inhibited at doses that did not impair motor performance.

IV. VARIABLES THAT MAY DETERMINE THE EFFECTS OF DRUGS ON MURICIDE

Paul, Miley and Baenninger (13) reported that deprivation state does not affect the maintenance of established mouse-killing. In their study, initial deprivation increased the number of rats that killed mice, however, subsequent changes in deprivation did not alter killing behavior in "experienced" rats. Malick (personal communication) found a decrease in mouse-killing after isolated

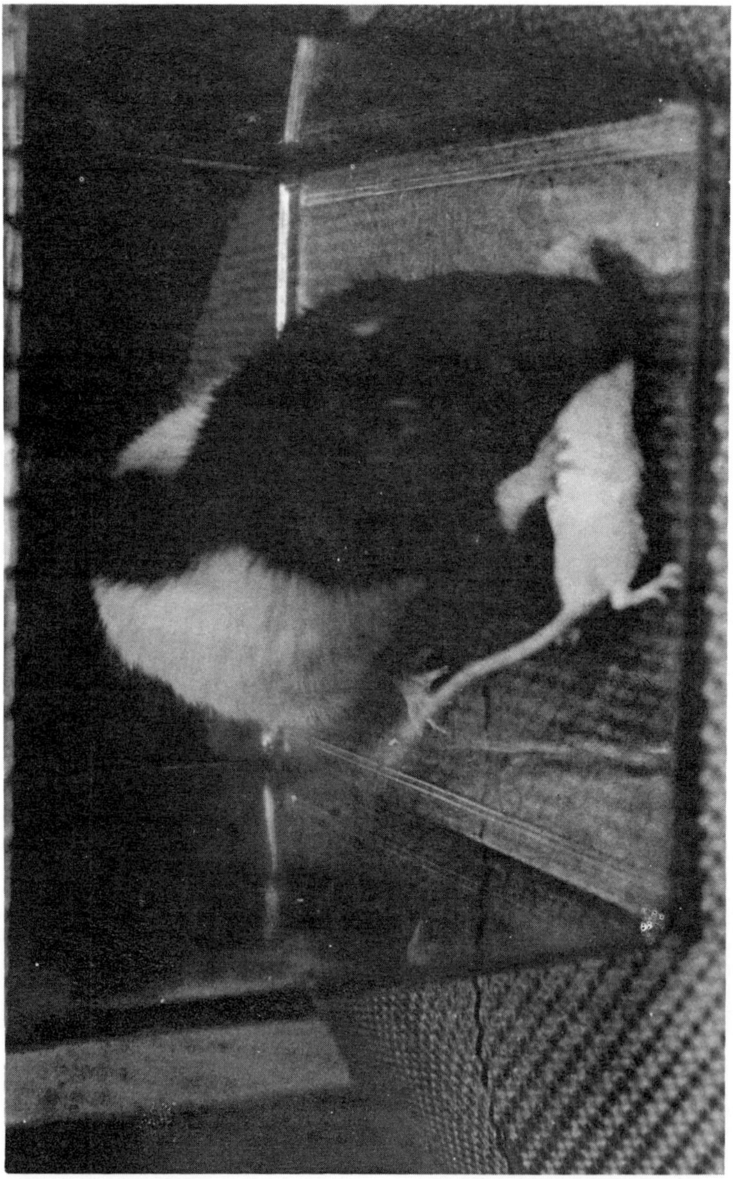

FIGURE 1 Typical attack-response pattern of the hooded rat directed at an albino mouse. A similar response pattern is obtained with albino rats. See text for further description.

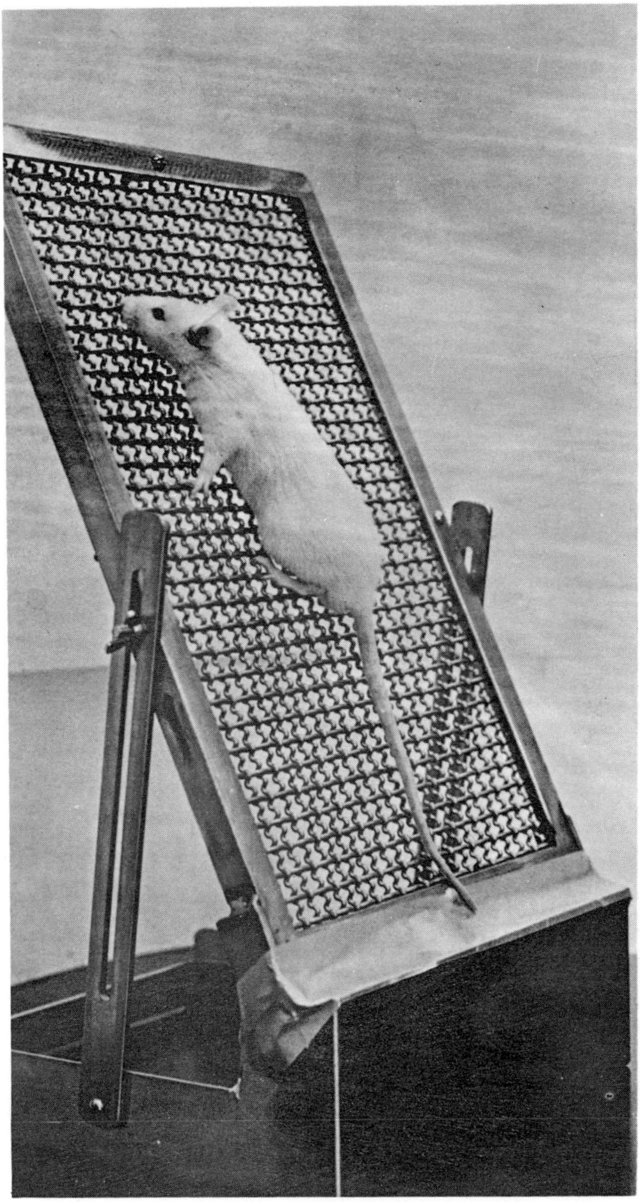

FIGURE 2 Inclined screen apparatus used for measuring grip strength. The screen is set at an angle of 60° and subjects are rated on their ability to grip and hold onto the screen.

TABLE I
Effects of *d*-Amphetamine and Amitriptyline on Muricide in Food-Deprived and Non-Deprived Rats

Drug	Ad libitum ED_{50} (mg/kg)	20 Grams per Day ED_{50} (mg/kg)
d-Amphetamine	1.4	3.0
Amitriptyline	13.5	27.5

"killer" rats were switched from restricted (7.5 g) to *ad libitum* feeding. The interaction between food deprivation and inhibition of muricide by drugs is currently underway in our laboratory (Vogel & Nathan, unpublished study). Preliminary results obtained with two drugs, *d*-amphetamine sulfate and amitryptyline, indicate that larger doses of these drugs were required to inhibit mouse-killing by food deprived rats than by non-deprived rats. As shown in Table I, the ED_{50}'s for inhibition of mouse-killing by rats who were given 20 g of food per day were greater than twice those for rats fed *ad libitum*. These preliminary data are based on a relatively small number of subjects and no conclusion should be drawn from them; however, they do suggest that the food deprived rat may be less sensitive to the antimuricide effects of drugs.

Route of administration may be another critical variable in determining the effects of drugs on mouse-killing. This author knows of no published reports of selective inhibition of mouse-killing by oral administration of a drug. Malick (personal communication) compared the effects of oral vs. intraperitoneal administration of various drugs on muricide. In general, oral administration of drugs drastically reduced their antimuricide activity. Other behavioral procedures demonstrated that these drugs were active following oral administration and there was no obvious reason why antimuricide activity was selectively attenuated.

V. EFFECTS OF DRUGS ON MURICIDE

Because the amygdala appears to control mouse-killing by rats (7-11) and antidepressant drugs block some functions of the amygdala, Horovitz, Ragozzino and Leaf (6) tested the antidepressant drugs iproniazid and imipramine in "killer" rats. They reported that these drugs block the mouse-killing response at dose levels that did not impair rotarod performance. Therefore, this effect could not be attributed to a general neurological impairment. The tranquilizers, chlordiazepoxide and chlorpromazine were also tested. Unlike the antidepressants, these drugs blocked muricide only at doses that impaired rotarod performance as well.

Two major studies reported the effects of several classes of psychotropic drugs on muricide. The first of these was reported by Horovitz, Piala, High, Burke and Leaf (8) and the second was reported by Sofia (18, 19). Horovitz and co-workers used Holtzman, female, albino rats that were food deprived during initial testing for mouse-killing behavior and fed *ad libitum* during testing with drugs. Rats that killed mice consistently within 5 minutes were given drugs. The experimental drugs were administered once a week to these "killers" and mouse-killing was tested at various intervals beginning 15 minutes after injection. Additional rats were trained on a rotarod and tested with the experimental drugs.

Sofia maintained rats on a daily ration of 15 grams of food which was placed on the cage floor each morning. Sofia reported (personal communication) that food was usually present on the cage floor at the time of testing with a mouse; however, these rats did not obtain the body weight expected for this strain. Prior to initial testing with the mouse, Sofia's rats were housed individually for six to eight weeks. At the end of the isolation period, the subjects were tested with mice. Rats that killed mice within two minutes on each of three consecutive test sessions were retained for drug testing. These rats were tested with drugs at intervals of 30 and 60 minutes following intraperitoneal injection. Longer treatment-test intervals were used with more slowly acting monoamine oxidase inhibitors. The effects of these drugs on rotarod performance were determined in another group of rats.

The drugs tested and the results obtained by these authors are shown in Table II. The following classes of drugs were represented: antidepressants, psychostimulants, antihistamines, anticholinergics, and tranquilizers. The results obtained are expressed as ED_{50}'s for the inhibition of muricide and rotarod performance and ratios of muricide to rotarod ED_{50}'s. Some of these drugs inhibited mouse-killing at doses that did not impair rotarod performance; others inhibited mouse-killing only at doses that also impaired rotarod performance.

Among the tricyclic antidepressants, high ratios, which indicate selective antimuricide activity, were found with imipramine and desipramine in both studies. Horovitz, et al, also reported high ratios with amitriptyline and thiazesim. Similar results were obtained with imipramine, desipramine, amitriptyline, and thiazesim by Goldberg (20) and Kulkarni (21). The ratios obtained by Sofia with amitriptyline and thiazesim were somewhat lower. This difference may reflect an altered sensitivity to the antimuricide effect of drugs as a consequence of food deprivation. The high ratios that were obtained indicate that the inhibition of

TABLE II
Effects of Various Drugs on Mouse-Killing (Muricide) and Rotarod Performance

Drug	Horovitz et al. (8)			Sofia (18, 19)		
	Antimuricide ED_{50} (mg/kg)	Rotarod ED_{50} (mg/kg)	Ratio	Antimuricide ED_{50} (mg/kg)	Rotarod ED_{50} (mg/kg)	Ratio
Tricyclic Antidepressants						
Imipramine	8.0	24.0	3.0*	8.1	23.0	2.8*
Amitriptyline	5.1	14.5	2.8*	12.4	17.8	1.4
Desipramine	9.8	24.0	2.4*	11.9	36.0	3.0*
Thiazesim	14.8	32.0	2.2*	34.6	32.2	0.9
Protriptyline	Not tested	-	-	8.8	11.1	1.3
Monoamine Oxidase Inhibitors						
Gamfexine	Not tested	-	-	25.4	41.7	1.6
Parglyine	Not tested	-	-	127.6	149.8	1.2*
Tranylcypromine	Not tested	-	-	4.1	50.7	12.4*
Harmaline	Not tested	-	-	8.1	4.9	0.6
Ertryptamine	Not tested	-	-	9.7	18.2	1.9
Iproniazid	155.0	250.0	1.7*	216.9	125.4	0.6
Nialamide	Not tested	-	-	158.9	275.9	1.7
Isocarboxazide	Not tested	-	-	28.7	72.5	2.5
Phenelzine	5.0	26.0	5.2*	28.0	36.2	1.3
Psychostimulants						
Methamphetamine	Not tested	-	-	0.8	5.5	6.9*
d-Amphetamine	1.5	6.6	4.4*	0.8	4.2	5.2*
Pipradrol	15.0	32.0	2.1*	6.5	17.7	2.7
Methylphenidate	33.0	44.0	1.3	6.0	11.6	1.9

Caffeine	Not tested	-	-	74.0	63.5	0.9
Thozalinone	Not tested	-	-	34.2	85.3	2.5
Antihistamines						
Pyrathiazine	Not tested	-	-	86.8	51.7	0.6
Antazoline	Not tested	-	-	49.7	91.8	1.9
Tripelennamine	5.2	30.0	5.8*	13.2	25.7	2.0
Dimenhydrinate	Not tested	-	-	54.9	54.9	1.0
Diphenhydramine	17.5	28.5	1.7	66.4	22.7	0.4
Chlorpheniramine	23.0	45.0	1.9*	22.0	47.8	2.2*
Dimethindene	Not tested	-	-	34.5	31.9	0.9
Cyclizine	Not tested	-	-	34.4	24.6	0.7
Promethazine	Not tested	-	-	109.9	27.2	0.2
Cyproheptadine	Not tested	-	-	58.2	17.8	0.3
Minor Tranquilizers						
Chlordiazepoxide	30.0	5.3	0.2	20.2	8.8	0.4
Diazepam	1.9	1.5	0.8	219.0	4.0	0.02
Meprobamate	>200.0	66.0	-	301.8	85.0	0.3
Pentobarbital	10.0	7.3	0.7	25.3	10.4	0.4
Major Tranquilizers						
Chlorpromazine	5.5	3.7	0.7	9.0	1.7	0.2
Fluphenazine	0.15	0.23	1.5	Not tested	-	-
Anticholinergics						
Atropine	20.0	34.0	1.7	Not tested	-	-
Benztropine	18.0	20.0	1.1	Not tested	-	-

* ED_{50}'s Significantly different $P < 0.05$

mouse-killing by these drugs was not due simply to debilitation, i.e., they did not impair rotarod performance at doses that did inhibit mouse-killing.

Horovitz et al tested the monoamine oxidase inhibitors iproniazid and phenelzine. High ratios, which indicated selective inhibition of mouse-killing, were obtained with both of these drugs. The ratios obtained with these drugs by Sofia were again lower. Sofia did report selective antimuricide activity with the monoamine oxidase inhibitors, pargyline and tranylcypromine. Pargyline is used as an antihypertensive agent rather than as an antidepressant. However, it is essentially similar to the other monoamine inhibitors. Tranylcypromine is used for depression, but because of toxicity, this drug is restricted to hospitalized patients. Non-significant trends towards selective inhibition of muricide were obtained with three other monoamine oxidase inhibitors: ertryptamine, nialamide, and isocarboxazide. Isocarboxazide and nialamide are used for the treatment of depression; however, ertryptamine is no longer marketed.

Selective inhibition of muricide was obtained with several psychostimulant compounds. Methamphetamine, *d*-amphetamine, and, to a lesser extent, pipradrol inhibited mouse-killing at dose levels that did not impair rotarod performance. Amphetamine, while generally regarded as a psychostimulant, has been used in the treatment of certain types of depression (22). Sofia also obtained statistically insignificant trends in the direction of selective inhibition of muricide with the psychostimulants methylphenidate and thozalinone.

The antihistamines chlorpheniramine and tripelennamine selectively inhibited mouse-killing, and this effect was shared to a lesser extent by antazoline and diphenhydramine. These antihistamines are active in other laboratory antidepressant tests as well. Barnett, Taber and Roth (23) reported that chlorpheniramine, tripelennamine, and diphenhydramine prevented tetrabenazine-induced ptosis in mice. The antidepressants, imipramine and amitriptyline, were also active in this test. Additional antihistamines, dimethindene, promethazine, and cyproheptadine were not active in the tetrabenazine test and do not block mouse-killing by rats (see Table II). Antihistamines that are active in laboratory antidepressant tests may have antidepressant activity in man. Barnett et al cited one study in which 10 out of 13 depressed patients showed a significant improvement after administration of diphenhydramine.

The minor tranquilizers exhibited a selective impairment of rotarod performance rather than muricide and had correspondingly low ratios, as did the major tranquilizer chlorpromazine. Fluphenazine, another major tranquilizer, has less sedative properties and inhibited mouse-killing at a dose level that did not impair rotarod performance. The anticholinergic drug, atropine, led to a slight inhibition of mouse-killing. This may reflect the role of brain acetylcholine in mouse-killing that has been postulated by several authors (11, 24-28).

The results of these studies suggest that some classes of drugs, namely antidepressants, psychostimulants, and antihistamines, selectively block mouse-killing by rats. An interesting disparity between mouse-killing and human depression is the finding that a single dose of a drug blocks mouse-killing while repeated administration of the same drug is usually necessary to produce therapeutic effects in man. It has been postulated that antidepressant drugs may reverse depression by altering brain catecholamine activity (29). A related finding is that repeated administration of the drug imipramine to laboratory rats led to an increase in brain catecholamine activity (30). This effect was not observed following a single administration of the drug. It is possible that the antimuricide test measures some acute change produced by drugs which have antidepressant effects when they are repeatedly administered to humans.

VI. INHIBITION OF MURICIDE BY CHRONIC ADMINISTRATION OF ELECTROCONVULSIVE SHOCK

Electroconvulsive shock (ECS) is also an effective treatment for depression. Repeated administration of ECS has been reported to produce as high as an 80-85 percent recovery rate in depressed patients. If muricide is under the control of some mechanism analogous to human depression, ECS should also block this phenomenon. Vogel and Haubrich (31) administered ECS to rats that consistently killed mice. Treatments were given two or three times per day and rats were not exposed to mice during the period of ECS treatments. Rats who received ECS stopped killing mice. In general, about 14-21 treatments produced a marked effect. After ECS some rats killed with longer latencies while others failed to kill mice even when they were exposed to them for 30 minutes. The finding that repeated ECS treatments were required to produce an inhibition of mouse-killing is consistent with the clinical finding that repeated ECS treatments are required in order to produce an antidepressant effect. Clinically, the therapeutic effects of ECS persist following termination of treatments. ECS had a persistent effect on mouse-killing as well; at the end of 21 days of testing, 33 percent of the rats given ECS had not resumed killing mice.

VII. CONCLUSIONS

The preceding studies indicate that mouse-killing by rats is selectively blocked by antidepressant drugs and electroconvulsive shock. The antimuricide effect obtained with antidepressant drugs was not simply due to "behavioral depression" because: 1) other behaviors such as rotarod performance were not impaired at these dose levels and 2) other drugs, having primarily depressant effects, are not selective potent inhibitors of mouse-killing. The inhibition of mouse-killing by these drugs and the antimuricide effect observed with electroconvulsive shock, another treatment for human depression, suggest that inhibition of mouse-killing by rats may reflect possible antidepressant activity in drugs. Some antihistamines and psychostimulants also inhibited mouse-killing. These compounds are easily distinguished from potential antidepressants in other laboratory procedures. The antimuricide test is a simple procedure that may help to detect potential antidepressant activity in new drugs.

ACKNOWLEDGEMENTS

The author expresses thanks to Paul Gittelson, Zola Horovitz, Russell Leaf, Jeffrey Malick and Thomas Mulligan for their helpful suggestions and criticisms.

REFERENCES

1. Domenjoz, R. and Theobald, W.: Zur pharmakologie des tofranil, *Arch. Intern. Pharmacodyn.,* **120**:450-489, 1959.
2. Goddard, G. V.: Functions of the amygdala, *Psychol. Bull.,* **62**:89-109, 1964.
3. Horovitz, Z. P.: The amygdala and depression, *in* Garattini, S. and Dukes, M. N. G. (Eds.), *Excerpta Medica International Congress Series,* No. 122, pp. 121, Excerpta Medica Foundation, Maastricht, 1966.
4. Horovitz, Z. P., Furgiuele, A. R., Brannick, L. J., Burke, J. C., and Craver, B. N.: A new chemical structure with specific depressant effects on the amygdala and on the hyperirritability of the "Septal" rat, *Nature,* **200**:369-370, 1963.
5. Horovitz, Z. P.: The relationship of the amygdala to the mechanism of action of two types of antidepressants. *In* Wortis, J. (Ed.), *Recent Advances in Biological Psychiatry,* pp. 21-31, Plenum Press, New York, 1966.
6. Horovitz, Z. P., Ragozzino, P. W., and Leaf, R. C.: Selective block of rat mouse-killing by antidepressants, *Life Sci.,* **4**:1909-1912, 1965.
7. Karli, P.: The Norway rat's killing response to the white mouse: an experimental analysis, *Behavior,* **10**:81-103, 1956.
8. Horovitz, Z. P., Piala, J. J., High, J. P., Burke, J. C., and Leaf, R. C.: Effects of drugs on the mouse-killing (muricide) test and its relation-

ship to amygdaloid function, *Int. J. Neuropharmacol.,* **5**:405-411, 1966.

9. Horovitz, Z. P. and Leaf, R. C.: The effects of direct injections of psychotropic drugs on the amygdalae of rats and the relationship to antidepressant site of action. *In* Brill, H., Cole, J. O., Deniker, P., Hippuis, H. and Bradley, P. B. (Eds.), *Excerpta Medica International Congress Series,* No. 129, p. 1042, Excerpta Medica Foundation, Amsterdam, 1967.
10. Leaf, R. C.: Pharmacology, limbic regulation, and cortical function. *In* Smith, W. L. (Ed.), *Drugs and Cerebral Function,* pp. 201-213, Thomas, Springfield, 1970.
11. Leaf, R. C., Lerner, L., and Horovitz, Z. P.: The role of the amygdala in the pharmacological and endocrinological manipulation of aggression. *In* Garattini, S. and Sigg, E. B. (Eds.), *Aggressive Behavior,* pp. 120-131, Excerpta Medica Foundation, Amsterdam, 1969.
12. Korn, J. H. and Moyer, K. E.: Behavioral effects of isolation in the rat: the role of sex and time of isolation, *J. Genet. Psychol.,* **113**:263-273, 1968.
13. Paul, L., Miley, W. M., and Baenninger, R.: Mouse-killing by rats: Roles of hunger and thirst in its initiation and maintenance, *J. Comp. Physiol. Psychol.,* **76**:242-249, 1971.
14. Litchfield, J. T. and Wilcoxon, F.: A simplified method of evaluating dose-effect experiments, *J. Pharmacol. Exptl. Therap.,* **96**:99-113, 1949.
15. Finney, D. J.: *Probit analysis,* Cambridge University Press, London, 1964, pp. 238-245.
16. Miller, C. L. and Tainter, M. L.: Estimation of the ED_{50} and its error by means of logarithmic-probit graph paper, *Proc. Soc. Exptl. Biol. Med.,* **57**:261-264, 1944.
17. Kinnard, W. J., Jr. and Carr, C. J.: A preliminary procedure for evaluation of central-nervous system depressants, *J. Pharmacol. Exptl. Therap.,* **121**:354-361, 1957.
18. Sofia, R. D.: Effects of centrally active drugs on experimentally-induced aggression in rodents, *Life Sci.,* **8**:705-716, 1969.
19. Sofia, R. D.: Structural relationship and potency of agents which selectively block mouse-killing (muricide) behavior in rats. *Life Sci.,* **8**:1201-1210, 1969.
20. Goldberg, M. E.: Pharmacologic activity of a new class of agents which selectively inhibit aggressive behavior in rats, *Arch. Int. Pharmacodyn.,* **186**:287-297, 1970.
21. Kulkarni, A. S.: Muricidal block produced by 5-hydroxytryptophan and various drugs, *Life Sci.,* **7**:125-128, 1968.
22. Dunlop, E.: The use of antidepressants and stimulants, *Mod. Treatment,* **2**:543-568, 1965.
23. Barnett, A., Taber, R. I., and Roth, F. E.: Activity of antihistamines in laboratory antidepressant tests, *Int. J. Neuropharmac.,* **8**:73-79, 1969.
24. McCarthy, D.: Mouse-killing induced in rats treated with pilocarpine, *Fed. Proc.,* **25**:385, 1966, Abstract.
25. Bandler, R. J.: Facilitation of aggressive behavior in rat by direct cholinergic stimulation of the hypothalamus, *Nature,* **224**:1035-1036, 1969.
26. Smith, D. E., King, M. B., and Hoebel, B. G.: Lateral hypothalamic

control of killing: evidence for a cholinoceptive mechanism, *Science*, **167**:900-901, 1970.

27. Vogel, J. R. and Leaf, R. C.: Initiation of mouse-killing in non-killer rats by repeated pilocarpine treatment, *Physiol. and Behavior*, **8**:421-424, 1972.
28. Wnek, D. J. and Leaf, R. C.: Effects of cholinergic drugs on prey-killing by rodents, *Physiol. and Behavior*, **10**:1107-1113, 1973.
29. Schildkraut, J. J.: *Neuropsychopharmacology and the affective disorders*, Little Brown and Company, Boston, 1969.
30. Schildkraut, J. J., Winokur, A., Draskoczy, P. R., and Hensle, J. H.: Changes in norepinephrine turnover in rat brain during chronic administration of imipramine and protriptyline: A possible explanation for the delay in onset of clinical antidepressant effects, *Amer. J. Psychiat.*, **127**:1032-1039, 1971.
31. Vogel, J. R. and Haubrich, D. R.: Chronic administration of electroconvulsive shock: Effects on mouse-killing activity and brain monoamines in rats, *Physiol. and Behavior*, **11**:725-728, 1973.

5

Antidepressives and the Kindling Effect

RONALD G. BABINGTON, PH.D.

I. INTRODUCTION

A common problem in the search for truly effective psychoactive drugs is the absence of specific animal models for any of the various mental disease states. At present, the pharmacologic approach to predicting clinical efficacy is to test new chemical agents in a battery of procedures in which standard psychotropic drugs are active. An antidepressive profile, for example, would include antagonism of reserpine or tetrabenazine (1, 4, 6), potentiation of the central effects of amphetamine (3, 14), and inhibition of norepinephrine uptake (10). The major criticism of the profile approach, however, contends that compounds with similar clinical activities are exposed and unique entities are missed.

Laboratory testing for antidepressives presents several additional problems such as the difficulty in separating central stimulants from the tricyclics. Another problem is the existence of clinically-active agents which are inactive in one or more of the standard tests; and conversely, there have been numerous compounds extremely active in the laboratory, but failures in the clinic. In addition, the most effective treatment for endogenous depression, electroconvulsive shock (ECS), does not lend itself to testing in the standard procedures, making comparative studies impractical. Finally, there is the enigma that in all laboratory tests, the antidepressives are tested and activity determined immediately after dosing, whereas in the clinic, the delayed onset of action is a major feature.

Thus, a diligent search continues for new procedures to establish distinct mechanisms or sites of action for antidepressive drugs. In recent years, the limbic system has been extensively studied and substantial evidence has accumulated implicating various limbic structures as the site of action of psychoactive drugs (13). In the case of the antidepressives, the amygdala is particularly suspect (9, 11). Naturally, the description by Goddard et al. (8) of the "kindling" effect proved to be extremely interesting because kindling, too, has a strong predilection for the limbic system and the amygdala in particular. In this procedure, daily low-intensity electrical stimulation produces tardive seizures. The kindling seizures apparently differ from other experimental models of epilepsy, however, in that antiepileptic drugs are active, but only at doses producing severe overt motor debilitation and approaching lethality. In fact, two other classes of psychoactive drugs, the antidepressives and anxiolytics, are much more efficacious (2).

As a neuropharmacologic test system, the tardive seizure procedure possesses numerous desirable features, including the fact that the response is a pathologic entity, an attribute lacking in most test models. Other attributes include: (a) the seizure duration of each animal is remarkably consistent from trial to trial; (b) the response is easy to measure and has a clear endpoint; (c) the apparatus is simple and inexpensive; (d) the rats can be used repeatedly; (e) both increases and decreases in the duration of seizures can be measured; (f) various types of centrally-active agents have differential effects; (g) with experience, the testing can be carried out quickly; and (h) once a colony of kindled rats is established, the procedure can be utilized as a limited screening test.

II. METHOD

Adult female Holtzman rats are implanted with a stainless steel bipolar electrode (Plastic Products MS 303) in the amygdala, or epidurally on the sensorimotor cortex.

Beginning 10 days postoperatively, each animal is stimulated electrically once daily for one minute with a 50μA, 60-Hz constant current sine wave (Bio-Medical Electronics Model LS 112 stimulator). With the exception of a few of the cortically-implanted rats, none of the animals exhibit seizures during the first few stimulation sessions. After eight to ten days, bilateral, clonic seizures begin to develop during the stimulation period. Once sensitization has been established, stimulation is continued only until the animal begins to show signs of seizure, whereupon the current is shut off and the duration of the seizure measured. Within four weeks, sensitization progresses so that according to individual animals, five to seven seconds of stimulation elicits seizures that last from 45-75 seconds.

On drug day, two control measurements are made 15 minutes apart. If the durations of the seizures do not vary by more than ten percent, the pair of control values is averaged to serve as the baseline value. The test drug is then administered intraperitoneally as a solution in saline or a suspension in saline-Tween 80. Each rat is then challenged at 15- and 30-minutes intervals after injection with the same length of stimulation needed to produce the control seizures.

The data reported represent the results obtained at 30 minutes after dosing. The duration of the postdrug seizures is expressed as a percent of baseline duration. The results obtained from groups of seven to nine rats each were averaged to determine each point on the dose-response curve. Whenever possible, the same group of rats was used for the various doses of a single drug. Occasionally, however, animals died or pulled the electrode out, and these were replaced with a new animal. An estimation of the median effective dose (ED_{50}), regression, and parallelism for drugs altering seizure durations were determined by linear regression analysis (5).

III. EFFECTS OF ANTIDEPRESSIVE DRUGS

The effects of three antidepressive agents on the duration of amygdaloid- and cortical-induced tardive seizures are illustrated in Figure 1. As can be seen, amitriptyline was quite potent in inhibiting kindled seizures elicited from the amygdala. Cortically-induced seizures were also suppressed, but at higher dose levels. Similarly, Figure 1 shows that nortriptyline and imipramine were more active in suppressing amygdaloid, as opposed to cortical, tardive seizures. However, neither was as potent against amygdaloid-induced seizures as amitriptyline; and the separation of the activity curves was least manifest with imipramine. With all three antidepressives, the difference in the slope of the amygdaloid and cortical dose-response curves was significantly different ($P<0.05$). Although not illustrated in Figure 1, the dose-response curves of all three antidepressives against seizures originating from kindled sites in the septum fall slightly to the right of the cortical dose-response curves (15). At the dose levels represented, blockade of the seizures was not complete; but even at higher doses where overt signs of CNS depression were observed, there was never a 100 percent suppression of the seizures.

To date, the only antidepressive with clinically-proven activity that has been ineffective against kindled seizures has been iprindole, a compound that does not behave like the other tricyclic antidepressives in the standard laboratory tests (7). Thyrotropin-releasing hormone has also been reported to relieve depression in man (12) but was inactive over a wide range of doses against tardive seizures. Another type of antidepressive, the monoamine

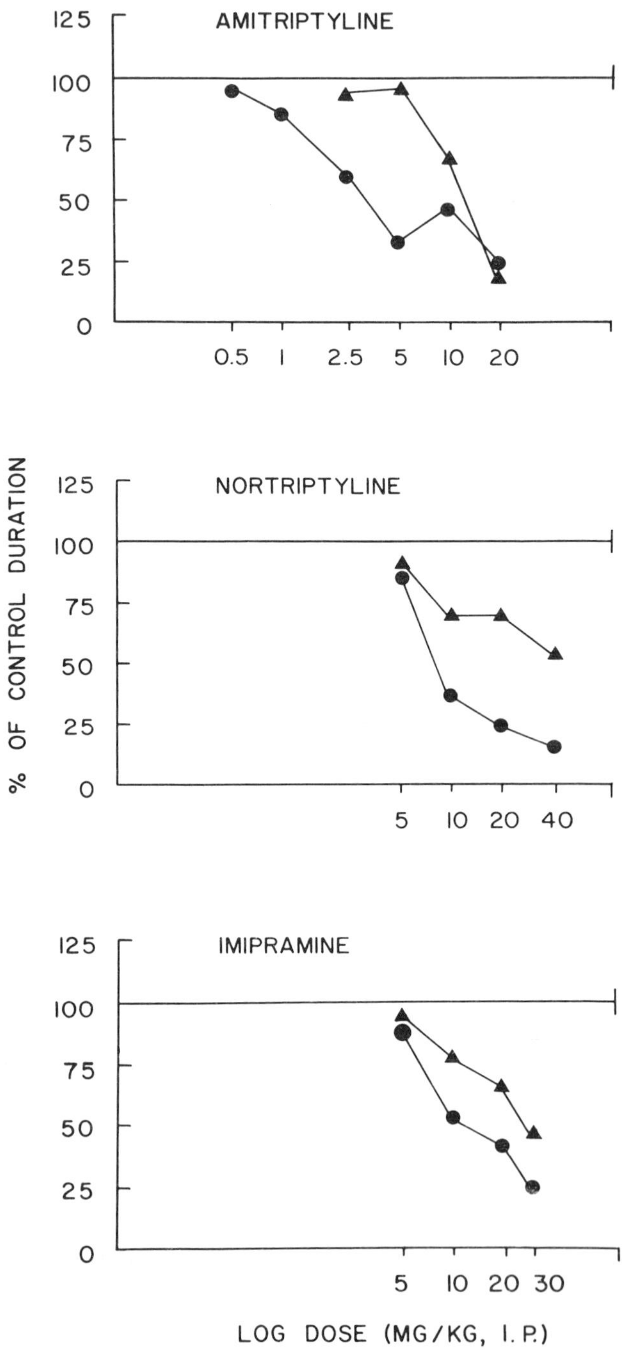

FIGURE 1 Effects of three antidepressive agents on the duration of tardive seizures elicited from the amygdala (•) or neocortex (▲).

oxidase inhibitors, had activity but the effect was one of slight potentiation rather than blockade of seizure duration (Babington, unpublished data).

Figure 2 presents the results of an experiment designed to determine the effects of chronic dosing with an antidepressive. Two groups of eight rats with amygdaloid tardive seizures were dosed with one mg amitriptyline/kg, a dose that has little or no effect on seizure duration. Two other groups of eight rats received ten mg amitriptyline/kg, a dose that effectively blocks seizures. One group from each dose level was administered drug daily for 14 days while the remaining two groups received amitriptyline only on the seventh and fourteenth days. On test days, all animals were electrically stimulated 30 minutes after drug dosing with the same length of stimulation required to produce seizures on day 0.

In both groups treated with ten mg amitriptyline/kg, seizures were suppressed when the animals were challenged with amygdaloid stimulation. Similarly, seizure duration was blocked to nearly the same extent in the group receiving a 1-mg/kg daily dose. However, 1 mg amitriptyline/kg was not sufficient for suppressing tardive seizures unless administered chronically. Note on the other hand, that chronic treatment with the higher dose of amitriptyline was no more effective than a single dose administered 30 minutes prior to amygdaloid stimulation.

IV. THE EFFECTS OF ECS

As mentioned above, direct comparison of the effects of antidepressive agents vs. ECS is difficult in the standard laboratory testing procedures. The tardive seizure model, however, readily accommodates such a collation. Figure 3 illustrates the effect of a single ECS treatment on the duration of seizures kindled from the amygdala, septum, or cortex. In this experiment, each animal received a 0.25 sec transpinnal train of 60-Hz current at 50 ∓ 2 ma. This current was sufficient to produce tonic limb extension. Groups of 8 rats were challenged at the various time intervals after ECS with each rat receiving the same length of stimulation used to produce the control kindled seizures.

Note that like the antidepressive drugs, ECS suppressed the duration of elicited seizures, and the most profound reduction was against the amygdaloid-induced response. Not only was the magnitude of the suppression greater, but the duration of the effect on the amygdaloid tardive seizures was much longer, lasting five to six hours after ECS treatment.

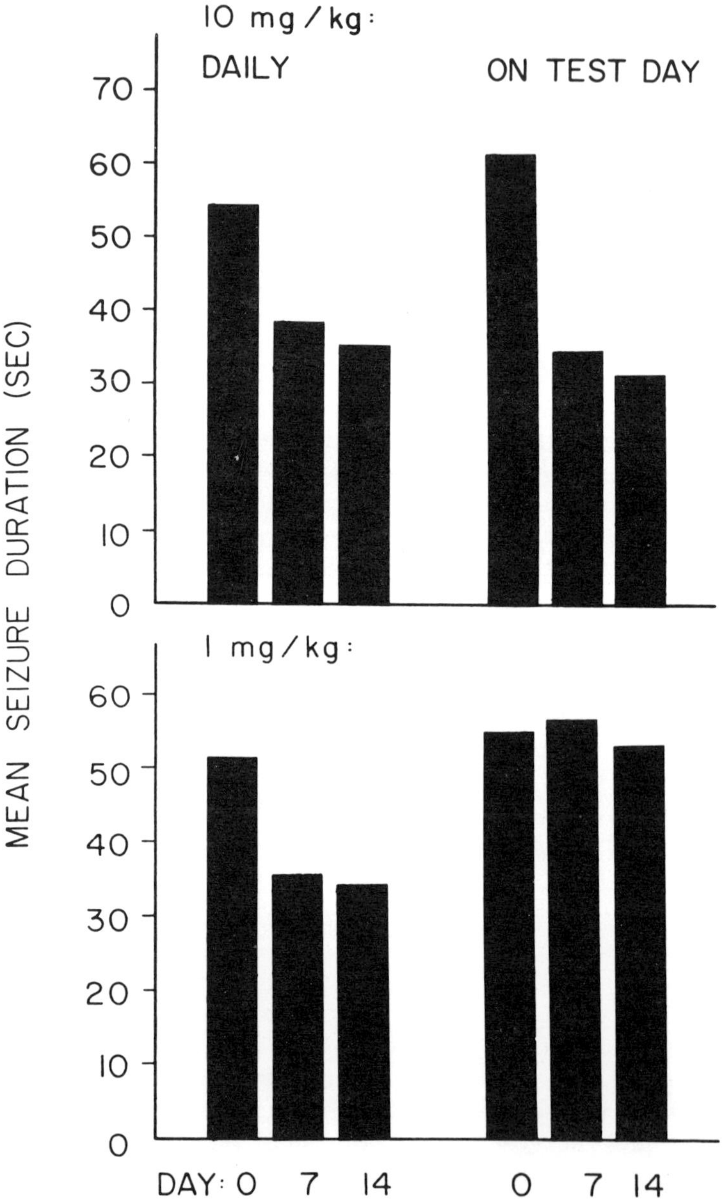

FIGURE 2 Effect of acute or chronic treatment with amitriptyline on the duration of seizures kindled in the amygdala. Two dose levels were studied—acutely effective (10 mg/kg) and acutely subeffective (1 mg/kg)—and each dose level was administered either daily for 14 days or only on test days (days 7 and 14). On test days, each animal was challenged 30 min after dosing with the same length of stimulation required to produce seizures on day 0 (Babington, unpublished data).

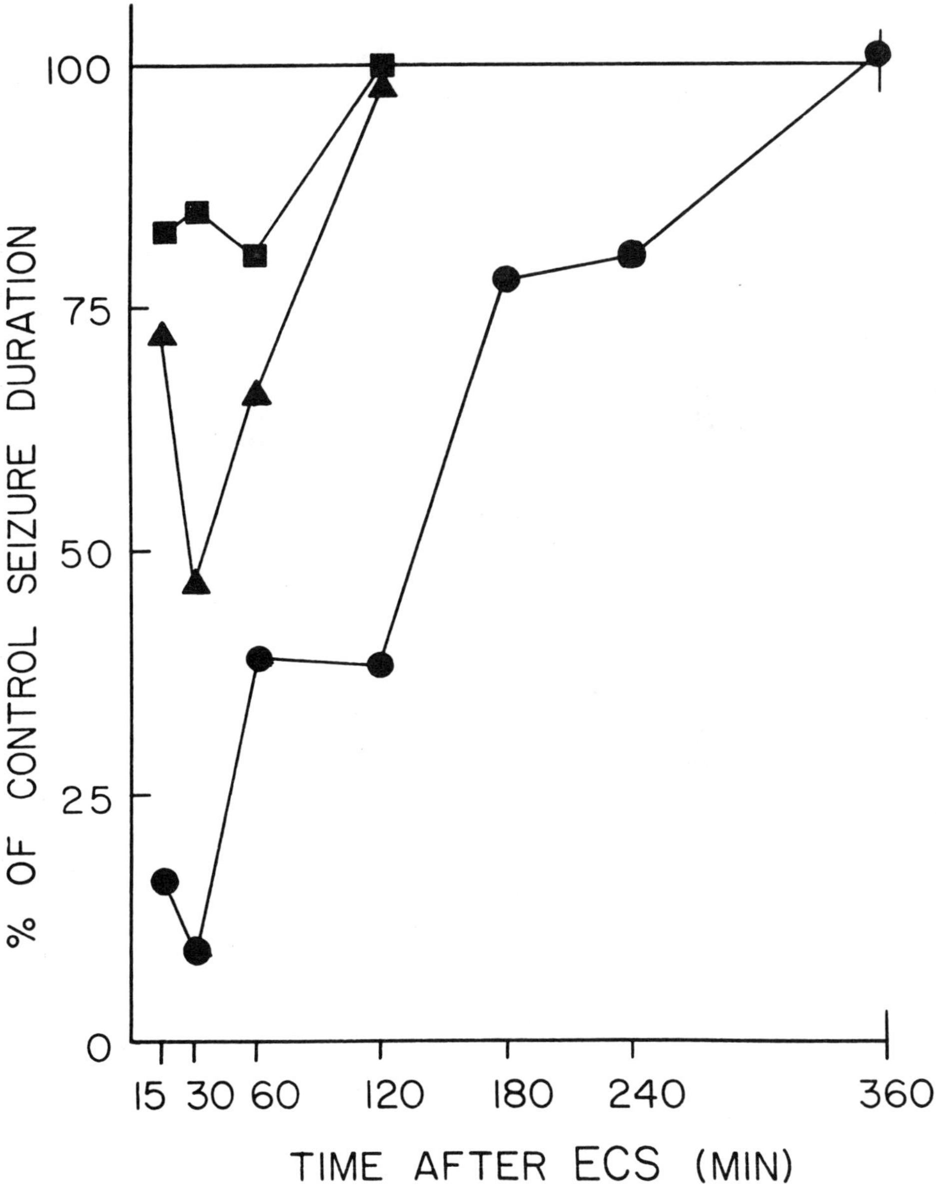

FIGURE 3 Effect of a single electroconvulsive shock (ECS) on the duration of tardive seizures elicited from the amygdala (●), neocortex (▲) or septum (■). Groups of 8 rats were tested at the various time intervals after ECS (Babington, unpublished data).

V. EFFECTS OF OTHER CNS-ACTIVE DRUGS

Figure 4 presents the activity against tardive seizures of four antianxiety drugs: chlordiazepoxide, diazepam, oxazepam, and meprobamate. A characteristic common to all four drugs was the marked potency in suppressing seizures. Although the antianxiety agents produce hypokinesia at effective dose levels in many neuropharmacologic tests in rats, none of the animals were debilitated at doses completely blocking kindled seizures. In addition, excepting chlordiazepoxide, the activity curves of the antianxiety drugs against cortical tardive seizures were to the left of the amygdaloid curve, but the separation was insignificant in all instances.

Among the drugs that effectively suppressed kindled seizures, a characteristic of the antiepileptic drugs was juxtaposition of the two dose-response curves. As can be seen in Figure 5, the amygdaloid and cortical activity for diphenylhydantoin, phenacemide, phenobarbital, or pentobarbital was, in each case, virtually indistinguishable. In contrast to the antianxiety drugs, diphenylhydantoin and phenacemide were much less potent in blocking tardive seizures, and depressed motor activity and ataxia were prominent at the higher dose levels. On the other hand, pentobarbital and phenobarbital were relatively potent—as might be expected for an anxiolytic. Both barbiturates, in fact, are used clinically for their anxiety-suppressing activity.

Two drugs that exert stimulatory effects on behavior in rats, *d*-amphetamine and methylphenidate both prolonged seizures elicited from either amygdaloid or cortical sites. Unexpectedly, the 20-25 percent increase in seizure duration attained at 2.5 mg/kg of either drug was the maximum despite obvious enhanced behavioral stimulation at higher doses.

Classes of centrally-active agents that proved to be ineffective at behaviorally-active doses include the neuroleptics, antihistamines, narcotic analgetics, and anticholinergics.

VI. CONCLUSIONS

Not only is the kindling procedure a new addition to the armamentarium of tests responsive to antidepressive agents, an additional dimension is the ability to differentiate several classes of CNS-active agents. In fact, the anti-anxiety agents are more potent and more active than the antidepressives. Yet the antidepressives are marked by an ability to selectively depress amygdaloid seizures. On the other, the anti-epileptic drugs are active in suppressing tardive seizures, but only at doses far exceeding those

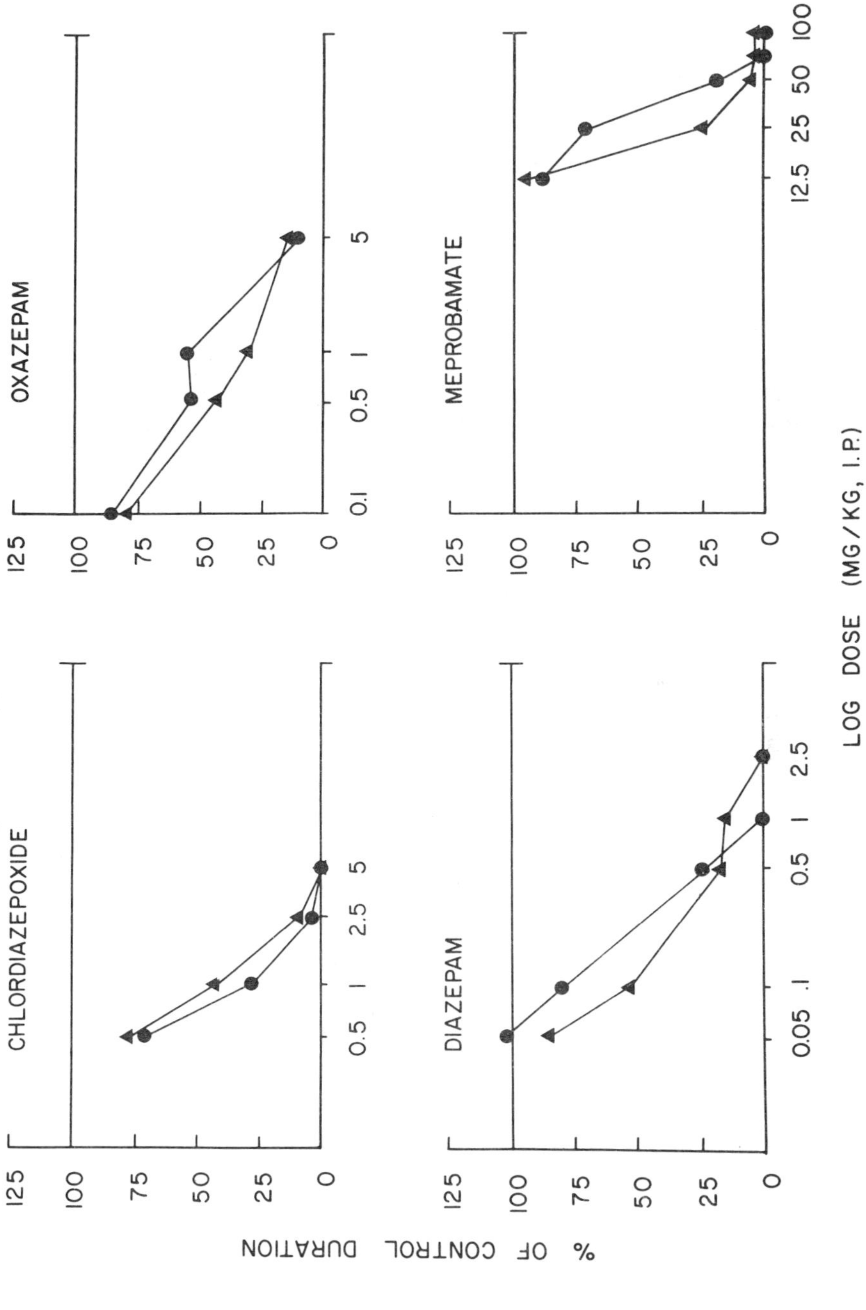

FIGURE 4 Effects of four antianxiety agents on the duration of kindled seizures elicited from the amygdala (●) or neocortex (▲).

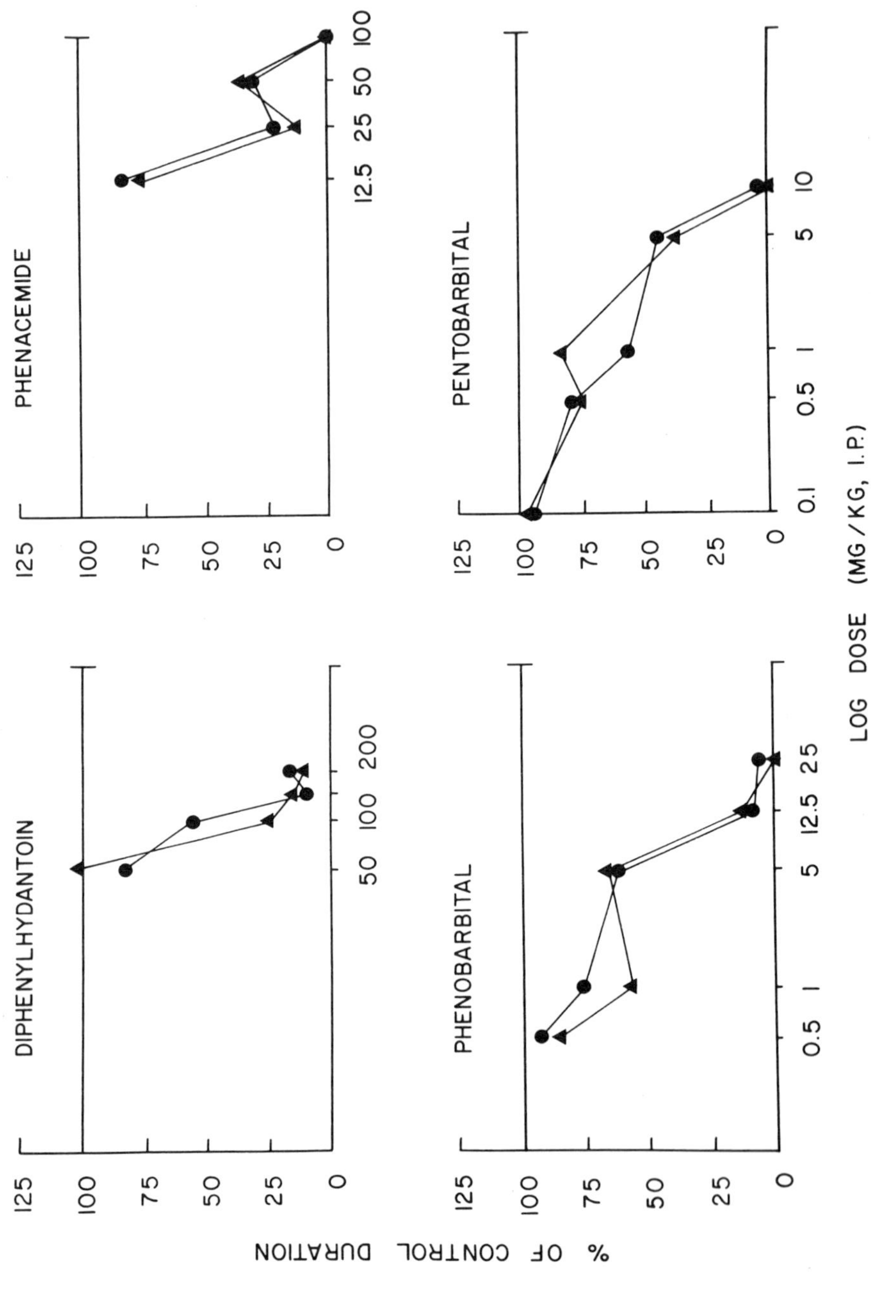

FIGURE 5 Effects of four agents with anticonvulsive activity in rats on the duration of tardive seizures elicited from the amygdala (●) or neocortex (▲).

necessary to block seizures in other animal models of epilepsy.

The tardive seizure test also enables the investigator to examine some of the problems peculiar to laboratory testing and clinical correlation of the antidepressives. The observation that the most effective therapeutic treatment of endogenous depression, ECS, not only suppresses tardive seizures, but like the antidepressives has a predilection for the amygdala lends strong support to the contention that the amygdala is the site of antidepressive action. Furthermore, the chronic studies with subactive doses of amitriptyline suggest that the delayed onset noted in the clinic might be due to the necessity to build up blood concentrations to effective therapeutic levels, and that massive initial dosing might result in immediate therapeutic benefits.

Another advantage of the tardive seizure test is the distinct separation of both behavioral stimulants and monoamine oxidase inhibitors from the tricyclic antidepressives.

To date, the procedure has reliably distinguished the currently available antidepressives and has proved to be an invaluable laboratory tool. Needless to say, it remains to be seen whether the test is another model that will continue to identify activity only associated with the tricyclics or whether it can identify new entities that have unique clinical vistas.

ACKNOWLEDGEMENTS

I wish to credit Mr. P. W. Wedeking who contributed immeasurably to all of the studies reported. I also wish to thank Dr. B. Beer for his suggestions and support.

REFERENCES

1. Askew, B. M.: A simple screening procedure for imipramine-like antidepressant agents, *Life Sci.,* **2**:725-730, 1963.
2. Babington, R. G. and Wedeking, P. W.: The pharmacology of seizures induced by sensitization with low-intensity brain stimulation, *Pharmacol. Biochem. Behav.,* **1**:461-467, 1973.
3. Carlton, P. L.: Potentiation of the behavioral effects of amphetamine by imipramine, *Psychopharmacologia,* **2**:364-376, 1961.
4. Costa, E., Garattini, S., and Valzelli, L.: Interactions between reserpine, chlorpromazine, and imipramine, *Experientia,* **16**:461-463, 1960.
5. Dixon, W. J. and Massey, Jr., F. J.: Introduction to statistical analysis, McGraw-Hill Book Company, New York 1969, pp. 300-302.
6. Garattini, S., Giachetti, A., Jori, A., Pieri, L., and Valzelli, L.: Effect of imipramine, amitriptyline, and their monomethyl derivatives on reserpine activity, *J. Pharm. Pharmacol.,* **14**:509-514, 1962.
7. Gluckman, M. I. and Baum, T.: The pharmacology of iprindole, a new antidepressant, *Psychopharmacologia,* **15**:169-185, 1969.

8. Goddard, G. V., McIntyre, D. C., and Leech, C. K.: A permanent change in brain function resulting from daily electrical stimulation, *Expl. Neurol.,* **25**:295-330, 1969.
9. Guerrero-Figueroa, R. and Gallant, D. M.: Effects of pinoxepin and imipramine on the mesencephalic reticular formation and amygdaloid complex in the cat: Neurophysiological and clinical correlations in human subjects, *Curr. Ther. Res.,* **9**:387-403, 1967.
10. Hertting, G., Axelrod, J., and Whitby, L. G.: Effect of drugs on the uptake and metabolism of H^3-norepinephrine, *J. Pharmacol. exp. Ther.,* **134**:146-153, 1961.
11. Horovitz, Z. P.: The amygdala and depression. Proceedings of the First International Symposium on Antidepressant Drugs, Milan. *Excerpta med. Int. Congr. Ser. No. 122,* 1966, pp. 121-129.
12. Prange, A. J., Wilson, I. C., Lara, P. P., Alltop, L. B., and Breese, G. R.: Effects of thyrotrophin-releasing hormone in depression, *Lancet,* Nov. 11:999-1002, 1972.
13. Schallek, W., Kuehn, A., and Jew, N.: Effects of chlordiazepoxide (Librium) and other psychotropic agents on the limbic system of the brain, *Ann. N. Y. Acad. Sci.,* **96**:303-312, 1962.
14. Stein, L. and Seifter, J.: Possible mode of antidepressive action of imipramine, *Science,* **134**:286-287, 1961.
15. Wedeking, P. W. and Babington, R. G.: Effects of neurological agents on seizures elicited by low-intensity brain stimulation in rats, *Pharmacologist,* **11**:279, 1969.

6

Differential Antagonism to Amphetamine-Induced Oxygen Consumption and Agitation by Psychoactive Drugs

CARLOS J. E. NIEMEGEERS, D.SC. and
PAUL A. J. JANSSEN, M.D.

I. INTRODUCTION

Amphetamine is a central stimulant with a wide range of pharmacological actions. Several of these actions are amphetamine-induced stereotyped behavior, agitation, and hyperthermia. It facilitates maze learning and conditioned reactions, and increases self-stimulation. It possesses anorexigenic properties and increases oxygen consumption.

In rats antagonism of amphetamine-induced phenomena with neuroleptics is well known (10, 11, 12, 13, 14, 15, 16, 17, 18, 19, 20, 21, 25, 26, 28, 29, 30, 31, 32, 33, 37). Interaction of various amphetamine-induced effects with the actions of antidepressants and monoamine-oxidase (MAO) inhibitors has also been extensively studied (1, 2, 3, 4, 5, 6, 7, 8, 9, 22, 23, 24, 26, 27, 28, 34, 35, 36, 37, 38, 39, 40, 41). In general, classical antidepressants and to a lesser extent MAO inhibitors potentiate several amphetamine-induced effects either in intensity or in duration.

In this chapter we will describe the antagonism of amphetamine-induced enhancement of oxygen consumption, brought about by 'antidepressants' without inhibition of concurrently heightened agitation. In contrast, neuroleptics, reduce simultaneously both amphetamine-induced agitation and increased oxygen consumption.

II. METHODOLOGICAL CONSIDERATIONS

A. Apparatus

The apparatus consists of a set of six identical animal chambers connected in parallel to an oxygen cylinder. One animal chamber with its connections to the manometer and to an oxygen cylinder is diagrammatically illustrated in Figure 1. The chamber consists of 2 main parts, a bottom and a cover, both made up of clear glass. The cover, containing a thermometer, is used to seal the chamber airtight. Inside the chamber is placed a metal frame, which holds a perforated plate to serve as an animal platform. Containers filled with calcium oxide (Calona®, soda lime: 4-10 mesh.) are placed below and above the animal holder.

An inlet into the chamber is connected to the oxygen cylinder through appropriate valves and pressure gauges. An outlet out of the chamber is devided by a glass T, one side of which is connected to a manometer and the other to a one way stop cork which opens to the air exhaust system of the room.

B. Procedure

The test animals are placed into the chamber and the chamber is closed airtight. The chamber is flushed with oxygen for 3 minutes by opening the oxygen inlet and the atmospheric outlet. The outlet is then closed and the oxygen pressure inside the chamber is allowed to stabilize at an overpressure of 50 units on the manometer, at which time the oxygen inlet is also closed. Thereafter the gastight chamber is connected only to the manometer. Any oxygen consumed by the animals causes proportional reduction in the

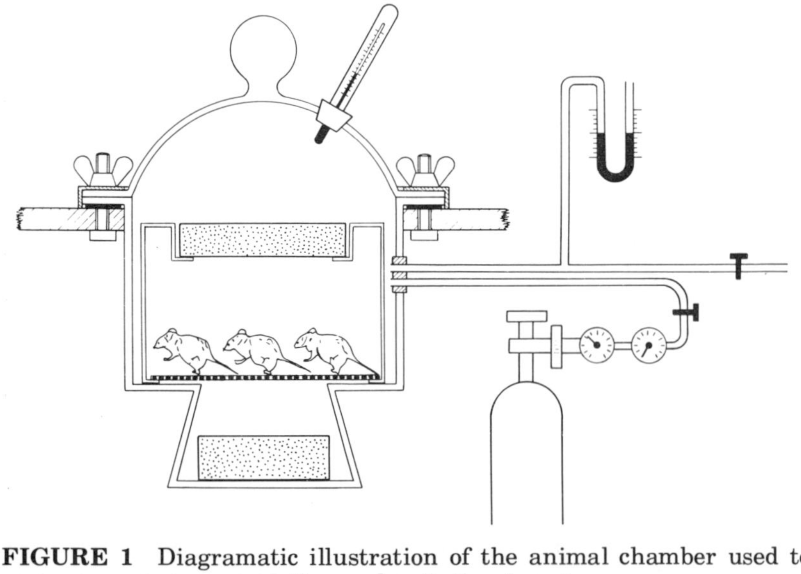

FIGURE 1 Diagramatic illustration of the animal chamber used to measure oxygen consumption and agitation in rats.

internal pressure and a drop in the manometer reading is recorded. The carbon dioxide produced by the animals is absorbed by the soda lime, which is replaced after each determination.

C. Animals

Experimental animals are inbred male Wistar rats, placed in groups of three in each chamber. Preliminary experiments have shown that the oxygen consumption of the rats depends upon the group weight of the animals (Fig. 2). Therefore, groups of 3 rats with the same total weight of 700 ± 10 g were selected (each individual rat weighing 235 ± 5 g). This way, body weight as a variable is adequately controlled and the resulting oxygen consumption provides a highly predictable base-line, as is demonstrated below.

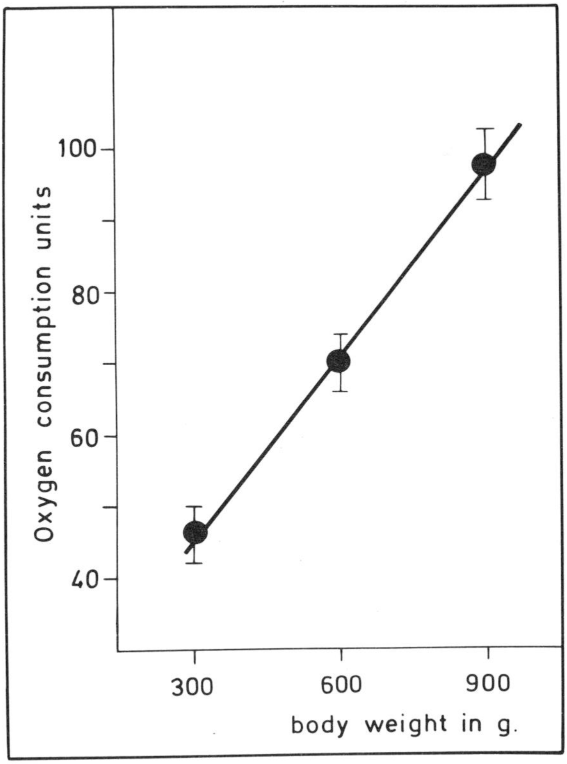

FIGURE 2 Effect of body weight (groups of 3 rats) on one hour oxygen consumption.

D. Drug administration

Route and time of drug administration are obviously important and may differ for different compounds. However, based on previously obtained results, all test drugs described in this chapter are injected subcutaneously 60 minutes before the animals are placed in the test chambers and 45 minutes before amphetamine is injected.

In order to select an appropriate dose of subcutaneously administered dl-amphetamine sulfate, a dose response curve of oxygen consumption was established first. A dose of 2.5 mg/kg was selected for routine use as it lies on the plateau portion of the dose-response curve and gives a consistently high stimulation of oxygen consumption. This dose of amphetamine also produces very pronounced agitation in all groups of rats.

In a single experiment on one day, one group of 3 rats is injected with saline, and the 5 other groups of 3 rats each are treated with one dose of five different test drugs, prior to the injection of amphetamine. This is repeated on additional five days and by the end each dose of the tested drug has been given to 6 groups of 3 rats in six different experiments.

E. Measurement

During the total observation period of one hour, manometer readings are taken in indicated units and agitation is scored every 15 minutes. To score agitation the following four point scoring scale is used by a trained observer:

- score 0: normal activity but no agitation.
- score 1: the presence of agitation is in doubt.
- score 2: presence of agitation but clearly less pronounced than maximal as described under score 3.
- score 3: very pronounced and continuous agitation, i.e. increased locomotion, rearing and sniffing.

As the animals are scored every 15 minutes, these 4 agitation scores are cumulated for each observation chamber and reaches 12 (4×3) if there is no antagonism to the amphetamine-induced hyperactivity. An agitation score of 0 will be obtained when the amphetamine-agitation in all 3 animals is completely abolished. Manometer readings for oxygen consumption are likewise cumulated over the 1 hour observation period. Thus each group of 3 animals in a test chamber is considered as a unit and both final readings after 1 hour testing in the chambers are computed, i.e. one for oxygen consumption (O.C.) and one for agitation (Ag.).

III. EFFECT OF TEST DRUGS

In order to illustrate actual working of the test as well as the method of computing data for comparison purposes, the results from two drugs are described below in detail. Desipramine is selected as a representative antidepressant, and haloperidol as a representative neuroleptic. For reason of simplicity the rats injected with amphetamine alone are called the 'control group', and the rats treated with amphetamine and test drug are the 'treated group'.

A. Normal oxygen consumption

In untreated rats (group of 3, combined weight 700 ± 10 g) oxygen consumption reaches 73.5 ± 4.5 units as shown in Figure 3. The mean agitation score is zero.

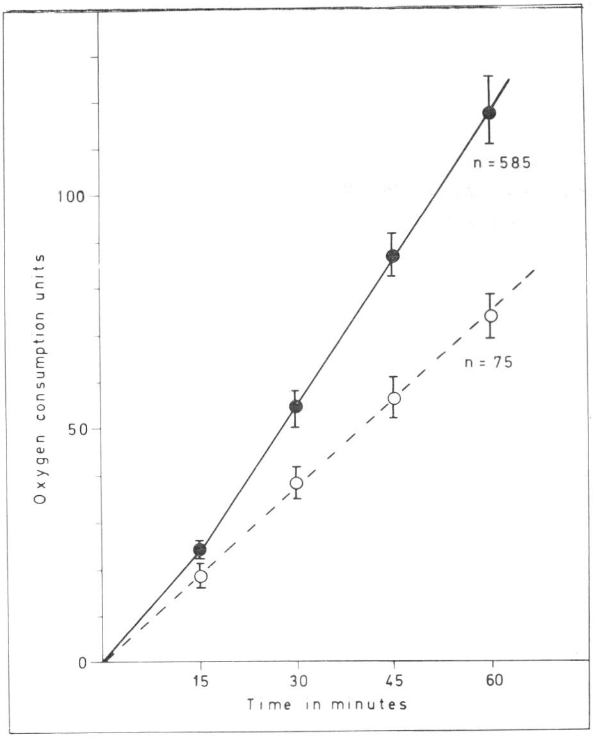

FIGURE 3 Oxygen consumption in manometer units expressed as mean values with standard error, obtained from saline treated rats (o) and rats treated s.c. with 2.5 mg/kg of amphetamine 15 minutes prior to the session.

B. Action of amphetamine 2.5 mg/kg s.c.

The same Figure 3 shows that in amphetamine-treated rats (groups of 3, combined weight 700 ± 10 g) oxygen consumption reaches 118 ± 6.45 units. A review of readings from the past 1,000 'control' determinations revealed that there were 5% of the readings below 110 units, and only 1 reading below 100 units.

The mean agitation score in amphetamine treated rats is 12. A score of less than 12 was observed only once in 1,000 'control' groups.

C. Action of desipramine on amphetamine-treated rats (Fig. 4)

Desipramine (DMI) was given in the following 9 doses: 0.08, 0.16, 0.31, 0.63, 1.25, 2.50, 5.00. 10.0, and 20.0 mg/kg. Each dose was given to 6 groups of 3 rats (solid points) and compared to as many different 'control' groups (open points) measured in the same experimental sessions.

1. Oxygen consumption

Actual readings of oxygen consumption from each chamber are plotted in Figure 4. Under the graph are given the number of readings obtained for different criteria of reduction in oxygen

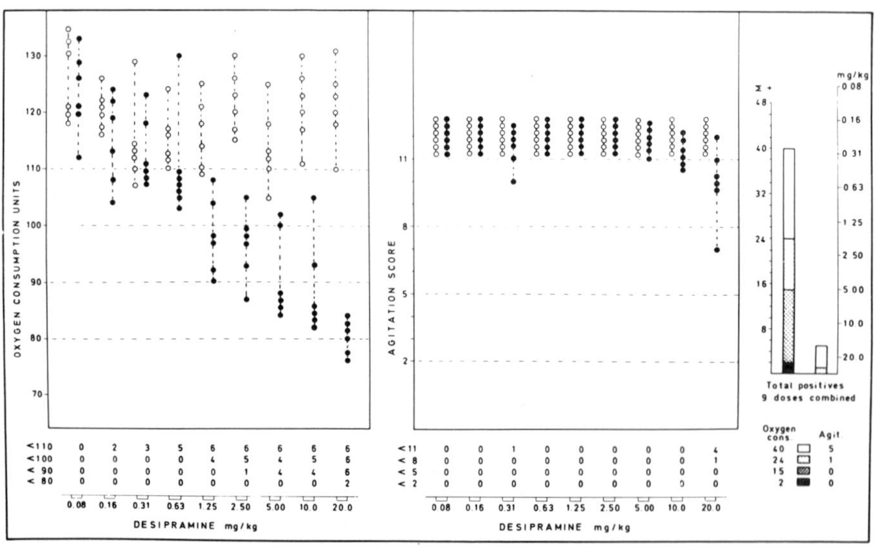

FIGURE 4 Effect of desipramine on oxygen consumption and agitation in amphetamine-treated rats. For explanation see text.

consumption. The selection of these criteria is based on a large number of 'control' readings and readings from normal rats (see above). For 'control' rats oxygen consumption less than 110 units, occurred in 5% of the animals. Oxygen consumption less than 110 units occurred in 0.1% of the 'controls', less than 90 units was never observed in controls. Less than 80 units is the amount of oxygen consumption found in normal rats without treatment of amphetamine. Based upon these observations 4 categories of amphetamine antagonism were evolved. The number of readings falling into each of these categories is then cumulated for all doses and is used to obtain a bar graph for rapid comparison among drugs and among drug-categories. The bar level roughly corresponds to the ED_{50} with respect to the category focussed; it can be estimated on the right ordinate, and subsequently will be referred to as the "estimated" ED_{50}. When the criterion of minimum effect is used (oxygen consumption less than 110 units), 40 out of a total of 54 readings fall into this category and are considered 'positives'. Considering the category of complete antagonism (oxygen consumption less than 80 units) only 2 out of 54 readings are found 'positive'. Twenty-four out of 54 and 15 out of 54 readings fall into the in-between categories of respectively less than 100 and less than 90 units. The bar graph based upon these readings is given on the right hand side of the figure and right above the sum of the 'positive' readings. These data show that desipramine is an active drug with respect to its antagonism of amphetamine-induced increase of oxygen consumption. Moreover, the DMI antagonism is dose-dependent.

2. Agitation

It may be recalled that agitation is scored in the same rats in which oxygen consumption is measured (Fig. 4). The agitation scores of the rats whose oxygen consumption is described above, are plotted against the different doses of DMI and compared with the corresponding 'control' readings. In addition, similarly to oxygen consumption, changes in agitation scores are also subdivided in four categories of intensity, on the basis of an 'all or none' effect, i.e. agitation scores less than 11, which occurred in 0.1 % of the controls, and agitation scores less than 8, less than 5 and less than 2, which were never observed in 'control' groups. The number of readings from the treated groups which fall into each of the four categories of agitation are given below the graph and the sum total of those readings obtained from all doses are given for each category of agitation on the right. It may be seen that 4 out of 54 readings fall into the category of minimal activity reduction (agitation score less than 11), none falls into the categories of highest activity reduction (less than 5 and less than 2). This shows that, unlike its effectiveness against amphetamine-induced increased oxygen consumption, DMI is a very poor antagonist of amphetamine-induced agitation. The differential effect of DMI on both amphetamine-induced activities is illustrated in the bar graphs given on the right hand side of the figure, right above the sum total of the 'positive' readings.

D. Action of haloperidol on amphetamine-treated rats (Fig. 5)

Haloperidol was given in the following 9 dose levels: 0.005, 0.01, 0.02, 0.04, 0.08, 0.16, 0.31, 0.63, and 1.25 mg/kg. Each dose was given to 6 groups of 3 rats (solid points) and compared to as many different 'control groups' (open points) measured in the same experimental sessions. Data obtained from the haloperidol-treated groups in the same way as those obtained with DMI in the preceeding section are described below.

1. Oxygen consumption

Figure 5 shows the dose-response curve of haloperidol antagonism to increased oxygen consumption induced by am-

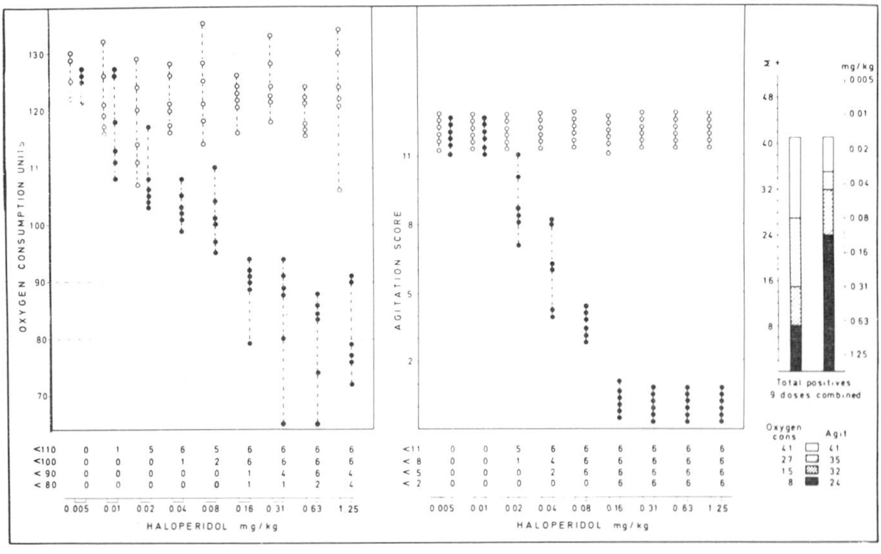

FIGURE 5 Effect of haloperidol on oxygen consumption and agitation in amphetamine-treated rats. For explanation see text.

phetamine. It is shown that the activity of the 9 haloperidol doses is comparable to that of the 9 DMI doses, i.e. oxygen consumption less than 110 gives 41 positive readings with haloperidol (with DMI: 40), oxygen consumption less than 100 gives 27 positive readings with haloperidol (with DMI: 24), oxygen consumption less than 90 gives 15 positive readings for both haloperidol and DMI, and for oxygen consumption less than 80 there are 8 positive readings with haloperidol and 2 with DMI. Thus as an antagonist of amphetamine-induced increase in oxygen consumption, haloperidol is approximately 16 times more potent than DMI on a mg/kg basis.

2. Agitation

The agitation scores of the rats which have been treated either with amphetamine (control groups) or with amphetamine in combination with haloperidol (treated groups) are also shown in Figure 5. The haloperidol data show that unlike DMI, haloperidol is very effective in antagonizing amphetamine-induced agitation. Whereas DMI showed some antagonism to amphetamine -induced agitation only at very high doses, haloperidol effects were seen at very low doses and in fact haloperidol seems to be actually more effective against amphetamine-induced agitation than against amphetamine-induced increase of oxygen consumption. The effect of haloperidol on both amphetamine-induced actions is clearly illustrated in the bar graphs given on the right hand side of the figure, right above the sum total of the 'positive' readings.

E. Comparison of 'antidepressant' and 'neuroleptic' drugs

In order to illustrate the similarities as well as the differences between the two classes of drugs under discussion, we have summarized the data from six representative antidepressants: desipramine, imipramine, nortriptyline, amitryptyline, norpropazepine, and propazepine (Fig. 6), and 6 representative neuroleptics from different chemical classes: benperidol, droperidol, trifluperidol, haloperidol, trifluoperazine and pimozide (Fig. 7). For each drug bar graphs were obtained in exactly the same way as described for DMI and haloperidol, using 9 consecutive dose levels and 6 groups of 3 rats per dose level. The dose range represented is selected in such a way, that out of the dose series (0.01, 0.02, . . . , 80, 160) 9 consecutive doses total 38 $\pm$ 3 positives according to the least severe criterion (oxygen consumption less than 110 units). An overall view of the data shows the similarity of action among the antidepressants and likewise a similarity of

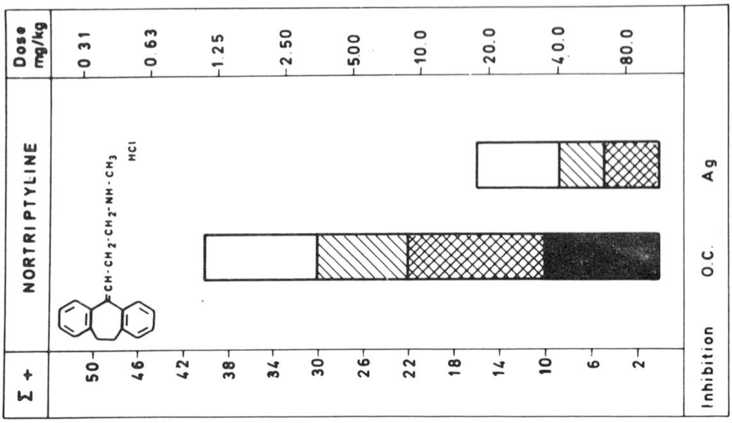
NORTRIPTYLINE
Σ +
Dose mg/kg
0.31
0.63
1.25
2.50
5.00
10.0
20.0
40.0
80.0
50
46
42
38
34
30
26
22
18
14
10
6
2
Inhibition
O.C.
Ag
HCl

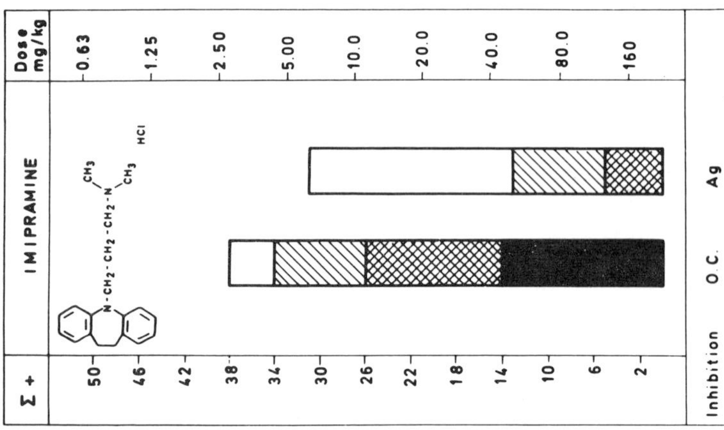
IMIPRAMINE
Σ +
Dose mg/kg
0.63
1.25
2.50
5.00
10.0
20.0
40.0
80.0
160
50
46
42
38
34
30
26
22
18
14
10
6
2
Inhibition
O.C.
Ag
HCl

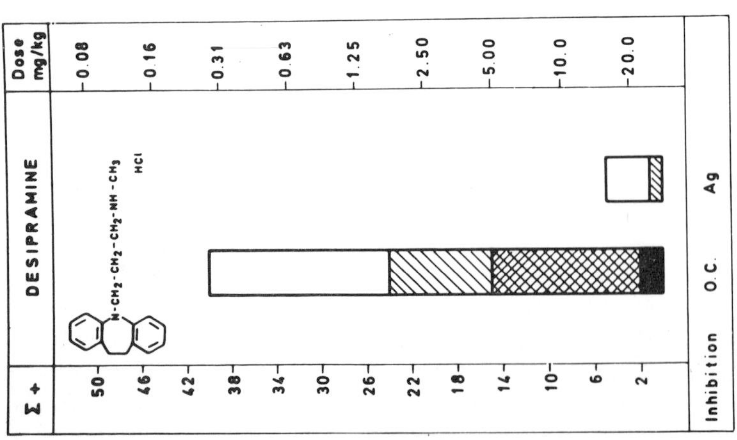
DESIPRAMINE
Σ +
Dose mg/kg
0.08
0.16
0.31
0.63
1.25
2.50
5.00
10.0
20.0
50
46
42
38
34
30
26
22
18
14
10
6
2
Inhibition
O.C.
Ag
HCl

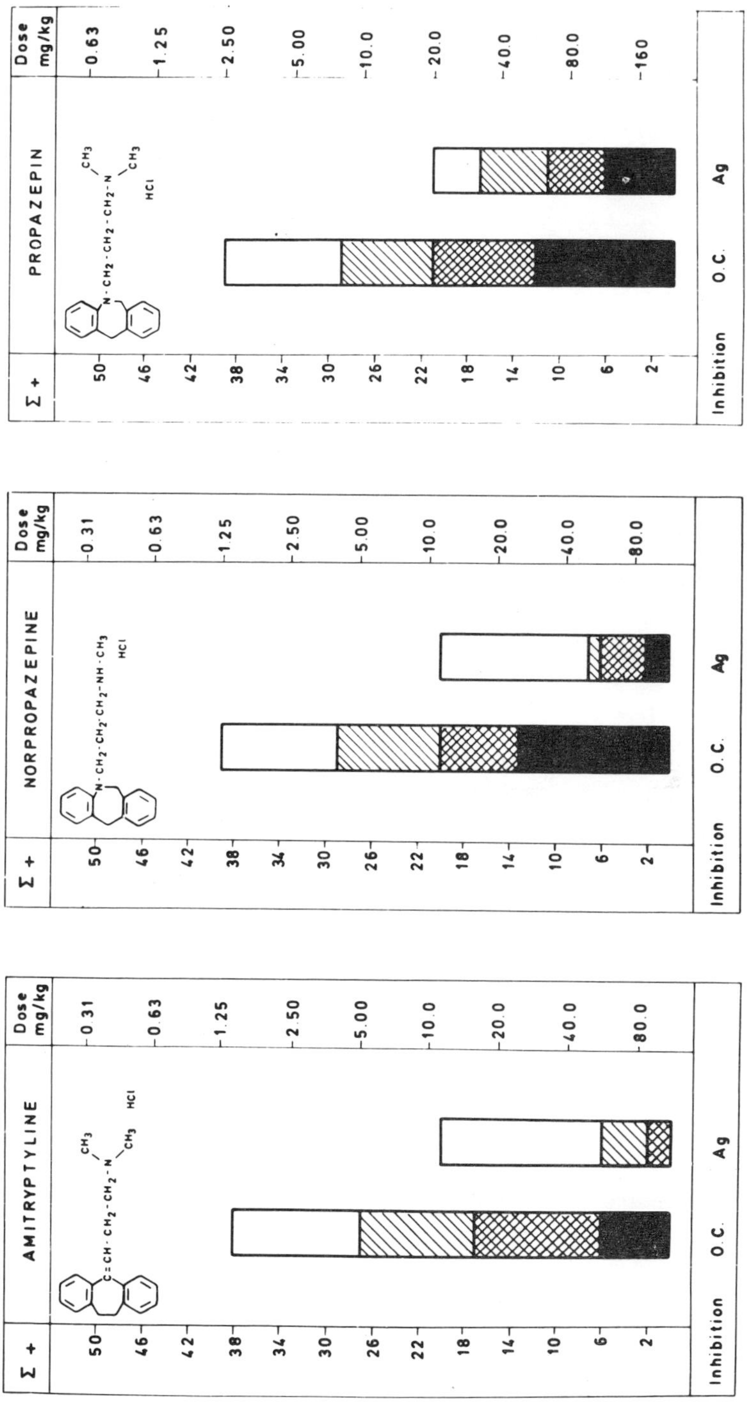

FIGURE 6 Comparison of the effects of six 'antidepressant' drugs on oxygen consumption and agitation in amphetamine-treated rats. For explanation see text.

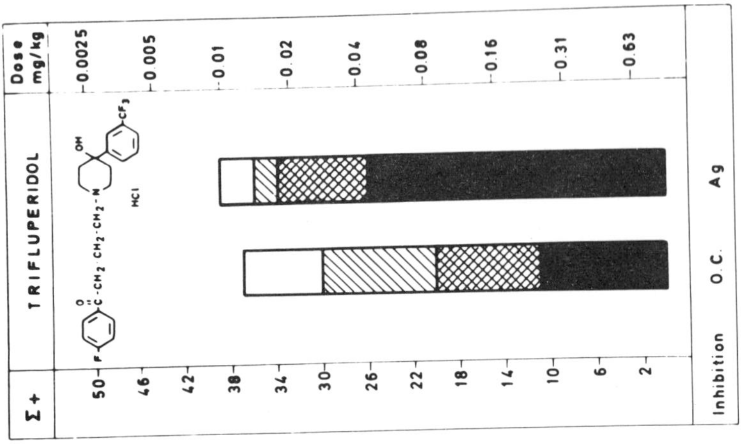
Σ+
Dose mg/kg
TRIFLUPERIDOL
HCl
50
46
42
38
34
30
26
22
18
14
10
6
2
0.0025
0.005
0.01
0.02
0.04
0.08
0.16
0.31
0.63
Inhibition
O.C.
Ag

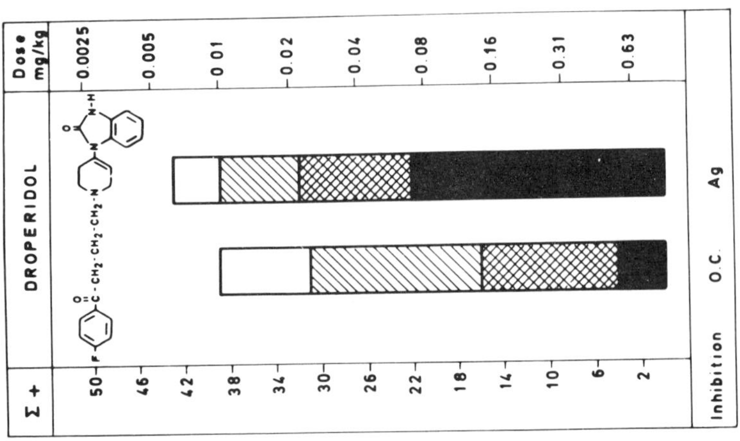
Σ+
Dose mg/kg
DROPERIDOL
50
46
42
38
34
30
26
22
18
14
10
6
2
0.0025
0.005
0.01
0.02
0.04
0.08
0.16
0.31
0.63
Inhibition
O.C.
Ag

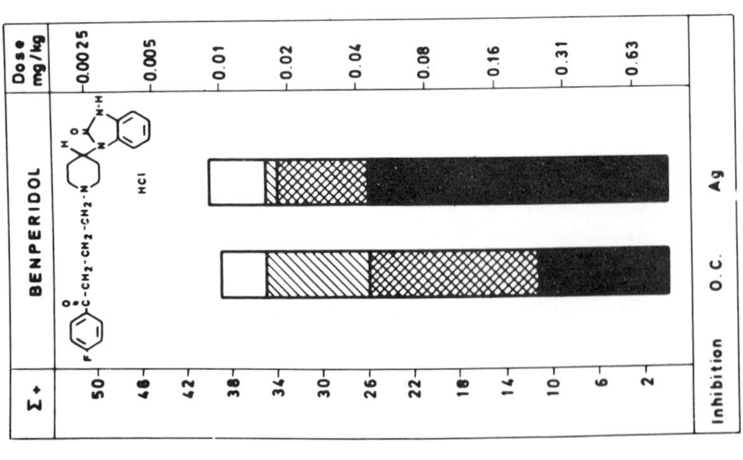
Σ+
Dose mg/kg
BENPERIDOL
HCl
50
46
42
38
34
30
26
22
18
14
10
6
2
0.0025
0.005
0.01
0.02
0.04
0.08
0.16
0.31
0.63
Inhibition
O.C.
Ag

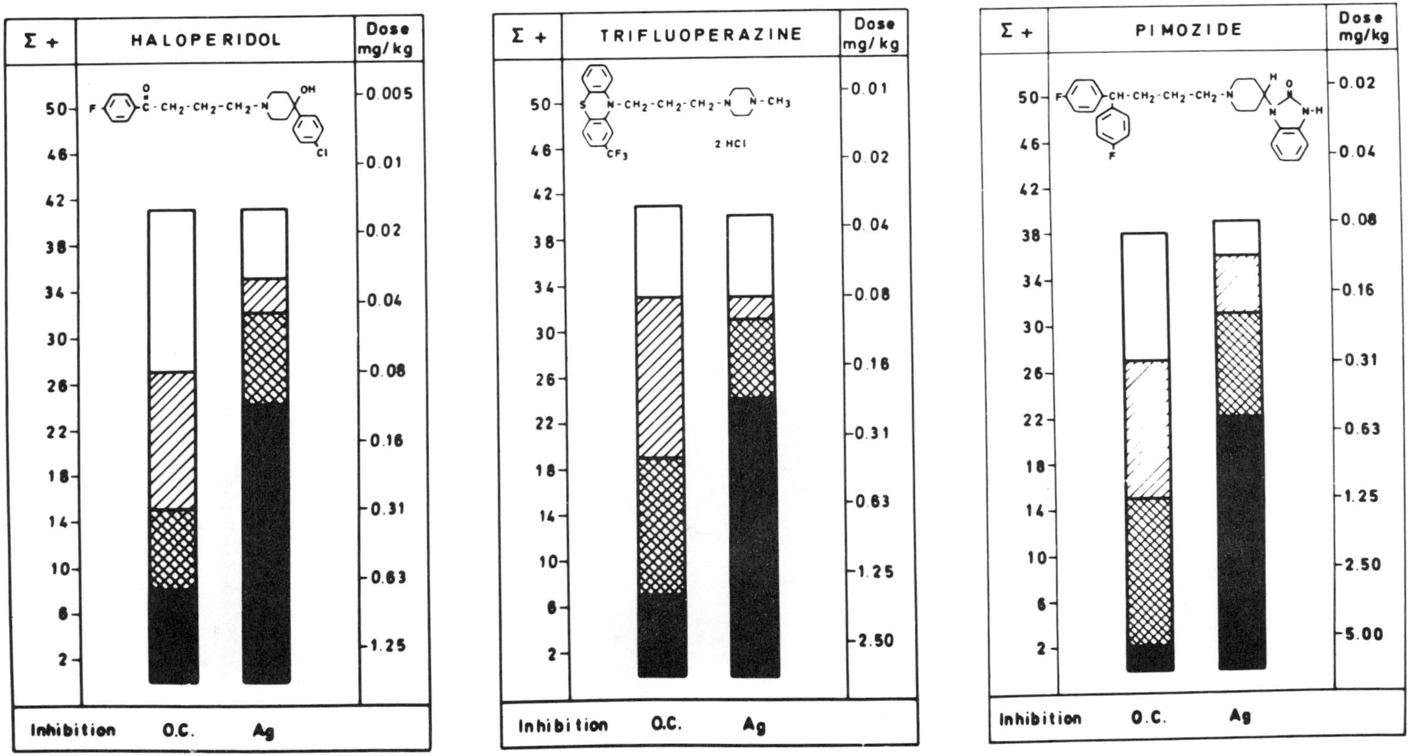

FIGURE 7 Comparison of the effects of six 'neuroleptic' drugs on oxygen consumption and agitation in amphetamine-treated rats. For explanation see text.

action among the compounds belonging to the neuroleptic series. One may also notice from the dose ranges employed, that the neuroleptics described are more potent drugs since far smaller doses are needed to produce their pharmacological action.

1. Antidepressants

All six drugs have a comparable activity against amphetamine-induced increase of oxygen consumption. The order of potency with the lowest estimated ED_{50} (criterion less than 110 units) in brackets is desipramine (0.31 mg/kg) more potent than nortriptyline (1.25 mg/kg), equal to amitryptyline, equal to norpropazepine, more potent than propazepine (2.50 mg/kg), which is equal to imipramine (2.50).

Antagonism of amphetamine-induced agitation is much less pronounced with all compounds, the lowest effective doses (score less than 11) being 5.00 to 10.0 mg/kg for imipramine, 10.0 mg/kg for amitryptyline and norpropazepine, 10.0 to 20.0 mg/kg for desipramine, and 20.0 mg/kg for nortriptyline and propazepine. With only 2 compounds, norpropazepine and propazepine, antagonism to amphetamine-induced agitation was obtained in all 4 criteria of antagonism.

The dissociation ratios, at the lowest criteria of antagonism, between amphetamine-induced increase of oxygen consumption and agitation are for desipramine (1:50), for nortriptyline (1:16), for amitryptyline, for norpropazepine and propazepine (1:8), and for imipramine (1:3). We have tested a number of other antidepressants and observed similar patterns.

2. Neuroleptics

All six neuroleptics described have a comparable activity against both amphetamine-induced effects. When the lowest criteria of activity are considered, i.e. less than 110 units for oxygen consumption and a score less than 11 for agitation, the lowest active doses are: 0.005 to 0.01 mg/kg for droperidol, 0.01 mg/kg for benperidol and trifluperidol, 0.01 to 0.02 mg/kg for haloperidol, 0.02 to 0.04 mg/kg for trifluoperazine, and 0.08 mg/kg for pimozide. Furthermore, the data show that when the most rigid criteria of activity are considered, i.e. less than 80 units for oxygen consumption and score less than 2 for agitation, all neuroleptics are more effective in antagonizing amphetamine-induced agitation, than in antagonizing amphetamine-induced increase of oxygen consumption. Evaluation of many other neuroleptics shows similar antagonism of amphetamine. They differ only in magnitude of their effective doses.

IV. CONCLUSION

Antidepressants are potent antagonists of amphetamine-induced increase in oxygen consumption and a significant number of 'positive' readings is obtained in all four categories of antagonism. Antagonism of amphetamine-induced agitation is either absent or is much less apparent. Neuroleptics are well-known amphetamine antagonists and, as expected, all neuroleptics described effectively antagonize amphetamine-induced increase in oxygen consumption. However, in contrast to antidepressants, all neuroleptics are even more effective against amphetamine-induced agitation. Because of the differential effects of neuroleptics and antidepressants in antagonizing amphetamine actions, the procedure described in this chapter may serve as a useful tool for preclinical evaluation of antidepressant drugs.

REFERENCES

1. Boissier, J., Dumont, C., and Ratonis, R.: Etude pharmacologique d'un nouvel antidépresseur tricyclique, *Thérapie,* **26**:459-479, 1971.
2. Carlton, P. L.: Potentiation of the behavioural effects of amphetamine by imipramine, *Psychopharmacologia,* **2**:364-367, 1961.
3. Claassen, V. and Davies, J. E.: Potentiation by tricyclic antidepressants of weight loss caused by amphetamine in rats, *Acta Physiol. Pharmacol. Neerlandica,* **15**:37-40, 1969.
4. Dolfini, E., Tansella, M., Valzelli, L., and Garattini, S.: Further studies on the interaction between desipramine and amphetamine, *Europ. J. Pharmacol.,* **5**:185-190, 1969.
5. Ernst, A. M.: Mode of action of apomorphine and dexamphetamine on gnawing compulsion in rats, *Psychopharmacologia,* **10**:316-323, 1967.
6. Gluckman, M. I. and Baum, I.: The pharmacology of iprindole, a new antidepressant, *Psychopharmacologia,* **15**:169-185, 1969.
7. Halliwell, G., Quinton, R. M., and Williams, F. E.: A comparison of imipramine, chlorpromazine and related drugs in various tests involving autonomic functions and antagonism of reserpine, *Brit. J. Pharmacol.,* **23**:330-350, 1964.
8. Herr, F., Voith, K., and Jaramillo, J.: The pharmacology of butriptyline, *J. Med.,* **2**:258-270, 1971.
9. Horovitz, Z. P., Furgiuele, A. R., High, J. P., and Burke, J. C.: Comparative activities of a substituted dibenzothiazepine, of imipramine and of desipramine, *Arch. Int. Pharmacodyn.,* **151**:180-191, 1964.
10. Janssen, P. A. J.: Vergleichende pharmakologische daten uber sechs neue basische 4'-fluorobutyrophenon-derivate: haloperidol, haloanison, triperidol, methylperidid, haloperidid und dipiperon, *Arzneim.-Forsch.,* **11**:819-832, 1961.

11. Janssen, P. A. J.: The evolution of the butyrophenones, haloperidol and trifluperidol from meperidine-like 4-phenylpiperidines, *Intern. Rev. Neurobiology,* **8**:221-263, 1965.
12. Janssen, P. A. J.: Haloperidol and related butyrophenones, *Psychopharmacological Agents,* **2**:199-248, 1967.
13. Janssen, P. A. J.: Chemical and pharmacological classification of neuroleptics, *Modern Problems of Pharmacopsychiatry,* **5**:33-44, 1970.
14. Janssen, P. A. J.: Chemical and pharmacological classification of neuroleptics, *Folia Pharmaceutica,* **59**:51-61, 1971.
15. Janssen, P. A. J.: Over de pharmakologie van neuroleptica, *Tijdschr. Geneesk.,* **14**:675-680, 1971.
16. Janssen, P..A. J., Niemegeers, C. J. E., Schellekens, K. H. L., Verbruggen, F. J., and Van Nueten, J. M.: The pharmacology of dehydrobenzperidol, a new potent and short acting neuroleptic agent, chemically related to haloperidol, *Arzneim.-Forsch.,* **13**:205-211, 1963.
17. Janssen, P. A. J., Niemegeers, C. J. E., and Schellekens, K. H. L.: Is it possible to predict the clinical effect of neuroleptic drugs (major tranquillizers) from animal data? Part I: 'Neuroleptic activity spectra' for rats, *Arzneim.-Forsch.,* **15**:104-117, 1965.
18. Janssen, P. A. J., Niemegeers, C. J. E., Schellekens, K. H. L., and Lenaerts, F. M.: Is it possible to predict the clinical effect of neuroleptic drugs (major tranquillizers) from animal data? Part IV: An improved experimental design for measuring the inhibitory effects of neuroleptic drugs on amphetamine or apomorphine-induced 'chewing' and 'agitation' in rats, *Arzneim.-Forsch.,* **17**:841-854, 1966.
19. Janssen, P. A. J., Niemegeers, C. J. E., Schellekens, K. H. L., Dresse, A., Lenaerts, F. M., Pinchard, A., Schaper, W. K. A., Van Nueten, J. M., and Verbruggen, F. J.: Pimozide, a chemically novel, highly potent and orally long-acting neuroleptic drug. Part I. The comparative pharmacology of pimozide, haloperidol and chlorpromazine, *Arzneim.-Forsch.,* **18**:261-279, 1968.
20. Janssen, P. A. J., Niemegeers, C. J. E., Schellekens, K. H. L, Lenaerts, F. M., Verbruggen, F. J., Van Nueten, J. M., and Schaper, W. K. A.: The pharmacology of penfluridol (R 16 341) a new potent and orally long-acting neuroleptic drug, *Europ. J. Pharmacol.,* **11**:139-154, 1970.
21. Janssen, P. A. J., Niemegeers, C. J. E., Schellekens, K. H. L., Lenaerts, F. M., Verbruggen, F. J., Van Nueten, J. M., Marsboom, R. H. M., Hérin, V. V., and Schaper, W. K. A.: The pharmacology of fluspirilene (R 6218), a potent long-acting and injectable neuroleptic drug, *Arzneim.-Forsch.,* **20**:1689-1698, 1970.
22. Johnson, M. E. and Goldberg, M. E.: A method for evaluating imipramine-like agents in rats, *J. Pharm. Pharmacol.,* **17**:54-55, 1965.
23. Lewander, T.: Effects of amphetamine on urinary and tissue catecholamines in rats after inhibition of its metabolism with desmethylimipramine, *Europ. J. Pharmacol.,* **5**:1-9, 1968.
24. Lwoff, J. M., Larousse, C., Simon, P., and Boissier, J. R.: Profil psychopharmacologique d'un antidépresseur potentiel, appartenant à la série pyridobenzodiazepine, *Thérapie,* **26**:451-457, 1971.
25. Maj, J., Sawinska, H., Kapturkiewicz, Z., and Sarnek, J.: The effect of L-dopa and (+)-amphetamine in the locomotor activity after pimozide

and phenoxybenzamine, *J. Pharm. Pharmacol.*, **24**:412-413, 1972.
26. Menge, H. G. and Brand, U.: Untersuchungen über die stereotypien nach amphetamine und apomorphin sowie deren pharmakologische beeinflussung, *Psychopharmacologia,* **21**:212-228, 1971.
27. Montanaro, N. and Babbini, M.: Interaction between iminodibenzyl-derivatives or phenothiazine-derivatives and methylamphetamine in the rat, *Psychopharmacologia,* **7**:321-333, 1965.
28. Morpurgo, C. and Theobald, W.: Influence of imipramine-like compounds and chlorpromazine on the reserpine-hypothermia in mice and amphetamine-hyperthermia in rats, *Med. Pharmacol. Exptl.,* **2**:226-232, 1965.
29. Niemegeers, C. J. E.: Kan de klinische waarde van een neuroleptikum voorspeld worden aan de hand van farmakologische proeven bij dieren? *Bulletin* **2**:38, 1969.
30. Niemegeers, C. J. E.: Preclinical neuropsychopharmacology of neuroleptics. Predictions of side effects in Fielding, S., and Lal, H., editors: *Neuroleptics* (Industrial Pharmacology, Vol. I). Futura Publishing Company, Mt. Kisco, N.Y., 1974, pp. 98-129.
31. Niemegeers, C. J. E., and Janssen, P. A. J.: Bromoperidol, a new potent neuroleptic of the butyrophenone series. Comparative pharmacology of bromoperidol and haloperidol, *Arzneim.-Forsch.,* **24**:45-52, 1974.
32. Niemegeers, C. J. E., Van Nueten, J. M., and Janssen, P. A. J.: Azaperone, a sedative neuroleptic of the butyrophenone series with pronounced anti-aggressive and anti-shock activity in animals, *Arzneim.-Forsch.,* 1974, (in press).
33. Randrup, A. and Munkvad, I.: Special antagonism of amphetamine-induced abnormal behaviour. Inhibition of sterotyped activity with increase of some normal activities, *Psychopharmacologia,* **7**:416-422, 1965.
34. Scheckel, C. L. and Boff, E.: Behavioral effects of interacting imipramine and other drugs with D-amphetamine, cocaine and tetrabenazine, *Psychopharmacologia,* **5**:198-208, 1964.
35. Schmitt, H. and Schmitt, H.: Valeur de la pharmacologie prévisionnelle dans le domaine des antidépresseurs dérivés de l'iminodibenzyle, *Thérapie,* **21**:653-674, 1966.
36. Simon, P.: Exploration pharmacologique des antidépresseurs, *Thérapie,* **20**:1123-1147, 1965.
37. Stein, L. and Seifter, J.: Possible mode of antidepressive action of imipramine, *Science,* **134**:286-287, 1961.
38. Sulser, F., Owens, M. L., and Dingell, J. V.: On the mechanism of amphetamine potentiation by desipramine (DMI), *Life Sci.,* **5**:2005-2010, 1966.
39. Theobald, W., Büch, O., Kunz, H. A., Morpurgo, C., Stenger, E. G., and Wilhelmi, G.: Vergleichende pharmakologische untersuchungen mit tofranil, pertofran und insidon, *Arch. int. Pharmacodyn.,* **148**:560-596, 1964.
40. Van Riezen, H., Van Der Berg, W. J., Berendsen, H., and Jaspar, M. L.: 0I77, a new tricyclic antidepressant, *Arzneim.-Forsch.,* **23**:1295-1301, 1973.
41. Voith, K. and Herr, F.: Psychopharmacological evaluation of a new antidepressant: butriptyline, *Arch. Int. Pharmacodyn.,* **182**:318-331, 1969.

7

Effects of Antidepressant Drugs on Brain Catecholamines and Serotonin

B. KENNETH KOE, PH.D.

I. INTRODUCTION

Investigation of the biochemical and pharmacological properties of drugs that are effective in the treatment of depression has led to the formulation of the catecholamine, biogenic amine, or monoamine hypothesis of depression and affective disorders. In addition to providing a rationale for the mode of action of antidepressant drugs, the biochemical indices of antidepressant activity derived from this hypothesis hopefully would also have predictive or confirmatory value in the discovery of novel antidepressants. It is of interest to compare such efforts in the search for new antidepressants with those for antipsychotic drugs. Neuroleptic drugs, despite several different chemical structural types and different modes of principal actions (i.e. receptor blockers or monoamine depletors), all share a common phenomenon of eliciting a "striatal dopamine deficiency syndrome". This characteristic is readily recognized biochemically by the marked acceleration of dopamine synthesis in dopaminergic neurons in response (negative feedback) to the decreased receptor activity induced by neuroleptic drugs (Koe, 73). There is not an analogous unifying theme for drugs used to treat depression. Biochemical parameters of antidepressant activity have been modified and increased in number as new clinically active drugs are discovered. Moreover, the predictive value of current biochemical, behavioral, and pharmacological criteria for antidepressant activity has been questioned by some investigators (Gershon et al., 51; Freeman and Sulser, 44; Lahti and Maickel, 76).

The clinically important tricyclic family of antidepressants constitute a subgroup in a remarkable continuum of drugs that contain the "diphenylalkylamine" moiety. A wide spectrum of pharmacological actions is displayed by this continuum, encompassing antihistaminic, anticholinergic, antiparkinsonian, antidepressant, and antipsychotic activities. Overlap of pharmacological properties between subgroups is common. The present chapter will focus on selected topics from the complex biochemistry and pharmacology of antidepressant drugs, namely their effects on catecholamine and serotonin metabolism in brain, with emphasis on those aspects involved in the discovery of new drugs (Coppen, 27; Davis, 34; Garattini and Dukes, 50; Kaiser and Zircle, 67, 68; Schildkraut, 115, 116; Schildkraut and Gershon, 117; Sigg, 129).

II. BIOCHEMICAL INDICES OF ANTIDEPRESSANT ACTIVITY

Three groups of drugs are commonly considered as antidepressants: 1) tricyclic and related blockers of norepinephrine (NE) uptake; 2) monoamine oxidase (MAO) inhibitors; and 3) psychomotor stimulants. Current research efforts in the discovery of new antidepressants are probably centered on uptake blockers. Historically, the pharmacotherapy of depression developed along a familiar outline: 1) drugs with antidepressant activity are initially identified by their clinical effects; 2) biochemical and pharmacological characteristics of such compounds, known before or determined after their classification, are then used to synthesize a hypothesis of antidepressant activity; and 3) the tenets of this hypothesis are then used as a basis for guiding the search for new drugs. The catecholamine hypothesis, formulated in this manner, suggests that some depressions are the result of a relative deficiency of NE at central receptors; antidepressants overcome this deficiency by increasing availability of NE at synapses (Table I). Norepinephrine is normally inactivated by oxidative deamination via MAO, by methylation via catecholamine O-methyltransferase (COMT), or by reuptake into the neuron via a membrane amine pump. Interference with these processes should counteract the deficiency of noradrenergic activity in depression and thereby provide methods for discovering new compounds with antidepressant activity. Furthermore, as suggested by electroconvulsive shock therapy, compounds which enhance NE turnover (as a primary action) should also exert antidepressant effects. Finally, noradrenergic activity at receptors may also be enhanced by a greater release of the neurotransmitter; this action apparently is a property of the psychomotor stimulant, amphetamine (the latter also blocks NE uptake). Since amphetamine exhibits limited clinical effects on severe depression (Davis et al., 35; Goodwin and Sack, 56), psychomotor stimulants will not be considered here. Attention will be directed towards the biochemical actions of

TABLE I

Catecholamine hypothesis of depression [a]

Drug	Actual or Assumed		Clinical Effects
	Neurochemical Action on Norepinephrine (NE)	Effect on NE Receptors in Brain [b]	
Tricyclics	Block neuronal uptake	↑	Antidepressant activity
MAO inhibitors	Inhibit oxidative deamination	↑	Some antidepressant activity
Amphetamine	Releases and blocks uptake	↑	Poor antidepressant; stimulant
Cocaine	Blocks neuronal uptake	↑	Poor antidepressant; stimulant
ECS therapy	Enhances turnover	↑	Antidepressant activity
Reserpine	Depletes stores	↓	Sedation (depression?)

[a] Sigg (127); Schildkraut and Kety (118); Schildkraut et al. (119); Davis (34); and Goodwin and Sack (56).
[b] Noradrenergic function: ↑, enhanced (activation); ↓, reduced (deactivation).

tricyclic uptake blockers, and, to a lesser extent, MAO inhibitors. Current psychotherapeutic drugs for depression do not include any which are COMT inhibitors.

Norepinephrine is the catecholamine considered to be principally involved in depression. Although a role for dopamine (DA) has been proposed (McClure, 86), it is noteworthy that virtually all tricyclic antidepressants do not inhibit uptake in dopaminergic neurons (Carlsson et al., 20; Fuxe and Ungerstedt, 49; Horn et al., 60); do not affect the rate of accumulation or disappearance of ^{14}C-DA formed in brain from intravenously administered ^{14}C-tyrosine (Schubert et al., 123); and do not alter the rate of dopa accumulation (i.e. DA synthesis) in corpus striatum of rats treated with a dopa decarboxylase inhibitor (Koe, unpublished data).

Clincial evidence for the catecholamine (NE) hypothesis comes from measurement of urinary excretion of 3-methoxy-4-hydroxyphenethylene glycol (MHPG), a metabolite originating in part from metabolism of NE in brain. The clinical subgroup of depressed patients suffering from primary affective disorders is characterized by low urinary MHPG excretion and good therapeutic response to desipramine (DMI), imipramine, and even amphetamine (Mass et al., 83).

A. Blocking Catecholamine Uptake

An important finding in the history of tricyclic antidepressant drugs has been the observation that they block NE uptake into the peripheral adrenergic neuron (Axelrod et al., 3), probably by competition with NE at the neuronal membrane pump (Berti and Shore, 6). Other studies have suggested that a reuptake mechanism accounts for the termination of the actions of NE released from adrenergic nerve endings by nerve stimulation (see Iversen, 64). These findings together explain certain peripheral adrenergic effects of tricyclic antidepressants, such as the potentiation of neurally released or exogenously administered NE (Stone, 136; Iversen, 64). The demonstration of blockade of ^{3}H-NE uptake in brain by tricyclic antidepressants has extended the mechanism of adrenergic potentiation via blockade of uptake to the central actions of tricyclics (Glowinski and Axelrod, 52; Sulser and Dingell, 139; Sulser et al., 141). Thus, if the signs elicited by reserpine-induced catecholamine depletion constitute a model of depression, then tricyclics counter depression by blocking an important natural pathway of neurotransmitter inactivation, thereby allowing more physiologically active NE to react with central receptors (Glowinski and Axelrod, 52).

A prodigious amount of research has been devoted to uptake studies (Iversen, 64,65). Such studies usually consist of measuring the uptake of radiolabeled catecholamine (^{3}H-NE or ^{3}H-DA) into various isolated, innervated tissues: perfused heart, aortic strip, atrium, salivary gland, ganglion, vas deferens, iride, heart slice, and brain slice (Iversen, 65). *In vivo* studies of uptake and the effect of drugs on this process are conducted by 1) measuring the direct accumulation in tissues of exogenously administered labeled NE (Hertting et al., 59) or metaraminol which is resistant to degradation by MAO (Carlsson and Waldeck, 23; Waldeck, 149); 2) measuring the secondary effects, usually depletion of endogenous NE stores, by related amines which are also transported into the nerve endings by the same neuronal membrane amine pump; e.g. guanethidine, metaraminol, 6-hydroxydopamine, and substituted metatyramine derivatives (Stone et al., 137; Carlsson, 17); or 3) histochemical fluorescence of (a) α-methylcatecholamines after their uptake into catecholaminergic neurons of rats pretreated with reserpine, or (b) catecholamines (administered directly or derived from dopa) after their neuronal uptake in rats pretreated with reserpine + nialamide (Hamberger, 57; Carlsson et al., 21; Fuxe and Ungerstedt, 49).

Compounds which release (deplete) NE will elicit reduced accumulation of labeled catecholamines because of degradation of the monoamine by MAO. Uptake of ^{3}H-metaraminol, a specific indicator of neuronal membrane uptake, may be used, although the metabolic stability of this amine may result in some extraneuronal retention (Waldeck, 149). In any event, tricyclic antidepressants do not cause release of NE as determined by prelabeling cardiac stores of this catecholamine with ^{3}H-NE (Axelrod et al., 2; Daly et al., 33).

A simple *in vivo* assessment of inhibiton of uptake consists of determining the effect of the test drug on the accumulation of ^{3}H-NE in heart (Hertting et al., 59). A comparison of some standard tricyclic drugs and newer compounds synthesized as potential antidepressant agents shows the following order of decreasing activity *in vivo* in rats (Table II; Fig. 1): 1) very potent blocker (ED_{50} 0.06 μmole/kg), mazindol; 2) potent blockers (ED_{50} 1 to 3.2 μmole/kg), Lu 3-010, DMI, protriptyline, and EXP-561; 3) strong blockers (ED_{50} 3.2 to 10 μmole/kg), fenazoxine, CP-24,441, imipramine, gamfexine, chlorpheniramine, and nortriptyline; 4) moderate blockers (ED_{50} 10 to 32 μmole/kg), methylphenidate, chlorpromazine, amitriptyline, doxepin, and mianserin; 5) weak blockers (ED_{50} 32 to 100 μmole/kg), tofenacine and orphenadrine; 6) inactive (ED_{50} 100 μmole/kg or greater), thioridazine,

TABLE II

Inhibition of heart uptake of ^{3}H-norepinephrine in rats [a]

		Phenylbutylamine Type				Phenylpropylamine Type	
Antidepressants		Neuroleptics and Others		Nontricyclics			
		ED$_{50}$ (μmole/kg)					
Imipramine	6	Chlorpromazine	19	EXP-561	3	Mazindol	0.06
Desipramine	1	Thioridazine	>100	CP-24,441	5	Gamfexine	8
Amitriptyline	24	Thiothixene	>100	Lu 3-010	1	Chlorpheniramine	9
Nortriptyline	10			Fenazoxine	4	Mianserin	29
Protriptyline	1	Cyproheptadine	>100	Orphenadrine	53		
Doxepin	26			Tofenacine	41		
Iprindole	>100						

[a] Doses (i.p.) of drugs required to block uptake of ^{3}H-NE (5 μCi/kg i.v.) in heart by 50% (ED$_{50}$) were estimated graphically from results of uptake studies such as those illustrated in Fig. 1 and 2. Sources of ^{3}H-NE uptake data: Koe and Constantine, 74; Sarges et al., 112; and B. K. Koe, unpublished data. The ED$_{50}$ value of methylphenidate, a phenethylamine compound, is 12 μmole/kg (Fig. 1).

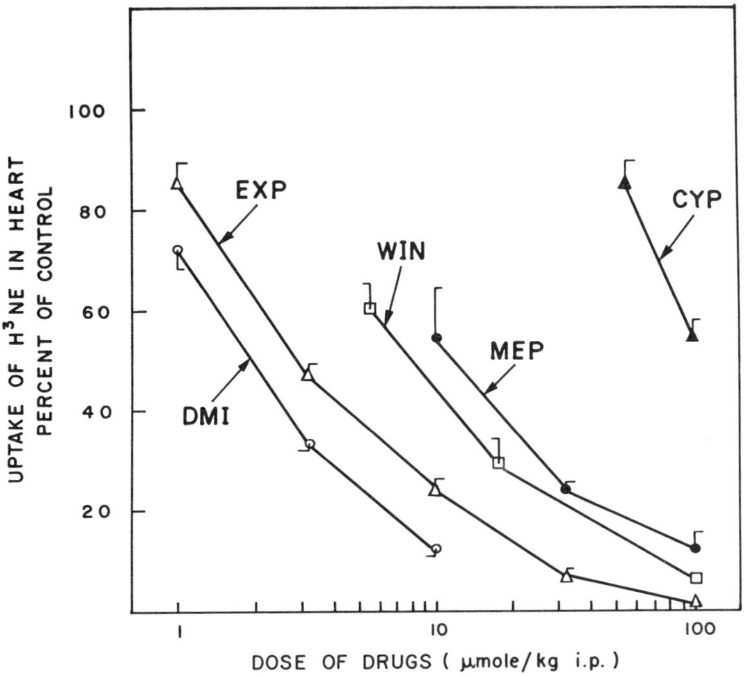

FIGURE 1 Relative specific activity of ^{3}H-norepinephrine (uptake as percent of control) in heart as a function of drug dose. Hearts were assayed 1 hr after the administration of DL-^{3}H-NE, 5 μCi/kg i.v., to rats pretreated 20 min earlier with the test drug (method of Koe and Constantine, 74). Each point is mean percent (N = 5-22). Vertical lines extend 1 S. E. from mean values. Specific activity (mean ± S.E. μCi/ mole) of heart ^{3}H-NE for control rats: 9.8 ±0.3 (N = 90). Abbreviations: DMI, desipramine; EXP, EXP-561; WIN, gamfexine; MEP, methylphenidate; CYP, cyproheptadine, B. K. Koe, unpublished data.

thiothixene, iprindole, and cyproheptadine (Koe and Constantine, 74; Sarges et al., 112; Koe, unpublished data). Similar comparisons are based on the prevention of NE depletion induced by the uptake of depleting/releasing amines, such as guanethidine, 6-hydroxydopamine, 4,α-dimethyl-m-tyramine, etc. (Stone et al., 137; Carlsson et al., 19; Carlsson, 17; Koe and Constantine, 74).

Although *in vivo* heart uptake measurements provide a facile means of ranking new drugs according to inhibitory activity, similar measurements for brain uptake should be more relevant to antidepressant activity. Studies of the accumulation of ^{3}H-NE following its intraventricular or intracisternal administration have, in general, shown blockade of uptake of the labeled catecholamine by tricyclic compounds. However, the extent of blockade in brain ascertained by this method is not impressive (Table III). Carlsson and co-workers (19) have determined the fol-

TABLE III

Inhibition of brain uptake of intracerebrally administered ^{3}H-norepinephrine in rats

Pretreatment hydrochloride	(i.p.) mg/kg	hr	Region	^{3}H-NE Content % control (*P*)	Reference
Imipramine	20	1	Whole brain	63 (<.001)	Glowinski and Axelrod (52)[a]
Desipramine	20	1	Whole brain	64 (<.001)	
Amitriptyline	10	1	Whole brain	77 (<.05)	
Chlorpromazine	40	1	Whole brain	91	
Imipramine	25	1.5	Whole brain	81 (<.001)	Schanberg et al. (114)[b]
Desipramine	25	1.5	Whole brain	70 (<.001)	
Chlorpromazine	25	1.5	Whole brain	81 (<.01)	
Imipramine	10	6	Whole brain	89 (<.01)	Schildkraut et al. (121)[d]
Imipramine	10	ch[c]	Whole brain	85 (<.01)	
Desipramine	20	1	Cerebellum	60 (<.01)	Glowinski et al. (53)[e]
			Medulla obl.	45 (<.001)	
			Hypothalamus	70	
			Striatum	125 (<.05)	
			Midbrain	80	
			Hippocampus	80 (<.05)	
			Cortex	115	
Desipramine	23	1	Hindbrain	74 (<.001)	B. K. Koe, unpublished data[f]
			Hypothalamus	82 (<.01)	
			Striatum	111	
			Cortex	110	

a Assayed 2 hr after DL-^{3}H-NE, 2 μCi/rat intraventricularly.
b Assayed 6 min after DL-^{3}H-NE, 6 μCi/rat intracisternally.
c Chronic administration of imipramine hydrochloride: 2 × 10 mg/kg daily for 3 weeks.
d Assayed 6 min after DL-^{3}H-NE, ~5 μCi/rat intracisternally.
e Assayed 1 hr after DL-^{3}H-NE, 6 μCi/rat intraventricularly.
f Assayed 6 min after L-^{3}H-NE, 5 μCi/rat intracisternally.

lowing uptake blocking activities of tricyclic drugs from their antagonism of the displacement (depletion) of brain (B) and heart (H) NE elicited by 4,α-dimethyl-m-tyramine (ED_{50} mg/kg): protriptyline, 4 (B), 4 (H); DMI, 15 (B), 6 (H); Lu 3-010, 40 (B), 3 (H); imipramine, >25 (B), 12 (H); amitriptyline >25 (B), 14 (H); nortriptyline, >25 (B), 15 (H); and chlorimipramine, >25 (B), 20 (H). A study of uptake in different tissues by various methods is detailed in the investigation of the properties of phthalane compounds related to Lu 3-010 (Carlsson et al., 21).

Uptake of ^{3}H-NE by synaptosomal preparations is an important *in vitro* method which has allowed rapid analysis of the kinetics of uptake (high and low affinity uptake), regional differences in uptake, and the relative inhibitory activity of a large number of compounds toward different monoamines (Snyder and Coyle, 132; Coyle and Snyder, 31; Horn et al., 60). This procedure has been extended to serotonin (Kannengiesser et al., 69; Wong et al., 152) and other putative neurotransmitters (Kuhar, 75). One interesting finding from synaptosomal uptake studies is that anticholinergic drugs, which are used for treating parkinsonian patients and for controlling extrapyramidal reactions to antipsychotic drugs, are potent inhibitors of ^{3}H-DA uptake (Coyle and Snyder, 30; Farnebo et al., 41; Fuxe et al., 48).

The search for improved drugs to treat depression has continued to generate new compounds which block catecholamine uptake (Kaiser and Zircle, 67,68). Other drug classes, such as antihistamines and antiparkinsonian agents also inhibit catecholamine uptake (Isaac and Goth, 63; Horn et al., 60). The latter two groups of agents suggest that the fused ring tricyclic (imipramine) or bicyclic (Lu 3-010) structure may not be necessary for inhibitory activity. A closer analysis discloses some common structural features of the different types of uptake blockers. In studies on the structure-activity relationships of uptake inhibitors, Maxwell and coworkers have attempted to overlap tricyclic and related structures with the extended phenethylamine molecule (Maxwell et al., 85; Salama et al., 110). Although superimposition with the phenethylamine or NE structure seems warranted for the sympathomimetic amine uptake blockers, there is no compelling reason why tricyclics and other compounds must do so. Studies in our laboratories using rigid molecules of known conformation as uptake blockers have led to a somewhat different active conformation than the one proposed by Maxwell and co-workers. A relatively simple rigid molecule with potent uptake blocking activity is 4-phenylbicyclo(2,2,2)octan-l-amine (EXP-561) (Gershon et al., 51). This compound is comparable to DMI in blocking heart uptake of ^{3}H-NE (Fig. 1) and surpasses DMI in potency as an inhibitor of serotonin uptake into synaptosomes (Table VI). The relative position of the benzene ring and amino group in EXP-561 is well-defined and may be a necessary structural requirement for inhibiting the membrane pump mechanism. That is, tricyclic and bicyclic uptake blockers containing the "phenylbutylamine" moiety must be able to assume the conformation of 1,4-phenylcyclohexylamine with equatorial phenyl and amino groups. Additional stereochemical requirements have been deduced from the synthesis of the four stereoisomers of N-methyl-4-phenyl-1,2,3,4-tetrahydro-1-naphthylamine (Sarges et al., 112). Only one isomer of this set shows marked blockade of heart uptake of ^{3}H-NE *in vivo* (Fig. 2). The molecular conformation of this active isomer, CP-24,441 (*trans* 1R,4S) (1aα in Fig. 3), has been ascertained by X-ray crystallography; models indicate the same distance between

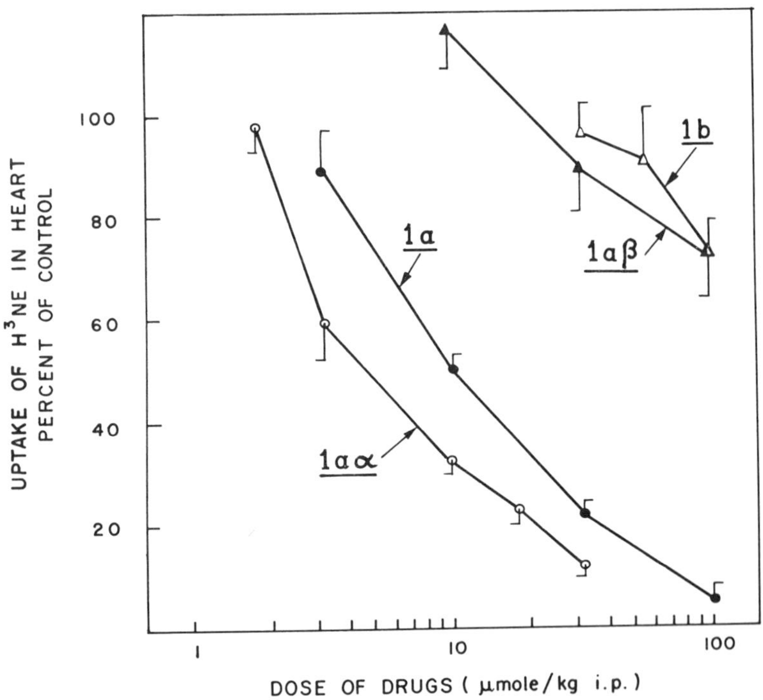

FIGURE 2 Relative specific activity of ^{3}H-norepinephrine (uptake as percent of control) in rat heart after N-methyl- 4-phenyl-1,2,3,4-tetrahydro-1-naphthylamines (same method as in Fig. 1). Conformation: 1aα (CP-24,441), *trans* 1R,4S; 1aβ, *trans* 1S,4R; 1a, *trans* enantiomeric pair; and 1b, *cis* enantiomeric pair. (From R. Sarges, B. K. Koe, A. Weissman, and J. P. Schaefer: *J. Pharmacol. Exp. Ther.*, **191**:393-402, 1974)

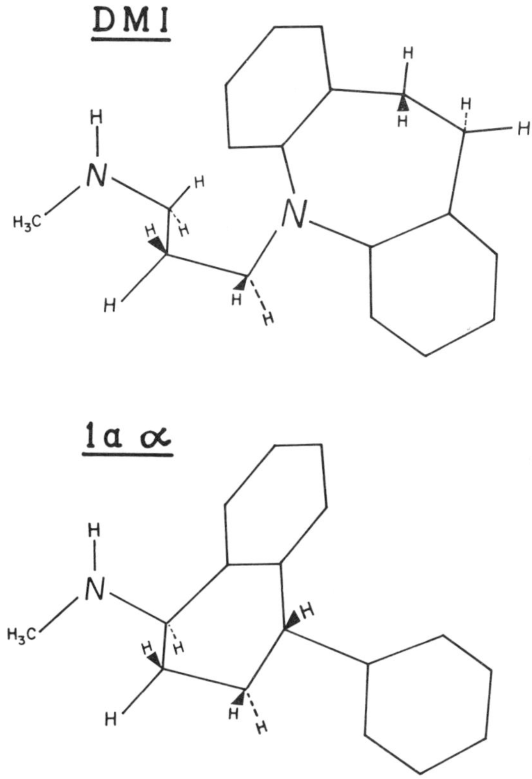

FIGURE 3 Active conformation proposed for desipramine (DMI). The aminoalkyl side chain of the tricyclic compound is folded towards the aromatic ring system in such a way that one benzene ring and the aminoalkyl residue can be superimposed on the corresponding atoms in CP-24,441 (1aα). (From R. Sarges, B. K. Koe, A. Weissman, and J. P. Schaefer: *J. Pharmacol. Exp. Ther.*, **191**:393-402, 1974)

phenyl and amino groups as in EXP-561. By superimposition with CP-24,441, the active conformation of DMI may be approximated (CP-24,441 is 1aα in Fig. 3). Supporting evidence of these proposals include 1) the relative inactivity of cyproheptadine as an uptake blocker (Fig. 1; Table II); and 2) the potent blocking activity of N,N-dimethylspiro[5H-dibenzo-[a, d]-cycloheptene-5,1′-cyclohexan]-4′-amine and the corresponding spiro[dibenzo-cycloheptene-cyclohex-2-en]-4′-amine (compounds "18" and "11", respectively, in Carnmalm et al., 24). The requisite phenylcyclohexane moiety is present in the latter compounds, and this portion of the molecular structure is superimposable over that of EXP-561, CP-24,441, or DMI. Other rigid uptake blockers N-methylspiro[5H-dibenzo[a,d]cycloheptene-5,1′-cyclopentan]

-3′-amine (compound "31" in Carnmalm et al., 24) and the related spiro[dibenzocycloheptane-tetrahydrofuran]-methylamine (Monkovic et al., 92) exhibit the same separation between phenyl and amino groups as in EXP-561. The fused ring tricyclic and bicyclic uptake blockers (Lu 3-010 and Lu 5-003 [Carlsson et al., 21]; amedalin and daledalin [Cañas-Rodriguez and Leeming, 15]) presently known all appear to be capable of assuming the active conformation proposed for DMI (Sarges et al., 112) (cf. first set of structures depicted in this chapter).

Antihistaminic and antiparkinsonian drugs, which exhibit NE uptake blocking activity, can assume the active conformation of CP-24,441 or DMI; e.g. diphenhydramine (Issac and Goth, 63), orphenadrine (Story and Story, 138), tofenacine (Van der Zee and Hespe, 145), and fenazoxine (Bassett et al., 5). Other antihistaminic uptake blockers, however, contain a "phenylpropylamine" moiety: promethazine, recipavrin, chlorpheniramine, and brompheniramine (Carlsson, 17; Horn et al., 60). Gamfexine (Davis, 34), a strong inhibitor of uptake (Fig. 1), is related structurally to the phenylpropylamine antihistaminics. Mianserin, a tetracyclic antidepressant (Fell et al., 42), contains a phenylpiperazine moiety which approximates the phenylpropylamine structure; it is not surprising that mianserin exerts uptake blocking activity (Table II). Mazindol, an appetite suppressant (Gogerty et al., 55), is an extremely potent blocker of ^{3}H-NE uptake in the heart (Table II). This drug may be visualized as a phenylpropylamine in which the "diphenylpropylamino" residue is fixed. In view of the high potency and rigid structure of mazindol, the active conformation of gamfexine, chlorpheniramine, and related uptake blockers may approximate that of this unusually active compound. (cf. second set of structures depicted in this chapter).

Still other antihistamines and anticholinergics contain a 4-benzyloxypiperidine ("phenylpentylamine") moiety. These drugs appear to be especially active antagonists of catecholamine uptake in the corpus striatum; e.g. benztropine and diphenpyraline (Horn et al., 60). Models of benztropine and EXP-561 demonstrate superimposability of the two structures, both of which possess the identical distance between phenyl ring and amino nitrogen. The membrane uptake mechanism for NE also transports into neurons other amines, including therapeutic drugs like guanethidine. Blockade of uptake of the latter by the tricyclic antidepressants, imipramine, DMI, and protriptyline, elicits reversal of the antihypertensive effect of guanethidine (Mitchell et al., 91). Antagonism of guanethidine uptake may be assessed in

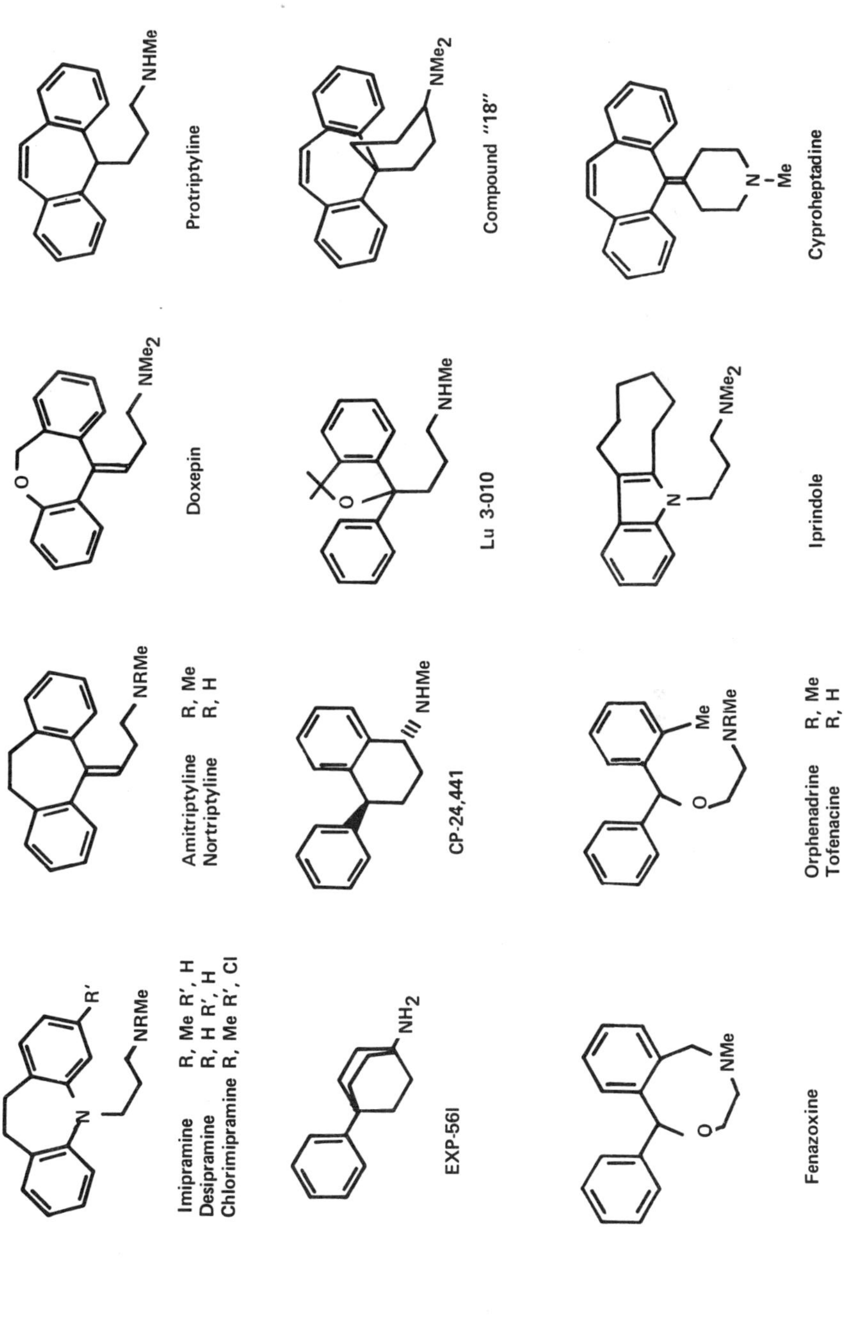
Imipramine R, Me R', H
Desipramine R, H R', H
Chlorimipramine R, Me R', Cl
Amitriptyline R, Me
Nortriptyline R, H
Doxepin
Protriptyline
EXP-561
CP-24,441
Lu 3-010
Compound "18"
Fenazoxine
Orphenadrine R, Me
Tofenacine R, H
Iprindole
Cyproheptadine

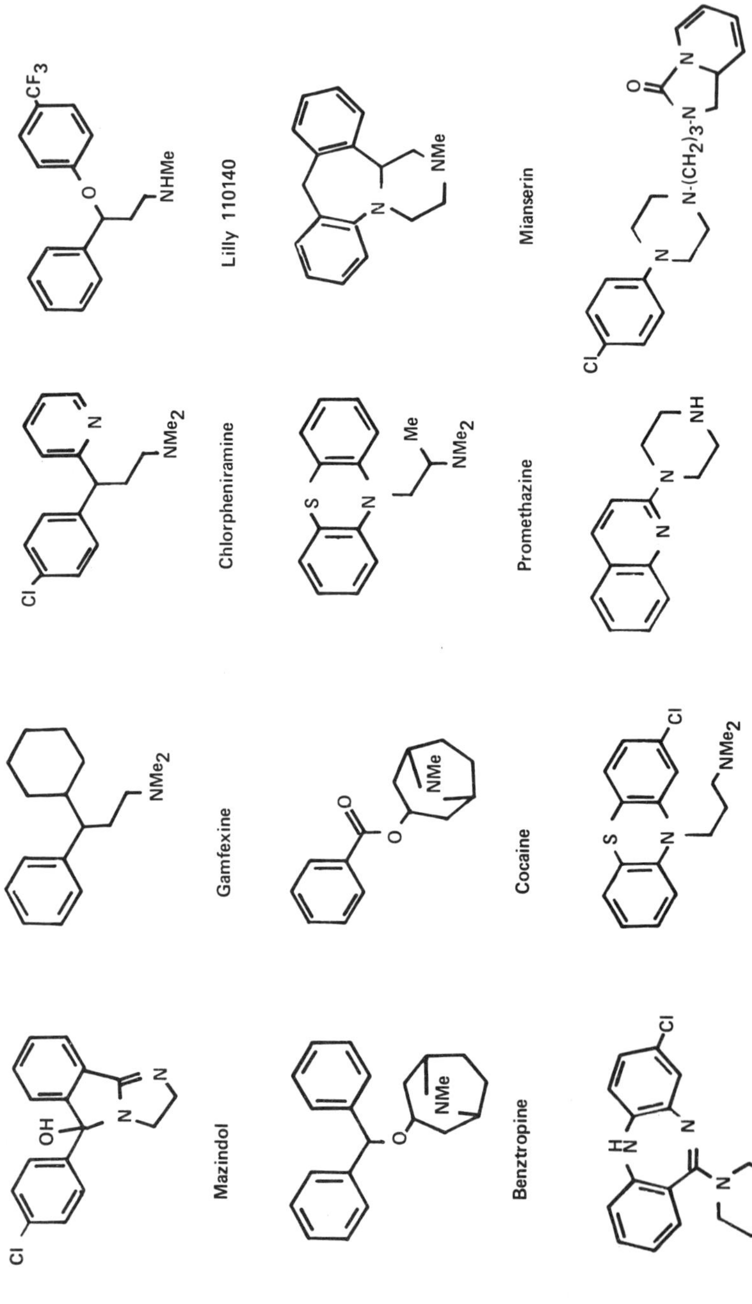
Mazindol
Gamfexine
Chlorpheniramine
Lilly 110140
Benztropine
Cocaine
Promethazine
Mianserin
Clozapine
Chlorpromazine
Quipazine
Trazodone

rats by the diminished depletion of heart NE stores induced by guanethidine (Koe and Constantine, 74).

B. Blocking Serotonin Uptake

In 1962 Sigg (128) reported that serotonin (5HT)-induced contractions of the cat nictitating membrane are potentiated more by imipramine than DMI, whereas NE-induced contractions are potentiated more by DMI than imipramine. It is noteworthy that chlorimipramine, a potent 5HT uptake blocker *in vitro*, exerts considerably less 5HT potentiation in this test than either imipramine or DMI (Sigg et al., 130). Because of the emphasis on the NE hypothesis of depression (Sigg, 127), interest in the effects of tricyclic antidepressants on central 5HT metabolism has developed only in the last few years.

The neuronal uptake of 5HT in brain is also characterized by a high affinity uptake process, associated with uptake into serotoninergic neurons, and a low affinity uptake system, associated with 5HT uptake into catecholaminergic neurons (Snyder et al., 133). The destruction of serotoninergic neurons in rat forebrain by lesions in midbrain raphe greatly reduces the high affinity synaptosomal uptake without affecting the low affinity uptake (Kuhar, 75).

The study of drug effects of 5HT uptake into serotoninergic neurons has assumed importance following the demonstration by histochemical fluorescence that imipramine, but not DMI or protriptyline, administered to rats, blocks the uptake of intraventricularly injected 5HT (i.e. for inhibiting 5HT uptake tertiary amines > secondary amines). This effect of tricyclics is opposite to that observed in central noradrenergic neurons in which blockade of NE uptake by secondary amines is greater than by tertiary amines (Carlsson et al., 20; Carlsson et al., 18; Fuxe and Ungerstedt, 49).

Confirmation of this structure activity relationship for closely related tricyclics is provided by 1) *in vitro* studies of 5HT uptake using (a) brain slices (Carlsson, 16; Shaskan and Snyder, 125) and (b) synaptosomal preparations (Kannengiesser et al., 69; Koe and Corkey, unpublished data in Table VI); 2) *in vivo* studies of the effect of tricyclics on 5HT displacement (depletion) in brain by 4-methyl-α-ethyl-m-tyramine (Carlsson et al., 18) or by p-chloromethamphetamine (Meek et al., 88); and 3) *in vivo* studies of tricyclics on the firing rate of raphe neurons (enhancing central serotoninergic activity, by inhibition of MAO or blockade of uptake, depresses the firing rate of raphe units via a negative feedback mechanism) (Sheard et al., 126). All of these studies give about the same order of potency for the tricyclic antidepressants (Table IV). It has been reported that blockade of uptake of ^{3}H-5HT, intracisternally administered, by imipramine (25 mg/kg) is not detectable (Schildkraut et al., 120); the relatively low sensitivity of a similar method for ascertaining antagonism of brain ^{3}H-NE uptake in rats has been referred to in the preceding section (Table III).

The marked inhibition of 5HT uptake in brain by the antihistamine chlorpheniramine (Tables IV and VI), has elicited speculation about its antidepressant activity (Carlsson and Lindqvist, 22). Structurally related phenylpropylamines, which are potent and selective inhibitors of 5HT uptake, include Lilly 110140 [3-(p-trifluoromethylphenoxy)-N-methyl-3-phenylpropylamine] (Wong et al., 151; Fuller and Perry, 47) and methadone (Ciafolo, 25).

The view that tricyclic secondary amines (R_2NH) are more po-

TABLE IV

Inhibition of brain uptake of serotonin in rats by drugs in decreasing order of potency [a]

A. *In vitro*

(1) Uptake of ^{14}C-5HT into whole brain synaptosomes[b]:
CIM > IMI ~ AMI > NOR ~ PRT ~ DMI
(2) Uptake of ^{14}C-5HT into striatal synaptosomes[c]:
CIM > IMI > AMI ~ NOR ~ PRT > DMI ~ DOX
(3) Uptake of ^{3}H-5HT into striatal slices[d]:
CIM > IMI ~ NOR ~ PRT ~ CPZ > DMI

B. *In vivo*

(1) Displacement of 5HT by 4-methyl-α-ethyl-m-tyramine[e]:
CPR ~ CIM > AMI > IMI ~ NOR > PRT ~ DMI
(2) Displacement of 5HT by p-chloromethamphetamine[f]:
CPR ~ CIM > IMI > DMI ~ MPD > PRT
(3) Depression of firing rate of midbrain raphe neurons[g]:
CIM > IMI ~ AMI > DMI ~ PRT

[a] Abbreviations: CIM, chlorimipramine; IMI, imipramine; AMI, amitriptyline; NOR, nortriptyline; PRT, protriptyline; DMI, desipramine; CPZ, chlorpromazine; DOX, doxepin; CPR, chlorpheniramine; MPD, meperidine.
[b] Kannengiesser et al. (69).
[c] B. K. Koe and R. F. Corkey, Jr., unpublished data (see Table VI).
[d] Shaskan and Snyder (125).
[e] Carlsson (17).
[f] Meek et al. (88).
[g] Sheard et al. (126).

tent than tertiary amines (R_3N) as inhibitors of NE uptake (Callingham, 14; Maxwell et al., 85; Bickel and Brodie, 7), while the latter compounds are stronger blockers of serotonin uptake than the former (Carlsson et al., 18), is widely held, the classic example being imipramine vs. DMI. Notable exceptions to this rule occur for tricyclic and nontricyclic uptake blockers: 1) amitriptyline (R_3N) is more potent than nortriptyline (R_2NH) in blocking ^{3}H-catecholamine uptake into rat hypothalamic synaptosomes (Horn et al., 60) (however, the reverse is true for mouse midbrain slices [Carnmalm et al., 24]); 2) N-methylation or N-demethylation of protriptyline (R_2NH) does not diminish the inhibitory activity towards ^{3}H-NE uptake in rat cortical slices (Salama et al., 110); 3) tofenacine (R_2NH) and its N-demethyl derivative (RNH_2) are better blockers of 5HT uptake than orphenadrine (R_3N) in rat cortical slices (Van der Zee and Hespe, 145); 4) in the spiro [dibenzocycloheptene-cyclohexen or cyclohexan]-4-amine series, tertiary amines are more potent inhibitors of ^{3}H-NE uptake than secondary amines in mouse midbrain slices (Carnmalm et al., 24); 5) as mentioned above Lilly 110140 (R_2NH) and methadone (R_3N) are both potent inhibitors of 5HT uptake; and 6) EXP-561, quipazine, and p-chloramphetamine, none containing N-methyl groups, are potent blockers of 5HT uptake in synaptosomal preparations of corpus striatum (Table VI). In view of this inconsistancy about the extent of substitution on the amino group, the search for novel uptake blockers and antidepressant drugs should include synthesis and study of the primary, secondary, and tertiary amines of a given compound.

C. Enhancing Monoaminergic Activity

According to the monoamine hypothesis of depression, compounds exert antidepressant activity because they are capable of enhancing central noradrenergic and/or serotoninergic function. In previous sections of this chapter one important method for achieving this goal has been discussed, i.e. blocking reuptake of the monoamine transmitter. Enhancing monoaminergic effects by blockade of uptake should induce a compensatory decrease in monoamine turnover in brain. This is observed in the 5HT system: 1) imipramine and amitriptyline, but not DMI or nortriptyline, decelerate the disappearance from mouse brain of ^{3}H-5HT formed from intravenously administered ^{3}H-tryptophan (Schubert et al., 123); 2) imipramine retards the disappearance of ^{3}H-5HT following intracisternal administration of the monoamine to rats (Schildkraut et al., 120); 3) chlorimipramine (Meek and Werdinius, 89) and Lilly 110140 (Perry and Fuller, 97) decrease the rate of probenecid-induced accumulation of 5-hydroxy-3-indoleacetic acid (5-HIAA) in rat brain; and 4) imipramine decreases the normal accumulation of 5-hydroxytryptophan (5HTP) in rat brain following the inhibition of 5HTP decarboxylase (Koe, 72). In contrast, tricyclic antidepressants do not alter the rate of disappearance of ^{14}C-NE formed from intravenously administered ^{14}C-tyrosine (Schubert et al., 123; Nybäck et al., 95), even though these agents, especially the secondary amines, block NE uptake. On the other hand, intracisternally administered ^{3}H-NE appears to disappear more slowly from brain in rats treated with imipramine (single dose) (Schildkraut et al., 121). Conclusions about the effects of drugs on neuronal function based on monoamine synthesis and turnover rates should be viewed with caution because of the possible overlap of several neurochemical or pharmacological events induced by the drug (Koe, 73).

Other methods to increase monoaminergic function at central synapses include: 1) blocking monoamine metabolism via monoamine oxidase (MAO) inhibitors, and 2) accelerating monoamine synthesis and turnover via (a) electroconvulsive shock; (b) chronic treatment with tricyclic antidepressants; (c) combination of the latter with thyroid hormone; and (d) administration of amino acid precursors (tryptophan). Several experimental treatments (rubidium and thyrotropin releasing hormone) also appear to involve enhancement of monoaminergic activity at central receptors.

1. *Monoamine Oxidase Inhibitors*

Inhibition of MAO, the enzyme catalyzing oxidative deamination of monoamines, elevates the concentration of the latter in brain. Leakage of excess monoamines into synapses could enhance monoaminergic activity at receptors. The early encouraging therapeutic effects of MAO inhibitors in depressed patients contributed to the formulation of the catecholamine hypothesis of affective disorders. Blockade of MAO, unfortunately, also enhances systemic levels of exogeneously-derived monoamines with potentially dangerous consequences (Blackwell, 8). Although MAO inhibitors are not considered to be very efficacious in treating endogenous depression, beneficial effects are obtained in "mixed anxiety-depression" types of syndromes (Tyrer, 142; Goodwin and Sack, 56; Pare, 96; Davis et al., 35; Raskin, 107). Tranylcypromine and phenelzine are MAO inhibitors currently approved by the FDA for antidepressant therapy (Morris and Beck, 93). The efficacy of MAO inhibitors as antidepressants appears to correlate better with inhibiting metaraminol uptake (chopped rat cerebral cortex) than inhibiting MAO (whole rat brain) (Hendley and Snyder, 58). These authors propose that the antidepressant action of clinically effective MAO inhibitors (tranylcypromine, phenelzine, and pargyline) may also involve blockade of NE reuptake. However, the absence of a tricyclic antidepressant standard in this study makes it difficult to assess the relevance of the data.

The occurrence of multiple forms of MAO with differential localization, substrate specificity, and sensitivity to inhibitors presents the theoretical possiblity of synthesizing selective inhibitors to preferentially affect a given monoamine or a given location of the monoamine (Youdim, 153; Fuller, 46). This possibility may rekindle interest in searching for new selective MAO inhibitors as psychotherapeutic agents. In current drug discovery programs, blockade of MAO is generally not considered to be a useful attribute in a potential therapeutic drug. Inhibition of MAO might be responsible in part for the antidepressant activity reported for dexamisole (Bobon et al., 9).

2. Electroconvulsive Shock

Electroconvulsive shock (ECS) therapy is generally considered to be the most effective treatment of depression (Kety et al., 71; Davis et al., 35; Davis, 34). An increase in the turnover rate of brain NE in rats receiving chronic ECS treatment (inferred from the accelerated disappearance of intracisternally administered ^{3}H-NE) seemingly is in accord with expectations of the catecholamine hypothesis of depression (Kety et al., 71; Schildkraut et al., 119). Tyrosine hydroxylase activity of brain is also enhanced in rats receiving multiple ECS treatments (Musacchio et al., 94). However, Laudisch and co-workers (77) have questioned whether the increased synthesis and utilization of NE suggested by these studies necessarily imply that the NE reaches receptor sites. Some experiments in rats suggest that ECS may share some similarities with lithium treatment (Matussek and Laudisch, 84). Although lithium is a psychotherapeutic agent for mania, it is also effective in certain depressions (Goodwin and Sack, 56). These laboratory and clinical findings, though consistent with each other, are somewhat paradoxical, since lithium is considered to reduce central noradrenergic function. It is of interest that chronic ECS treatment antagonizes mouse-killing (muricide) in mouse-killing rats (Vogel and Haubrich, 148). Clinical antidepressants also inhibit rat muricidal behavior; moreover, this behavioral antagonism has been proposed as a method for predicting antidepressant activity in new compounds (Horowitz et al., 61). It is difficult to relate these effects on muricide to NE turnover, since acute administration of tricyclics, in contrast to the ECS treatment, retards NE turnover.

3. Chronic Imipramine and Protriptyline

Schildkraut and co-workers have attempted to relate the delayed onset of action of tricyclic antidepressants to the apparent acceleration of NE turnover in brain induced by chronic administration of the drugs (Schildkraut et al., 121, 122). Since blockade of NE uptake and elevation of normetanephrine levels in brain, two characteristic effects of acute imipramine or protriptyline treatment, persist after chronic administration of drug, the increase in NE turnover rate presumably contributes to therapeutic efficacy by magnifying noradrenergic activity at central receptors. The complications of overlapping neurochemical events and their priorities make the interpretation of these experiments difficult (Koe, 73). The deceleration of NE turnover after acute treatment may be the consequence of negative feedback compensation for the enhanced noradrenergic function caused by the blockade of NE reuptake. Since the latter process is not diminished on chronic administration of drug, some loss of endogenous stores of NE is not unexpected and is observed (Schildkraut et al., 121). This reduction of endogenous NE then leads to disinhibition of tyrosine hydroxylase and, as a result, normal or accelerated turnover rate of the monoamine. Thus, the effects of tricyclics on NE metabolism after either acute or chronic treatment appear to be initiated by the primary drug action of inhibiting NE reuptake. The reason for the delayed onset of therapeutic effects of tricyclics remains unknown. Faster-acting agents continue to be the goal of antidepressant drug discovery research.

4. Thyroid Hormone

Administration of L-triiodothyronine or thyroid stimulating hormone with imipramine accelerates the recovery process in depression (Prange et al., 102; Coppen et al., 29). Similar effects of thyroid hormone have been reported with amitriptyline therapy (Wheatley, 150) and other tricyclics (Earle, 37). Two explanations have been advanced for this acceleration of the therapeutic effects of tricyclic antidepressants: 1) thyroxine shortens the time required to attain the equivalent effects of chronic imipramine treatment (from 3 weeks to 10 days in rats); i.e. thyroxine apparently reverses the retardation of NE turnover characteristic of shorter term imipramine treatment (see previous section) (Schildkraut et al., 122); or 2) thyroid hormone treatment enhances catecholaminergic receptor sensitivity in brain, thereby enhancing the effect of imipramine in depressed patients (who may be viewed as having a deficit in receptor sensitivity) (Prange et al., 101; Breese et al., 12). These two viewpoints are not easily reconciled. The former rationale seems to be somewhat circuitous; the effects of imipramine on the disappearance rate of ^{3}H-NE from brain may be merely secondary ones (see previous section). The second explanation is based on the following: a) the synthesis rate of labeled DA and NE from ^{14}C-tyrosine in brain is decreased by thyroxine treatment; increased receptor activity is inferred from negative feedback consideration (Prange et al., 98); b) combined thyroxime + imipramine treatment gives maximal response in the dopa + pargyline behavioral response test (Everett, 39) at doses at which either drug alone exhibits only minimal effects (Breese et al., 13). It is of interest that lithium appears to lower thyroid function in man and rats via diminished release of thyroid hormone (Sedvall et al., 124). The therapeutic effects of lithium in mania is attributed to the diminished catecholaminergic activity induced by the ion. Since hypothyroid rats are considered to be deficient in monoaminergic receptor activity, in view of the increased catecholamine synthesis and turnover observed in such rats (Lipton et al., 82), one may speculate that the effects of lithium on mania (beneficial) and the thyroid (decreased function) might be related.

5. *Hypothalamic Regulatory Hormones (Schally et al., 113)*

a. *Melanocyte stimulating hormone release inhibiting factor (MIF).*

This tripeptide (L-prolyl-L-leucylglycine amide) elicits marked potentiation of dopa in the dopa + pargyline response test (Plotnikoff et al., 103) and antagonizes the central and peripheral effects of oxotremorine (Plotnikoff et al., 104). Both effects occur in normal and hypophysectomized mice, suggesting that these CNS actions are extrapituitary. Moreover, MIF exerts only weak potentiation of 5HTP-induced temors, indicating that its effects are mainly catecholaminergic (Huidobro-Toro et al., 62). The central effects might be mainly dopaminergic, since DA synthesis in striatal slices from MIF-treated rats is enhanced, whereas NE synthesis in hypothalamic slices is unaffected (Friedman et al., 45). However, these biochemical findings may be dissociated from behavioral effects, since hypophysectomized rats fail to show enhanced DA synthesis. Antiparkinsonian activity has been observed for MIF (Kastin and Barbeau, 70).

b. Thyrotropin releasing hormone (TRH)

This tripeptide (L-glutamyl-L-histidyl-L-proline amide) also potentiates behavioral effects of dopa in the dopa + pargyline response test in normal and hypophysectomized mice (Plotnikoff et al., 105) and in thyroidectomized rats (Plotnikoff et al., 106). Although TRH appears to enhance central catecholaminergic activity, dose-response comparisons on mouse behavior show the following potency ranking: for dopa potentiation, MIF > TRH; for 5HTP potentiation, TRH >> MIF (Huidobro-Toro et al., 62). Thus, TRH effects may be mostly serotoninergic. An interesting spectrum of clinical activity is emerging for TRH ("the effects of a single injection are rapid, occurring within a few hours, and lasting no more than a few days" [Prange et al., 100]). In normal women THR elicits relaxant and euphoric effects; in female patients, TRH exerts therapeutic effects in depression and schizophrenia (see Plotnikoff et al., 106 and Prange et al., 100 for references to clinical studies). The biochemical mechanisms underlying these CNS activities of TRH are unknown. Definitive effects of TRH on brain DA, NE, and 5HT metabolism have not been observed, except for the brain dopa or DA sparing effect of TRH (and triiodothyronine): either substance will enhance the increase in DA concentration elicited by pargyline + dopa in mice (Breese et al., 11, 12). Neither TRH nor MIF alters the metabolism of endogenous or exogenously administered dopa in rats as determined by analyses of 24 hour urinary metabolites (Sandler et al., 111).

6. Tryptophan

Treating depressed patients by loading with precursor amino acids has been characterized by contention and controversy over the real efficacy of this relatively direct method for enhancing central monoaminergic function by increasing supplies of neurotransmitters (various authors, 147). Three precursors have been studied extensively: dopa, 5HTP, and tryptophan; the findings with the first two precursors have been termed "disappointing" and "inconclusive", respectively, whereas the status of tryptophan appears to be slightly better (Prange et al., 99). One study indicates that tryptophan is as effective as imipramine in improving moderately severe depression; unlike the latter the efficacy of tryptophan is not potentiated by thyroid hormone (Coppen et al., 29). The therapeutic effect of the MAO inhibitor, tranylcypromine, is potentiated by including tryptophan in the treatment (Coppen et al., 28). It has been suggested that the antidepressant effects of tryptophan may be diminished by its diversion from the production of 5HT to formation of other metabolites by the pathway catalyzed by tryptophan pyrrolase. This enzyme is inducible by administration of the amino acid or by high pituitary-adrenal activity, a condition which might be associated with some depressions. A corollary of this hypothesis is that pyrrolase inhibitors might exert a direct antidepressant effect or potentiate that of tryptophan (Curzon, 32).

7. Rubidium

Rubidium accelerates brain NE synthesis and turnover and facilitates the formation of normetanephrine formed from this monoamine (Stolk et al., 135; Eichelman, 38). These data suggest that the cation might enhance noradrenergic activity or accelerate physiological release of NE at synapses (alerting or arousing EEG effects). In rats rubidium facilitates shock-induced aggression (Stolk et al., 134). In man rubidium exhibits a long half-life (50-60 days); some indication of antidepressant activity has been observed after chronic administration of rubidium (Fieve et al., 43). It is notable that rubidium and lithium ions apparently exert opposite neurochemical and behavioral effects (Stolk et al., 135; Fieve et al., 43).

D. Blocking Amphetamine Metabolism

Interaction of tricyclic antidepressants with amphetamine in rats results in pronounced potentiation and prolongation of amphetamine stimulation. This has been attributed originally to the phenomenon of uptake blockade, whereby inactivation of the catecholamines released by amphetamines is prevented. Consolo and coworkers (26) and Lewander (81) have shown that DMI and related tricyclics inhibit the metabolism of amphetamine in the rat, probably by blocking para hydroxylation, thereby eliciting increased accumulation of amphetamine in brain. Consequently, the behavioral potentiation of amphetamine by tricyclics is probably caused by a metabolic rather than neurochemical interaction (Dolfini et al., 36; Lew et al., 80). This conclusion is supported by the antidepressant iprindole which does not inhibit uptake of catecholamines or serotonin (Ross et al., 109) but strongly potentiates amphetamine. This behavioral potentiation is correlated with the high amphetamine levels in brain elicited by iprindole (Lemberger et al., 78; Miller et al., 90; Freeman and Sulser, 44). Enhanced accumulation of amphetamine in brain and increased urinary excretion of unchanged amphetamine in rats occur after administration of tricyclic neuroleptics (chlorpromazine, chlorprothixene, prochlorperazine, and propericiazine) and tricyclic antidepressants (DMI, imipramine, amitriptyline, nortriptyline, protriptyline, Lu 3-010, and dibenzepine) (Lewander, 81; Valzelli et al., 144). The behavioral and pharmacological effects of the enhanced brain accumulation of amphetamine after chlorpromazine are masked (except for low doses of chlorpromazine) by the adrenergic blocking action of the neuroleptic (Sulser and Dingell, 140; Borella et al., 10; Lemberger et al., 79). Thioridazine and promethazine also elevate amphetamine accumulation in rat brain (Table V). Thioridazine, like chlorpromazine, antagonizes amphetamine stimulation, whereas promethazine, a non-neuroleptic, potentiates amphetamine. Nontricyclic drugs such as diazepam, nialamide, and cocaine also inhibit amphetamine metabolism (Lewander, 81). It is noteworthy that potent NE uptake blockers like EXP-561, fenazoxine, and CP-24,441 do not enhance accumulation of amphetamine in brain (Table V). The findings of the various studies discussed here lead to the conclusion that potentiation of amphetamine, via blockade of its metabolism, is dissociated from 1) inhibition of monoamine reuptake, and 2) antidepressant activity.

The structural requirements for inhibiting amphetamine metabolism are obscure. A survey of representative tricyclic and bicyclic CNS drugs for this activity using standard experimental conditions (Table V) offers the following pertinent observations: 1) the proposed conformation of DMI and tricyclics necessary for uptake blocking activity, as exemplified by that of CP-24,441, is not the one for inhibiting the metabolism of amphetamine, because CP-24,441 is noticeably devoid of effect on brain amphetamine levels; 2) cyproheptadine, a very poor uptake blocker which cannot assume the CP-24,441 conformation, however, does enhance amphetamine accumulation in brain. These findings suggest that the aminoalkyl group attached to the diphenylmethyl or diphenylamino moiety must be more or less perpendicular to the common edge (convex side) of the dihedral angle formed by the two benzene rings.

E. Discovering New Antidepressant Drugs

The question which comes to mind after analysis of the biochemical features of antidepressant drugs is whether new antidepressants discovered on the basis of these biochemical indices of activity will offer any major advantages over those presently in clinical use? Blockade of monoamine reuptake is probably the most important test for confirming the "antidepressant activity" suggested in

TABLE V
Amphetamine accumulation in rat brain [a]

Tricyclics				Nontricyclics	
Antidepressants		Neuroleptics and Others			
	% control		% control		% control
Imipramine	1425 ± 139	Chlorpromazine	666 ± 54	EXP-561	118 ± 24
Desipramine	944 ± 55	Thioridazine	773 ± 83	CP-24,441	96 ± 10
Chlorimipramine	191 ± 19	Promethazine	610 ± 43	Lu 3-010	1426 ± 120
Amitriptyline	273 ± 22	Clozapine	155 ± 18	Fenazoxine	202 ± 46
Nortriptyline	749 ± 49	Cyproheptadine	480 ± 20	Gamfexine	176 ± 41
Doxepin	204 ± 18	Mianserin	73 ± 19	Quipazine	115 ± 23
Iprindole	1247 ± 140			Trazodone	88 ± 11

[a] Rats received test drug (32 μmole/kg i.p.) or water (control) 1 hr before labeled amphetamine sulfate (15 μmole/kg; 25 μCi/kg i.p.) and 5 hr before sacrifice. Whole brain was assayed for amphetamine content by the method of Glowinski et al. (53). Contemporary controls were always run. Entries are mean relative concentrations ± S.E. for groups of 5 to 10 rats. Amphetamine concentration in brain of control rats: 1.64 ± 0.12 nmole/g (N = 55). B. K. Koe, unpublished data.

new compounds by behavioral or pharmacological studies. In addition, it may be used for primary biochemical screening of novel structures for potential antidepressant activity. By employing synaptosomal preparations for assessing uptake of monoamines, the inhibitory activity of large numbers of compounds can be readily determined. Since blocking 5HT reuptake in brain may be important for the therapeutic effects of tricyclic drugs in depression, inhibition of synaptosomal uptake of this indolealkylamine has been proposed as a criterion of antidepressant activity (Kannengiesser et al., 69). Tricyclic antidepressants exhibit IC_{50} values for blocking synaptosomal uptake of 5HT in the range of 0.09 to 4 μM (Table VI). The IC_{50} values for a group of nontricyclic compounds reported to have some antidepressant activity, however modest, fall into this range (Table VI). Perhaps an answer to the question posed above will be forthcoming when the antidepressant properties of the nontricyclic agents in Table VI and other specific 5HT uptake blockers like methadone (Ciafolo, 25) and Lilly 110140 (Wong et al., 151) have been adequately evaluated. It has been recognized that the relationship of blockade of neuronal reuptake to antidepressant activity is not a straightforward one: cocaine, a strong inhibitor of uptake (Table VI), is a "poor antidepressant" (Goodwin and Sack, 56), whereas iprindole, an effective antidepressant, is a poor inhibitor of uptake (Table VI) (Ross et al., 109; Fann et al., 40).

A modified amine hypothesis states that 1) "the activities of amine-mediated synapses in brain are modified in affective illness either as a result of altered input into the neuronal systems [low output depression] or as a result of altered sensitivity of the postsynaptic receptors [low sensitivity depression]"; 2) "functional recovery of these systems in depression will follow either a rise in receptor sensitivity or a rise in transmitter output or both"; and 3) "we must reexamine our therapies to consider effects on postsynaptic as well as presynatic events" (Ashcroft et al., 1). Design of drugs to enhance postsynaptic receptor sensitivity, if practical, offers an alternative approach to novel antidepressants. Almost all of the drug discovery research to date have focused on actual or presumed presynaptic events. Postsynaptic changes might be involved in the facilitation of imipramine's antidepressant effects by thyroid hormone. Prange and co-workers (101) attribute this potentiation to enhancement of receptor sensitivity induced by thyroid hormone. Perhaps the psychotherapeutic activity of the hypothalamic regulatory hormones is also derived from similar mechanisms.

An important property of the tricyclic antidepressant drugs not discussed in this chapter is their central anticholinergic effects.

TABLE VI
Inhibition of serotonin uptake into synaptosomes of rat corpus striatum [a]

Clinically Active Antidepressants		Potential Antidepressants	
	$IC_{50} \times 10^6 M$ [b]		
Imipramine	0.8	EXP-561 [c]	0.035
Desipramine	4.0	Fenazoxine [d]	0.37
Chlorimipramine	0.09	Tofenacine [e]	1.5
Amitriptyline	1.8	Gamfexine [c]	1.1
Nortriptyline	1.6	Chlorpheniramine [f]	0.45
Protriptyline	2.1	Cocaine [g]	0.8
Doxepin	3.1	Quipazine [h]	0.58
		Trazodone [i]	1.3
Iprindole	25	p-Chloramphetamine [j]	0.6
		Lu 3-010 [k]	7
		Mianserin [l]	17

[a] B. K. Koe and R. F. Corkey, Jr., unpublished data.
[b] Concentrations of drug required to inhibit uptake of ^{14}C-5HT by 50% (IC_{50}) were estimated on log probit paper (Horn et al., 60). Crude synaptosomes, prepared by homogenizing rat corpus striatum in 0.32M sucrose followed by differential centrifugation, were incubated with ^{14}C-5HT (0.1 μM) at 30° for 10 min (see Wong et al., 152). The pellet of an aliquot of the incubation mixture collected on a Millipore filter was dried and counted in scintillation fluid.
[c] Davis (34).
[d] Bassett et al. (5).
[e] Van der Zee and Hespe (145).
[f] Carlsson and Lindqvist (22); Carlsson (17).
[g] Goodwin and Sack (56).
[h] Medon et al. (87); Rodriguez and Pardo (108).
[i] Silvestrini et al. (131); Udabe (143).
[j] Van Praag and Korf (146).
[k] Carlsson et al. (21).
[l] Fell et al. (42).

According to the cholinergic-adrenergic hypothesis of mania and depression: 1) "a given affective state may represent a balance between central cholinergic and adrenergic neurotransmitter activity in those areas of the brain which regulate affect, with depression being a disease of cholinergic dominance and mania being the converse"; and 2) "tricyclic antidepressants block central cholinergic activity, as well as increasing functionally available adrenergic neurotransmitters . . this would shift the . . . balance towards adrenergic predominance" (Janowsky et al., 66). Theoretically, one might be able to adjust the relative degree of anticholinergic vs. adrenergic activities in a given compound by suitable manipulations in chemical structure and thereby synthesize the optimal molecules for treating various depressions. Reducing this approach to practice may be a difficult task.

Iprindole stands out as an anomaly in the biochemical pharmacology of antidepressants. As stated previously, this compound inhibits the uptake of NE and 5HT very weakly *in vitro* or *in vivo*. Moreover, it is not as active as the tricyclic drugs in most pharmacological tests of antidepressant activity (Gluckman and Baum, 54). On the other hand, iprindole is regarded as being comparable to imipramine clinically, including a similar time of onset of therapeutic effects (Ayd, 4; Fann et al., 40). Ascertaining the mechanism of action of iprindole should provide new insights into the parameters of antidepressant activity. On the basis of current knowledge about the biochemical pharmacology of antidepressant drugs, one might speculate whether iprindole, an agent whose main characteristic in the laboratory is potentiating amphetamine-induced stimulation in rats—apparently by inhibiting the metabolism of amphetamine, would be advanced to clinical trial for depressed patients today?

III. SUMMARY

The most prominent biochemical property of tricyclic antidepressants is their potent blockade of the neuronal reuptake of monoamines. Antidepressant activity is assumed to result from the enhancement of central monoaminergic function, regarded to be deficient in depressed patients, by the excess monoamines now available at receptors. The important monoamines in depression are norepinephrine and serotonin. The increase in drive and the brightening of mood elicited in depressed patients by the tricyclic drugs are postulated to be associated with antagonism of the membrane concentrating mechanisms for norepinephrine and serotonin, respectively (Carlsson et al., 18). However, blockade of monoamine uptake may be only one facet of the complex biochemical requirements for antidepressant activity. Iprindole, a poor inhibitor of uptake, is effective in treating depression by an as yet unknown mechanism. At the same time, clinical efficacy has not been definitely established for potent uptake blockers like EXP-561 and gamfexine (Davis, 34). Other established therapies (electroconvulsive shock, monoamine oxidase inhibitors) and the newer experimental treatments of depression (tryptophan, rubidium, thyroid homone + tricylics, thyrotropin releasing hormone) also appear to be based on the enhancement of central monoaminergic function, although different mechanisms are expected to be involved.

REFERENCES

1. Ashcroft, G. W., Eccleston, D., Murray, L. G., Glen, A. I. M., Crawford, T. B. B., Pullar, I. A., Shields, P. J., Walter, D. S., Blackburn, I. M., Connechan, J., and Lonergan, M.: Modified amine hypothesis for the aetiology of affective illness, *Lancet,* **II**:573-577, 1972.
2. Axelrod, J., Hertting, G., and Potter, L.: Effect of drugs on the uptake and release of ^{3}H-norepinephrine in the rat heart, *Nature,* **194**:297, 1962.
3. Axelrod, J., Whiteby, L. G., and Hertting, G.: Effect of psychotropic drugs on the uptake of ^{3}H-norepinephrine by tissues, *Science,* **133**:383-384, 1961.
4. Ayd, F. J. Jr.: Clincal evaluation of a new tricyclic antidepressant iprindole, *Dis. Nerv. Syst.,* **30**:818-823, 1969.
5. Bassett, J. R., Cairncross, K. D., Hacket, N. B., and Story, M.: Studies on the peripheral pharmacology of fenazoxine, a potential antidepressant drug, *Br. J. Pharmacol.,* **37**:69-78, 1969.
6. Berti, F. and Shore, P. A.: A kinetic analysis of drugs that inhibit the adrenergic neuronal membrane amine pump, *Biochem. Pharmacol.,* **16**:2091-2094, 1967.
7. Bickel, M. H. and Brodie, B. B.: Structure and antidepressant activity of imipramine analogues, *Int. J. Neurophamacol.,* **3**:611-621, 1964.
8. Blackwell, B.: Hypertensive crisis due to monoamine-oxidase inhibitors, *Lancet,* **II**:849-851, 1963.
9. Bobon, J., Bobon, D. P., Bourdouxhe, S., and Pinchard, A.: A pilot open trial of dexamisole (R 12.563) in retarded depression: preliminary results, *J. Int. Med. Res.,* **2**:171-174, 1974.
10. Borella, L., Herr, F., and Wojdan, A.: Prolongation of certain effects of amphetamine by chlorpromazine, *Can. J. Physiol. Pharmacol.,* **47**:7-13, 1969.
11. Breese, G. R., Cooper, B. R., Prange, A. J. Jr., Cott, J. M., and Lipton, M. A.: Interactions of thyrotropin-releasing hormone with centrally acting drugs, *in* Prange, A. J. Jr., editor: *The thyroid axis, drugs and behavior,* Raven Press, New York, 1974, pp. 115-127.
12. Breese, G. R., Prange, A. J. Jr., and Lipton, M. A.: Pharmacological studies of thyroid-imipramine interactions in animals, *in* Prange, A. J. Jr., editor: *The thyroid axis, drugs and behavior,* Raven Press, New York, 1974, pp. 29-48.
13. Breese, G. R., Traylor, T. D., and Prange, A. J. Jr.: The effect of triiodothyronine on the disposition and actions of imipramine, *Psychopharmacologia,* **25**:101-111, 1972.
14. Callingham, B. A.: The effects of imipramine and related compounds on the uptake of noreadrenaline into sympathetic nerve endings, *in* Garattini, S. and Dukes, M. N. G., editors: *Antidepressant drugs,* Excerpta Medica Foundation, New York, 1967, pp. 35-43.
15. Cañas-Rodriguez, A. and Leeming, P. R.: N-Phenyl-2-indolinones

and N-phenylindolines. A new class of antidepressant agents, *J. Med. Chem.*, **15**:762-770, 1972.

16. Carlsson, A.: Structural specificity for inhibition of [^{14}C]-5-hydroxytryptamine uptake by cerebral slices, *J. Pharm. Pharmacol.*, **22**:729-732, 1970.
17. Carlsson, A.: Effect of drugs on amine uptake mechanisms in the brain, *in* Schümann, H. J. and Kroneberg, G., editors: *New aspects of storage and release mechanisms of catecholamines*, Springer-Verlag, Berlin, 1970, pp. 223-233.
18. Carlsson, A., Corrodi, H., Fuxe, K., and Hökfelt, T.: Effect of antidepressant drugs on the depletion of intraneuronal brain 5-hydroxytryptamine stores caused by 4-methyl-α-ethyl-meta-tyramine, *Eur. J. Pharmacol.*, **5**:357-366, 1969.
19. Carlsson, A., Corrodi, H., Fuxe, K., and Hökfelt, T.: Effects of some antidepressant drugs on the depletion of intraneuronal brain catecholamine stores caused by 4, α-dimethyl-meta-tyramine, *Eur. J. Pharmacol.*, **5**:367-373, 1969.
20. Carlsson, A., Fuxe, K., Hamberger, B., and Lindqvist, M.: Biochemical and histochemical studies on the effects of imipramine-like drugs and (+)-amphetamine on central and peripheral catecholamine neurons, *Acta Physiol. Scand.*, **67**:481-497, 1966.
21. Carlsson, A., Fuxe, K., Hamberger, B., and Malmfors, T.: Effect of a new series of bicyclic compounds with potential thymoleptic properties on the reserpine-resistant uptake mechanism of central and peripheral monoamine neurones *in vivo* and *in vitro*, *Br. J. Pharmacol.*, **36**:18-28, 1969.
22. Carlsson, A. and Lindqvist, M.: Central and peripheral monoaminergic membrane-pump blockade by some addictive analgesics and antihistamines, *J. Pharm. Pharmacol.*, **21**:460-464, 1969.
23. Carlsson, A. and Waldeck, B.: Inhibition of ^{3}H-metaraminol uptake by antidepressive and related agents, *J. Pharm. Pharmacol.*, **17**:243-244, 1965.
24. Carnmalm, B., Jacupovic, E., Johansson, L., DePaulis, T., Rämsby, S., Stjernström, N. E., Renyi, A. L., Ross, S. B., and Ögren, S. O.: Antidepressant agents. 1. Chemistry and pharmacology of amino-substituted spiro [5H-dibenzo[a, d]cycloheptene-5,1′-cycloalkanes], *J. Med. Chem.*, **17**:65-72, 1974.
25. Ciofalo, F. R.: Methadone inhibition of ^{3}H-5-hydroxytryptamine uptake by synaptosomes, *J. Pharmacol. Exp. Ther.*, **189**:83-89, 1974.
26. Consolo, S., Dolfini, E., Garattini, S., and Valzelli, L.: Desipramine and amphetamine metabolism, *J. Pharm. Pharmacol.*, **19**:253-256, 1967.
27. Coppen, A.: The biochemistry of affective disorders, *Br. J. Psychiatry,* 113:1237-1264, 1967.
28. Coppen, A., Shaw, D. M., and Farrell, M. B.: Potentiation of the antidepressive effect of a monoamine-oxidase inhibitor by tryptophan, *Lancet,* **I**:79-81, 1963.
29. Coppen, A., Whybrow, P. C., Noguera, R., Maggs, R., and Prange, A. J. Jr.: The comparative antidepressant value of 1-tryptophan and imipramine with an without attempted potentiation by liothyronine, *Arch. Gen. Psychiatry.*, **26**:234-241, 1972.
30. Coyle, J. T. and Snyder, S. H.: Antiparkinsonian drugs: inhibition of

dopamine uptake in the corpus striatum as a possible mechanism of action, *Science,* **166**:899-901, 1969.
31. Coyle, J. T. and Snyder, S. H.: Catecholamine uptake by synaptosomes in homogenates of rat brain: stereospecificity in different areas, *J. Pharmacol. Exp. Therm.,* **170**:221-231, 1969.
32. Curzon, G.: Tryptophan pyrrolase—a biochemical factor in depressive illness? *Brit. J. Psychiatry,* **115**:1367-1374, 1969.
33. Daly, J. W., Creveling, C. R., and Witkop, B.: The chemorelease of norepinephrine in mouse hearts. Structure-activity relationships. II. Drugs affecting the sympathetic and central nervous systems, *J. Med. Chem.,* **9**:280-284, 1966.
34. Davis, J. M.: Theories of biological etiology of affective disorders, *Int. Rev. Neurobiol.,* **12**:145-175, 1970.
35. Davis, J. M., Klerman, G. L., and Schildkraut, J. J.: Drugs used in the treatment of depression, *in* Efron, D. H., editor: *Psychopharmacology. A review of progress 1957-1967,* U.S. Government Printing Office, Washington, D. C., 1968, pp. 719-747.
36. Dolfini, E., Tansella, M., Valzelli, L., and Garattini, S.: Further studies on the interaction between desipramine and amphetamine, *Eur. J. Pharmacol.,* **5**:185-190, 1969.
37. Earle, B. V.: Thyroid hormone and tricyclic antidepressants in resistant depressions, *Am. J. Psychiatry,* **126**:1667-1669, 1970.
38. Eichelman, B., Thoa, N. B., and Perez-Cruet, J.: Rubidium and cesium: effects on aggression, adrenal enzymes and amine turnover, *Fed. Proc.,* **31**:289, 1972.
39. Everett, G. M.: The dopa response potentiation test and its use in screening for antidepressant drugs, *in* Garattini, S. and Dukes, M. N. G., editors: *Antidepressant drugs,* Excerpta Medica Foundation, Amsterdam, 1967, pp. 164-167.
40. Fann, W. E., Davis, J. M., Janowsky, D. S., Kaufmann, J. S., Griffith, J. D., and Oates, J. A.: Effect of iprindole on amine uptake in man, *Arch. Gen. Psychiatry,* **26**:158-162, 1972.
41. Farnebo, L.-O., Fuxe, K., Hamberger, B., and Ljungdahl, H.: Effect of some antiparkinsonian drugs on catecholamine neurons, *J. Pharm. Pharmacol.,* **22**:733-737, 1970.
42. Fell, P. J., Quantock, D. C., and Van der Burg, W. J.: The human pharmacology of GB 94—a new psychotropic agent, *Eur. J. Clin. Pharmacol.,* **5**:166-173, 1973.
43. Fieve, R. R., Meltzer H., Dunner, D. L., Levitt, M., Mendlewicz, J., and Thomas, A.: Rubidium: biochemical, behavioral and metabolic studies in humans, *Am. J. Psychiatry,* **130**:1, 1973.
44. Freeman, J. J. and Sulser, F.: Iprindole-amphetamine interactions in the rat: the role of aromatic hydroxylation of amphetamine in its mode of action, *J. Pharmacol. Exp. Ther.,* **183**:307-315, 1972.
45. Friedman, E., Friedman, J., and Gershon, S.: Dopamine synthesis: stimulation by a hypothalamic factor, *Science,* **182**:831-832, 1973.
46. Fuller, R. W.: Selective inhibition of monoamine oxidase, *Adv. Biochem. Psychopharmacol.,* **5**:339-354, 1972.
47. Fuller, R. W. and Perry, K. W.: Blockade of 4-chloroamphetamine-induced depletion of brain serotonin by 3-(p-trifluoromethylphenoxy)-N-methyl-3-phenylpropylamine hy-

drochloride (Lilly 110140), a specific inhibitor of uptake by serotonin neurons, *Fed. Proc.*, **33**:255, 1974.
48. Fuxe, K., Goldstein, M., and Ljungdahl, A.: Antiparkinsonian drugs and central dopamine neurons, *Life Sci.*, **9**:811-824, 1970.
49. Fuxe, K. and Ungerstedt, U.: Histochemical studies on the effect of (+)-amphetamine, drugs of the imipramine group and tryptamine on central catecholamine and 5-hydroxytryptamine neurons after intraventricular injection of catecholamines and 5-hydroxytryptamine, *Eur. J. Pharmacol.*, **4**:135-144, 1968.
50. Garattini, S. and Dukes, M. N. G. (editors): *Antidepressant drugs,* Excerpta Medica Foundation, Amsterdam, 1967.
51. Gershon, S., Hekimian, L. J., and Floyd, A.: Non-correlation of preclinical-clinical evaluation of a proposed antidepressant, 4-phenyl-bicyclo-(2,2,2)-octan-1-amine hydrochloride monohydrate. Exp. 561, *Arzneimittel-Forschung,* **18**:243-245, 1968.
52. Glowinski, J. and Axelrod, J.: Inhibition of uptake of tritiated-noradrenaline in the intact rat brain by imipramine and structurally related compounds, *Nature,* **204**:1318-1319, 1964.
53. Glowinski, J., Axelrod, J., and Iversen, L. L.: Regional studies of catecholamines in the rat brain. IV. Effects of drugs on the disposition and metabolism of H^3-norepinephrine and H^3-dopamine, *J. Pharmacol. Exp. Ther.*, **153**:30-41, 1966.
54. Gluckman, M. I. and Baum, T.: The pharmacology of iprindole, a new antidepressant, *Psychopharmacologia,* **15**:169-185, 1969.
55. Gogerty, J. H., Houlihan, W., Galen, M., Eden, P., and Penberthy, C.: Neuropharmacological studies on a imidazo-isoindole derivative, 42-548, *Fed. Proc.*, **27**:501, 1968.
56. Goodwin, F. K. and Sack, R. L.: Affective disorders: the catecholamine hypothesis revisited, *in* Usdin, E. and Snyder, S. H., editors: *Frontiers in catecholamine research,* Pergamon Press, Inc., New York, 1973, pp. 1157-1164.
57. Hamberger, B.: Reserpine-resistant uptake of catecholamines in isolated tissues of the rat, *Act Physiol. Scand.*, (Suppl.) **295**:1-56, 1967.
58. Hendley, E. D. and Snyder, S. H.: Relationship between the action of monoamine oxidase inhibitors on the noradrenaline uptake system and their antidepressant efficacy, *Nature,* **220**:1330-1331, 1968.
59. Hertting, G., Axelrod, J., and Whitby, L. G.: Effect of drugs on the uptake and metabolism of H^3-norepinephrine, *J. Pharmacol. Exp. Ther.*, **134**:146-152, 1961.
60. Horn, A. S., Coyle, J. T., and Snyder, S. H.: Catecholamine uptake by synaptosomes from rat brain, *Mol. Pharmacol.*, **7**:66-80, 1971.
61. Horovitz, Z. P., Piala, J. J., High, J. P., Burke, J. C., and Leaf, R. C.: Effects of drugs on the mouse-killing (muricide) test and its relationship to amygdaloid function, *Int. J. Neuropharmacol.*, **5**:405-411, 1966.
62. Huidobro-Toro, J. P., Scotti DeCarolis, A., and Longo, V. G.: Action of two hypothalamic factors (TRH, MIF) and of angiotensin II on the behavioral effect of L-dopa and 5-hydroxytryptophan in mice, *Pharmacol. Biochem. Behav.*, **2**:105-109, 1974.
63. Isaac, L. and Goth, A.: The mechanism of the potentiation of norepinephrine by antihistaminics, *J. Pharmacol. Exp. Ther.*, **156**:463-468, 1967.

64. Iversen, L. L.: *The uptake and storage of noradrenaline in sympathetic nerves,* Cambridge University Press, London, 1967.
65. Iversen, L. L.: The uptake of biogenic amines, *in* Biel, J. H. and Abood, L. G., editors: *Biogenic amines and physiological membranes,* Marcel Dekker, Inc., New York, 1971, pp. 259-327.
66. Janowsky, D. S., El-Yousef, M. K., Davis, J. M., and Sekerke, H. G.: A cholinergic-adrenergic hypothesis of mania and depression, *Lancet,* **II**:632-635, 1972.
67. Kaiser, C. and Zircle, C. L.: Antidepressives and stimulants, *in* Heinzelman, R. H., editor: *Annual reports in medicinal chemistry,* Vo. 7, Academic Press, New York, 1972. pp. 18-30.
68. Kaiser, C. and Zircle, C. L.: Antidpressive drugs and stimulants, *in* Heinzelman, R. H., editor: *Annual reports in medicinal chemistry,* Vol. 8, Academic Press, New York, 1973, pp. 11-19.
69. Kannengiesser, M. H., Hunt, P., and Raynaud, J.-P.: An *in vitro* model for the study of psychotropic drugs and as a criterion of antidepressant activity, *Biochem. Pharmacol.,* **22**:73-84, 1973.
70. Kastin, A. J. and Barbeau, A.: Preliminary clinical studies with L-prolyl-L-leucyl-glycine amide in Parkinson's disease, *Can. Med. Assoc. J.,* **107**:1079-1081, 1972.
71. Kety, S. S., Javoy, F., Thierry, A.-M., Julou, L., and Glowinski, J.: A sustained effect of electroconvulsive shock on the turnover of norepinephrine in the central nervous system of the rat, *Proc. Natl. Acad. Sci. USA.,* **58**:1249-1254, 1967.
72. Koe, B. K.: Dopa and 5-hydroxytryptophan (5HTP) accumulation in rat brain: a facile assessment of the effects of CNS drugs on dopamine (DA) and serotonin (5HT) synthesis, *Fed. Proc.,* **33**:467, 1974.
73. Koe, B. K.: Biochemical effects of neuroleptic drugs on brain catecholamines, *in* Fielding, S. and Lal, H., editors: *Neuroleptics,* Futura Publishing Co., New York, 1974, pp. 131-172.
74. Koe, B. K. and Constantine, J. W.: Blocking H^3-norepinephrine uptake and some guanethidine-induced effects with tricyclic psychotherapeutic drugs, *Arch. Int. Pharmacodyn. Ther.,* **195**:71-80, 1972.
75. Kuhar, M. J.: Neurotransmitter uptake: a tool in identifying neurotransmitter-specific pathways, *Life Sci. (II),* **13**:1623-1634, 1973.
76. Lahti, R. A. and Maickel, R. P.: The tricyclic antidepressants - inhibition of norepinephrine uptake as related to potentiation of norepinephrine and clinical efficacy, *Biochem. Pharmacol.,* **20**:482-486, 1971.
77. Laudisch, W., Steinhauff, N., and Matussek, N.: Chronic administration of electroconvulsive shock and norepinephrine metabolism in the rat brain, *Psychopharmacologia,* **15**:296-304, 1969.
78. Lemberger, L., Sernatinger, E., and Kuntzman, R.: Effect of desmethylimipramine, iprindole and dl-erythro-α-(3,4-dichlorophenyl)-β-(t-butylamino) propanol HCl on the metabolism of amphetamine, *Biochem. Pharmacol.,* **19**:3021-3028, 1970.
79. Lemberger, L., Witt, E. D., Davis, J. M., and Kopin, I. J.: The effects of haloperidol and chlorpromazine on amphetamine metabolism and

amphetamine stereotype behavior in the rat, *J. Pharmacol. Exp. Ther.,* **174**:428-433, 1970.

80. Lew, C., Iversen, S. D., and Iversen, L. L.: Effects of imipramine, desipramine and monoamine oxidase inhibitors on the metabolism and psychomotor stimulant actions of d-amphetamine in mice, *Eur. J. Pharmacol.,* **14**:351-359, 1971.
81. Lewander, T.: Influence of various psychoactive drugs on the *in vivo* metabolism of d-amphetamine in the rat, *Eur. J. Pharmacol.,* **6**:38-44, 1969.
82. Lipton, M. A., Prange, A. J. Jr., Dairman, W., and Udenfriend, S.: Increased rate of norepinephrine biosynthesis in hypothyroid rats, *Fed. Proc.,* **27**:399, 1968.
83. Mass, J. W., Dekirmenjian, H., and Jones, F.: The identification of depressed patients who have a disorder of NE metabolism and/or disposition, *in* Usdin, E. and Snyder, S. H., editors: *Frontiers in catecholamine research,* Pergamon Press, Inc., New York, 1973, pp.1091-1096.
84. Matussek, N. and Laudisch, W.: Chronic administration of electroconvulsive shock and norepinephrine metabolism in the rat brain, *Psychopharmacologia,* **15**:305-309, 1969.
85. Maxwell, R. A., Keenan, P. D., Chaplin, E., Roth, B., and Eckhardt, S. B.: Molecular features affecting the potency of tricyclic antidepressants and structurally related compounds as inhibitors of the uptake of tritiated norepinephrine by rabbit aortic strips, *J. Pharmacol. Exp. Ther.,* **166**:320-329, 1969.
86. McClure, D. J.: The role of dopamine in depression, *Can. Psychiatr. Assoc. J.,* **18**:309-312, 1973.
87. Medon, P. J., Leeling, J. L., and Phillips, B. M.: Influence of quipazine, a potential anti-parkinsonian agent on the uptake of ^{3}H-dopamine and ^{3}H-serotonin into rat striatal tissue *in vitro, Life Sci. (I),* **13**:685-691, 1973.
88. Meek, J. L., Fuxe, K., and Carlsson, A.: Blockade of p-chlorometh-amphetamine induced 5-hydroxytryptamine depletion by chlorimipramine, chlorpheniramine and meperidine, *Biochem. Pharmacol.,* **20**:707-709, 1971.
89. Meek, J. and Werdinius, B.: Hydroxytryptamine turnover decreased by the antidepressant drug chlorimipramine, *J. Pharm. Pharmacol.,* **22**:141-143, 1970.
90. Miller, K. W., Freeman, J. J., Dingell, J. V., and Sulser, F.: On the mechanism of amphetamine potentiation by iprindole, *Experientia,* **26**:863-864, 1970.
91. Mitchell, J. R., Cavanaugh, J. H., Arias, L., and Oates, J. A.: Guanethidine and related agents. III. Antagonism by drugs which inhibit the norepinephrine pump in man, *J. Clin. Invest.,* **49**:1596-1604, 1970.
92. Monkovic, I., Perron, Y. G., Martel, R., Simpson, W. J., and Gylys, J. A.: Substituted tetrahydrofurfurylamines as potential antidepressants, *J. Med. Chem.,* **16**:403-407, 1973.
93. Morris, J. B. and Beck, A. T.: The efficacy of antidepressant drugs, *Arch. Gen. Psychiatry,* **30**:667-674, 1974.
94. Musacchio, J. M., Julou, L., Kety, S. S., and Glowinski, J.: Increase in rat brain tyrosine hydroxylase activity produced by electroconvulsive shock, *Proc. Natl. Acad. Sci. USA.,* **63**:1117-1119, 1969.

95. Nybäck, H., Borzecki, Z., and Sedvall, G.: Accumulation and disappearance of catecholamines formed from tyrosine-^{14}C in mouse brain; effect of some psychotropic drugs, *Eur. J. Pharmacol.*, **4**:395-403, 1968.
96. Pare, C. M. B.: Clinical implications of monoamine oxidase inhibition, *Adv. Biochem. Psychopharmacol.*, **5**:441-444, 1972.
97. Perry, K. W. and Fuller, R. W.: Effect of 3-(p-trifluoromethylphenoxy)-N-methyl-3-phenylpropylamine hydrochloride (Lilly 110140), a specific inhibitor of serotonin uptake, on 5-hydroxyindole levels and turnover in rats, *Fed. Proc.*, **33**:560, 1974.
98. Prange, A. J. Jr., Meek, J. L., and Lipton, M. A.: Catecholamines: diminished rate of synthesis in rat brain and heart after thyroxine pretreatment, *Life Sci. (I)* **9**:901-907, 1970.
99. Prange, A. J. Jr., Sisk, J. L., Wilson, I. C., Morris, C. E., Hall, C. D., and Carman, J. S.: Balance, permission and discrimination among amines: a theoretical consideration of the actions of L-tryptophan in disorders of movement and affect, *in* Barchas, J. and Usdin, E., editors: *Serotonin and behavior,* Academic Press, New York, 1973, pp. 539-548.
100. Prange, A. J. Jr., Wilson, I. C., Breese, G. R., Plotnikoff, N. P., Lara, P. P., and Lipton, M. A.: Hypothalamic releasing hormones and catecholamines: a new interface, *in* Usdin, E. and Snyder, S. H., editors: *Frontiers in catecholamine research,* Pergamon Press, Inc., New York, 1973, pp. 1149-1155.
101. Prange, A. J. Jr., Wilson, I. C., Knox, A. E., McClane, T. K., Breese, G. R., Martin, B. R., Alltop, L. B., and Lipton, M. A.: Thyroid-imipramine clinical and chemical interaction: evidence for a receptor deficit in depression, *J. Psychiatr. Res.*, **9**:187-205, 1972.
102. Prange, A. J. Jr., Wilson, I. C., Knox, A., McClane, T. K., and Lipton, M. A.: Enhancement of imipramine by thyroid stimulating hormone: clinical and theoretical implications, *Am. J. Psychiatry,* **127**:191-199, 1970.
103. Plotnikoff, N. P., Kastin, A. J., Anderson, M. S., and Schally, A. V.: Dopa potentiation by a hypothalamic factor, MSH release-inhibiting hormone (MIF), *Life Sci. (I),* **10**:1279-1283, 1971.
104. Plotnikoff, N. P., Kastin, A. J., Anderson, M. S., and Schally, A. V.: Oxotremorine antagonism by a hypothalamic hormone, melanocyte-stimulating hormone release-inhibiting factor (MIF), *Proc. Soc. Exp. Biol. Med.,* **140**:811-814, 1972.
105. Plotnikoff, N. P., Prange, A. J. Jr., Breese, G. R., Anderson, M. S., and Wilson, I. C.: Thyrotropin releasing hormone: enhancement of dopa activity by a hypothalamic hormone, *Science,* **178**:417-418, 1972.
106. Plotnikoff, N. P., Prange, A. J. Jr., Breese, G. R., and Wilson, I. C.: Thyrotropin releasing hormone: enhancement of dopa activity in thyroidectomized rats, *Life Sci.,* **14**:1271-1278, 1974.
107. Raskin, A.: The prediction of antidepressant drug effects: review and critique, *in* Efron, D. H., editor: *Psychopharmacology. A review of progress 1957-1967,* U.S. Government Printing Office, Washington, D.C., 1968, pp. 757-765.
108. Rodriguez, R. and Pardo, E. G.: Quipazine, a new type of antidepressant agent, *Psychopharmacologia,* **21**:89-100, 1971.
109. Ross, S. B., Renyi, A. L., and Ögren, S.-O.: A comparison of the

inhibitory activities of iprindole and imipramine on the uptake of 5-hydroxytryptamine and noradrenaline in brain slices, *LifeSci, (II)*, **10**:1267-1277, 1971.
110. Salama, A. I., Insalaco, J. R., and Maxwell, R. A.: Concerning the molecular requirements for the inhibition of the uptake of racemic ^{3}H-norepinephrine into rat cerebral cortex slices by tricyclic antidepressants and related compounds, *J. Pharmacol. Exp. Ther.*, **178**:474-481, 1971.
111. Sandler, M., Goodwin, B. L., Leask, B. G. S., and Ruthren, C. R. J.: Melanocyte-stimulating hormone and parkinsonism: the role of hypothalamic releasing factors, *Lancet*, **I**:612, 1973.
112. Sarges, R., Koe, B. K., Weissman, A., and Schaefer, J. P.: Blockade of heart ^{3}H-norepinephrine uptake by 4-phenyl-1-aminotetralines: implications for the active conformation of imipramine-like drugs, *J. Pharmacol. Exp. Ther.*, **191**:393-402, 1974.
113. Schally, A. V., Arimura, A., and Kastin, A. J.: Hypothalamic regulatory hormones, *Science*, **179**:341-350, 1973.
114. Schanberg, S. M., Schildkraut, J. J., and Kopin, I. J.: The effects of psychoactive drugs on norepinephrine-^{3}H metabolism in brain, *Biochem. Pharmacol.*, **16**:393-399, 1967.
115. Schildkraut, J. J.: Neuropharmacology of the affective disorders, *Annu. Rev. Pharmacol.*, **13**:427-454, 1973.
116. Schildkraut, J. J.: Biogenic amines and affective disorders, *Annu. Rev. Med.*, **25**,:333-348, 1974.
117. Schildkraut, J. J. and Gershon, E. S.: Antidepressants and related drugs, *in* Lajtha, A., editor: *Handbook of neurochemistry*, Plenum Press, New York, 1971, pp. 357-386.
118. Schildkraut, J. J. and Kety, S. S.: Biogenic amines and emotion, *Science*, **156**:21-30, 1967.
119. Schildkraut, J. J., Schanberg, S. M., Breese, G. R., and Kopin, I.: Norepinephrine metabolism and drugs used in affective disorders: a possible mechanism of action, *Am. J. Psychiatry*, **124**:600-608, 1967.
120. Schildkraut, J. J., Schanberg, S. M., Breese, G. R., and Kopin, I. J.: Effects of psychoactive drugs on the metabolism of intracisternally administered serotonin in rat brain, *Biochem. Pharmacol.*, **18**:1971-1978, 1969.
121. Schildkraut, J. J. Winokur, A., and Applegate, C. W.: Norepinephrine turnover and metabolism in rat brain after long-term administration of imipramine, *Science*, **168**:867-869, 1970.
122. Schildkraut, J. J., Winokur, A., Draskóczy, P. R. and Hensle, J. H.: Changes in norepinephrine turnover in rat brain during chronic administration of imipramine and protriptylene: a possible explanation for the delay in onset of clinical antidepressant effects, *Am. J. Psychiatry*, **127**:1032-1039, 1971.
123. Schubert, J., Nybäck, H., and Sedvall, G.: Effect of antidepressant drugs on accumulation and disappearance of monamines formed *in vivo* from labelled precursors in mouse brain, J. Pharm. Pharmacol., **22**:136-139, 1970.
124. Sedvall, G., Jönsson, B., and Petterson, U.: Evidence of an altered thyroid function in man during treatment with lithium carbonate, *Acta Psychiatr. Scand.*, (suppl.) **207**:59-66, 1969.
125. Shaskan, E. G. and Snyder, S. H.: Kinetics of serotonin accumula-

tion into slices from rat brain: relationship to catecholamine uptake, *J. Pharmacol. Exp. Ther.,* **175**:404-418, 1970.

126. Sheard, M. H., Zolovick, A., and Aghajanian, G. K.: Raphe neurons: effect of tricyclic antidepressant drugs, Brain Res., **43**:690-694, 1972.
127. Sigg, E. B.: Pharmacological studies with tofranil, *Can. Psychiatr. Assoc. J.,* **4** (suppl.); 75-85, 1959.
128. Sigg, E. B.: The pharmacodynamics of imipramine, *in* Nodine, J. and Moyer, J. H., editors: *Psychosomatic medicine,* Lea & Febiger, Philadelphia, 1962, pp. 671-672.
129. Sigg, E. B.: Tricyclic thymoleptic agents and some newer antidepressants, *in* Efron, D. H., editor: *Psychopharmacology. A review of progress 1957-1967,* U.S. Government Printing Office, Washington, D.C., 1968, pp. 655-669.
130. Sigg, E. G., Soffer, L., and Gyermek, L.: Influence of imipramine and related psychoactive agents on the effect of 5-hydroxytryptamine and catecholamines on the cat nictitating membrane, *J. Pharmacol. Exp. Ther.,* **142**:13-20, 1963.
131. Silvestrini, B. and Lisciani, R.: Pharmacology of trazodone, *Curr. Ther. Res.,* (suppl.) **15**:749-754, 1973.
132. Snyder, S. H. and Coyle, J. T.: Regional differences in H^3-norepinephrine and H^3-dopamine uptake into rat brain homogenates, *J. Pharmacol. Exp. Ther.,* **165**:78-86, 1969.
133. Snyder, S. H., Shaskan, E. G., and Kuhar, M. J.: Serotonin uptake systems in brain tissue, *in* Barchas, J. and Usdin, E., editors: *Serotonin and behavior,* Academic Press, Inc., New York, 1973, pp. 97-108.
134. Stolk, J. M., Conner, R. L., and Barchas, J. D.: Rubidium-induced increase in shock-elicited aggression in rats, *Psychopharmacologia,* **22**:250-260, 1971.
135. Stolk, J. M., Nowack, W. J., and Barchas, J. D.: Brain norepinephrine: enhanced turnover after rubidium treatment, *Science,* **168**:501-503, 1970.
136. Stone, C. A.: Relationship of some autonomic actions to potential antidepressant activity among antidepressant drugs, *in* Garattini, S. and Dukes, M. N. G., editors: *Antidepressant drugs,* Excerpta Medica Foundation, Amsterdam, 1967, pp. 158-163.
137. Stone, C. A., Porter, C. C., Stavorski, J. M., Ludden, C. T., and Totaro, J. A.: Antagonism of certain effects of catecholamine-depleting agents by antidepressant and related drugs, *J. Pharmacol. Exp. Ther.,* **144**:196-204, 1964.
138. Story, D. F. and Story, M.: Inhibition by orphenadrine of ^{3}H-dl-noradrenaline and ^{14}C-tyramine uptake in atria, *Eur. J. Pharmacol.,* **5**:296-298, 1969.
139. Sulser, F. and Dingell, J. V.: Adrenergic mechanisms in the central action of tricyclic antidepressants and substituted phenothiazines, *Agressologie,* **9**:281-287, 1968.
140. Sulser, F. and Dingell, J. V.: Potentiation and blockade of the central action of amphetamine by chlorpromazine, *Biochem. Pharmacol.,* **17**,:634-636, 1968.
141. Sulser, F., Owens, M. L., Strada, S. J., and Dingell, J. V.: Modification by desipramine (DMI) of the availability of norepinephrine released by reserpine in the hypothalamus of the rat *in vivo, J. Pharmacol. Exp. Ther.,* **168**:272-282, 1969.

142. Tyrer, P.: Current status of monoamine oxidase inhibitors in psychiatry, *Br. J. Hosp. Med.,* **9**:795-802, 1973.
143. Udabe, R. U.: Clinical experience with a new psychotropic drug, trazodone: a review of literature, *Curr. Ther. Res.,* (suppl.) **15**:755-763, 1973.
144. Valzelli, L., Dolfini, E., Tansella, M. and Garattini, S.: Activity of centrally acting drugs on amphetamine metabolism, *J. Pharm. Pharmacol.,* **20**:595-599, 1968.
145. Van der Zee, P. and Hespe, W.: Influence of orphenadrine HCl and its N-dimethylated derivatives on the *in vitro* uptake of noradrenaline and 5-hydroxytryptamine by rat brain slices, *Neuropharmacology,* **12**:843-851, 1973.
146. Van Praag, H. M. and Korf, J.: 4-Chloramphetamines. Chance and trend in the development of new antidepressants, *J. Clin. Pharmacol.,* **13**:3-14, 1973.
147. Various authors: Human behavior: tests for serotonin utilization in humans and effects of precursor loading in various disorders, *in* Barchas, J. and Usdin, E., editors: *Serotonin and behavior,* Academic Press, New York, 1973, pp. 455-564.
148. Vogel, J. R. and Haubrich, D. R.: Chronic administration of electroconvulsive shock effects on mouse-killing activity and brain monoamines in rats, *Physiol. Behav.,* **11**:725-728, 1973.
149. Waldeck, B.: Inhibition of amine uptake in the mouse heart by some new "thymoleptic" drugs, *J. Pharm. Pharmacol.,* **20**:111-115, 1968.
150. Wheatley, D.: Potentiation of amitriptyline by thyroid hormone, *Arch. Gen. Psychiatry,* **16**:229-233, 1972.
151. Wong, D. T., Bymaster, F. P., Horng, J. S., and Molloy, B. B.: 3-(p-trifluoromethylphenoxy)-N-methyl-3-phenylpropylamine (Lilly 110140), a specific inhibitor of serotonin uptake into synaptosomes of rat brain, *Fed. Proc.,* **33**:255, 1974.
152. Wong, D. T., Horng, J. S., and Fuller, R. W.: Kinetics of serotonin accumulation into synaptosomes of rat brain—effects of amphetamine and chloroamphetamines, *Biochem. Pharmacol.,* **22**:311-322, 1973.
153. Youdim, M. B. H.: Multiple forms of monoamine oxidase and their properties, *Adv. Biochem. Psychopharmacol.,* **5**:67-77, 1972.

8

The Cardiovascular Pharmacology of Antidepressants

MICHAEL J. ANTONACCIO, PH.D.
and RONALD D. ROBSON, PH.D.

At the risk of oversimplification but for the sake of clarity, the antidepressants have been arbitrarily classified into three groups: tricyclics, monoamine oxidase inhibitors, and psychomotor stimulants. Not only do each of these groups have very different and profound effects on the cardiovascular system but, also, compounds within a group may vary significantly in their relative effects. Thus, although a particular chemical structure may be predictive of a particular action on the cardiovascular system, it would be unwise to assume *a priori* that other more serious effects are lacking. It is incumbent upon an industrial cardiovascular pharmacologist to test a new antidepressant in a very large number of cardiovascular tests because of the wide variety of effects observed with previous compounds, some of which are harmful, most of which are described below. It will become obvious that there is no simple test(s) to which a new antidepressant could be subjected to in order to clear it for cardiovascular safety; rather, a meticulous series of tests must be performed to be certain of a relative lack of side effects. On the positive side, the peripheral cardiovascular actions of the drug may help to clarify the central antidepressant mechanism and place it in a particular classification from a CNS point of view.

I. TRICYCLICS

The tricyclic antidepressants were originally synthesized as derivatives of phenothiazines and tested for their sedative and hypnotic properties. One of the tricyclics, imipramine, differs from the phenothiazines only by substitution of the sulfur with an ethylene linkage. The structure of chlorpromazine and representative antidepressants are shown in Figure 1. Although the cardiovascular effects of the tricyclics are similar to those of the pheno-

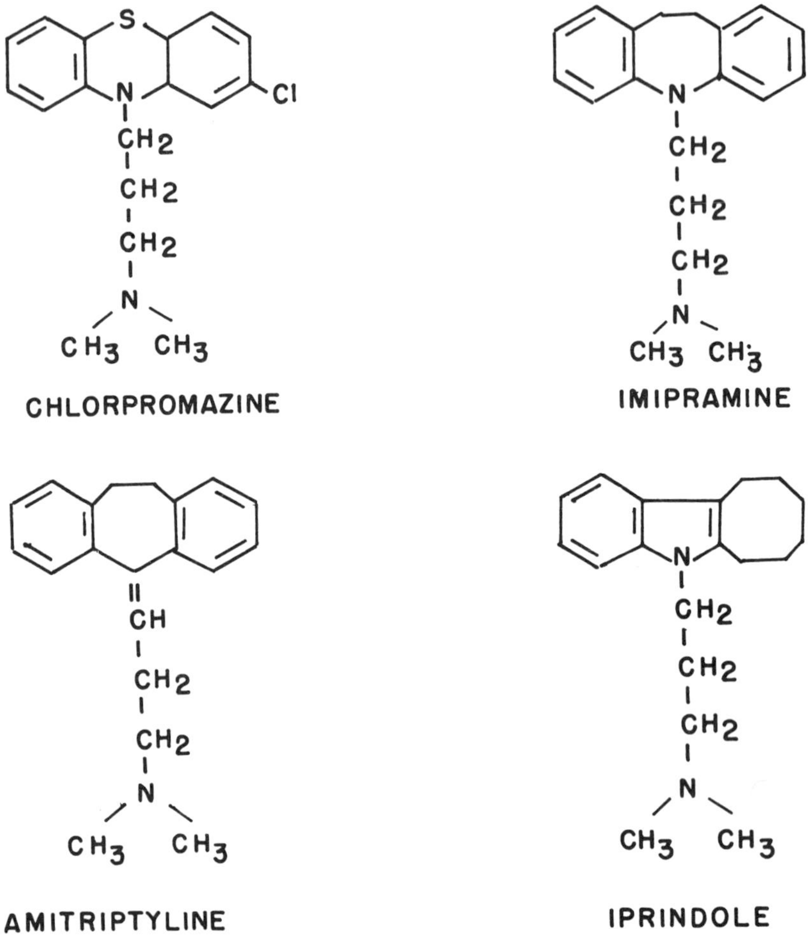

FIGURE 1 Structures of representative antidepressants.

thiazines—namely, hypotension and tachycardia (see Robson et al. (160))—it will become obvious that the mechanisms of these effects are different.

A. Effects on exogenous amines and sympathetic nerve stimulation

The most obvious pharmacological property of the imipramine—amitryptyline class of antidepressants is the ability to markedly potentiate the cardiovascular actions of norepinephrine while antagonizing the effects of indirectly-acting sympathomimetic amines such as tyramine (3, 7, 12, 18, 36, 66, 98, 101, 146, 147, 163, 171, 172, 177). These effects are characterized by a very rapid onset of action without the accompaniment of norepinephrine depletion which occurs with guanethidine or reserpine, drugs with the same effects on amine responses as the tricyclics (23, 124). In sharp contrast to norepinephrine, the effects of epinephrine and isoproterenol are not significantly modified by desmethylimipramine (DMI) (7, 101). Responses to 5-HT are also potentiated by DMI, imipramine, and chlorimipramine (173). The latter two compounds are the most effective enhancers of 5-HT and least effective enhancers of norepinephrine, whereas the relative order of enhancement for DMI is the reverse. The ratio of 5 HT/norepinephrine potentiation of these drugs is apparently related to their respective effects on neuronal uptake inhibition, chlorimipramine being relatively specific for 5-HT (27, 161, 169).

The effects of the tricyclics on the peripheral actions of sympathomimetic amines are undoubtedly due to the inhibitory effects of these compounds on the amine uptake pump of adrenergically innervated tissues (9, 12, 73, 86, 96, 97, 104, 110, 122, 123, 161, 176). However, a puzzling aspect of the effects of imipramine and DMI is the ability of these drugs to markedly potentiate both the duration and magnitude of the cardiovascular responses to exogenously administered norepinephrine while only prolonging the duration but not the magnitude of the response to stimulation of a variety of sympathetic nerves including the cervical (147), cardioaccelerator (3), lumbar chain (7), and entire spinal outflow (98). Kaumann et al (101) and Osborne and Sigg (147) reported that DMI and imipramine actually decreased responses to sympathetic nerve stimulation and carotid occlusion while potentiating responses to exogenously administered norepinephrine. Kaumann et al (101) suggested that the inhibitory effects of DMI on the sympathetic nervous system were due to blockade of release of norepinephrine in a manner akin to that of guanethidine. However, our own studies indicate that the inhibition of responses to cardiac nerve stimulation may be due to a non-specific inhibition of responses to catecholamines in general. Figure 2 shows the responses to post-ganglionic cardiac nerve stimulation in the anesthetized dog after non-cumulative doses of DMI (0.1-3 mg/kg i.v.). Low doses of DMI (0.1 and 0.3 mg/kg) caused only slight potentiation of the very low-frequency responses and slight depression of high-frequency responses. However, higher doses of DMI (1.0 and 3.0 mg/kg) caused only marked inhibition of responses to high-frequency nerve stimulation (Fig. 2). Table I shows the responses to norepinephrine, epinephrine, tyramine, and isoproterenol in

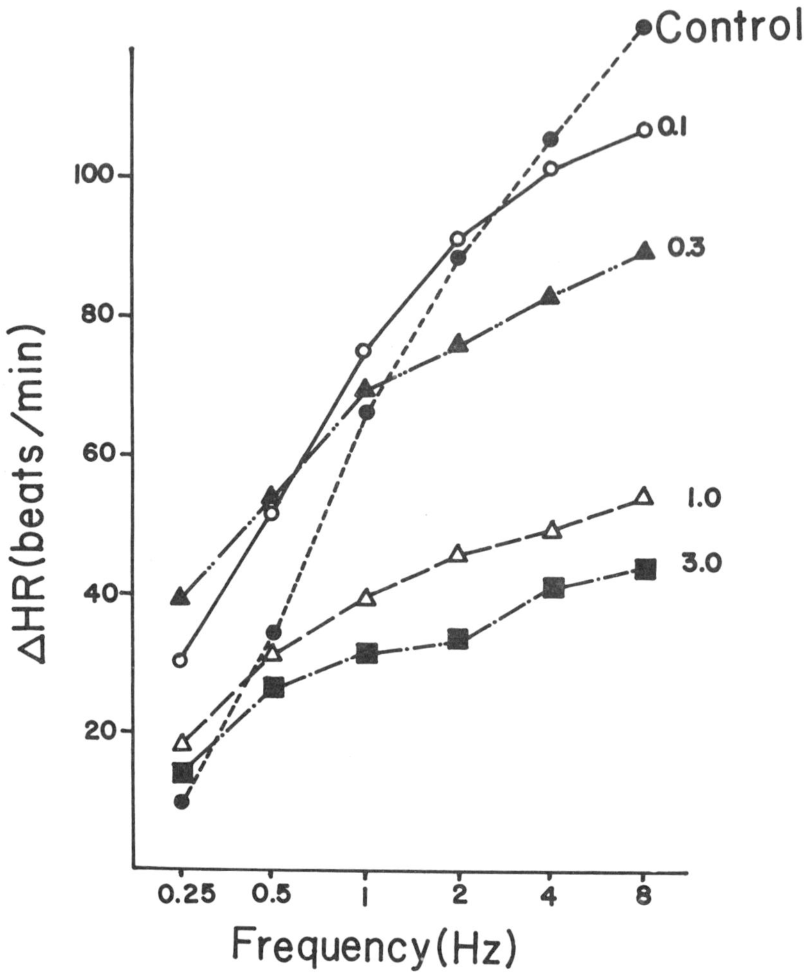

FIGURE 2 Effects of increasing doses of desipramine (mg/kg i.v.) on responses to postganglionic cardiac nerve stimulation in anesthetized dogs.

Stimulation (10 V, 5 msec duration) was maintained at each frequency until a stable response was obtained before proceeding to the next higher frequency (n = 5).

the same dogs used for cardiac nerve stimulation. DMI caused marked decreases in the response to tyramine and maximum potentiation of the response to norepinephrine between 0.1 and 0.3 mg/kg i.v. However, the chronotropic response to isoproterenol became progressively decreased. After 1.0 to 3.0 mg/kg i.v. of DMI, responses to norepinephrine became progressively smaller, though slightly higher than control values, and responses to tyramine and isoproterenol were very severely reduced (Table I).

TABLE I

Effect of DMI on Blood Pressure [BP, mm Hg], Heart Rate [HR, beats/min] and Responses to Sympathomimetic Amines In Anesthetized Dogs [n = 5]

	Dose [mg/kg i.v.]									
	Control		0.1		0.3		1.0		3.0	
BP	126.0 ± 4.8		127.2 ± 9.9		131.0 ± 5.3		118.0 ± 9.8		105.0 ±12.1	
HR		127.2 ± 9.9		125.4 ± 8.3		125.4 ± 6.4		127.2 ±16.7		111.0 ± 9.3
	Δ BP	Δ HR	Δ BP	Δ HR	Δ BP	Δ HR	Δ BP	Δ HR	Δ BP	Δ HR
NE 0.5	37.0 ± 2.0	16.2 ± 8.0	56.0 ± 7.1	36.0 ±14.5	82.0*** ± 7.3	45.0*** ±11.6	66.0* ±10.9	25.2 ± 7.1	54.0 ±14.5	21.0 ± 2.8
Epi 0.5	17.0 ± 2.0	12.6 ± 2.4	25.0 ± 2.7	13.8 ± 5.4	28.0 ± 4.6	12.6 ± 4.4	18.0 ± 7.5	5.4 ± 2.4	18.0 ± 6.0	4.8* ± 2.8
Tyr 100	75.0 ±11.3	32.4 ±11.7	44.0*** ± 7.5	17.4 ± 8.0	19.0** ± 5.3	6.6 ± 3.1	4.0*** ± 1.9	0*	4.0*** ± 2.9	5.4 ± 5.4
Iso 0.3	–42.0 ± 5.2	79.0 ±11.1	–43.0 ± 5.4	66.0 ±12.6	–39.0 ± 2.9	50.8** ±11.3	–34.0 ± 7.0	27.0* ± 7.5	–34.0 ± 8.3	19.8** ± 7.7

*$p < 0.05$; **$p < 0.02$; ***$p < 0.001$.
Shown are mean values ± the standard errors of the mean.

Thus, at low doses, DMI can cause maximum potentiation of responses to norepinephrine while markedly inhibiting those to tyramine, an effect apparently attributable to inhibition of the amine uptake pump. Under these conditions, responses to cardiac nerve stimulation and isoproterenol are not significantly affected. At high doses, DMI reduces the responses to nerve stimulation and to isoproterenol and thereby causes a reduction in the maximum responses to norepinephrine obtained at lower doses of DMI; responses to tyramine are totally abolished. The mechanism of the inhibitory effect of high doses of DMI is unknown but may be a result of a direct myocardial effect (33, 136, 164). An alternative explanation might be found in the report by Sigg et al (173) who found that imipramine and DMI could potentiate the magnitude of responses of nictitating membrane to sympathetic nerve stimulation in chloralose-urethane-but not pentobarbital-anesthetized cats.

B. Quality of effect on smooth muscle

Imipramine and DMI have a dual effect on responses of adrenergically innervated tissues to exogenous norepinephrine as indicated above. In low doses, they potentiate responses to exogenous norepinephrine but, as the dose of imipramine or DMI is increased, the potentiating effect becomes progressively masked by an inhibitory one (79, 90, 93, 165, 184). The dual effect of DMI on norepinephrine-induced contractions of isolated vascular smooth muscle has also been demonstrated (89, 90, 167, 180, 181, 183, 184). DMI produced a reversible but non-competitive antagonism of norepinephrine and barium-induced contractions which was not due to α-receptor blockade. Hrdina and Ling (90) attributed the antagonism to an interference by DMI with calcium availability for the contractile process. However, Toda (181) found that when rabbit aortic and pulmonary arterial strips were exposed to 3 times the normal calcium in the perfusion fluid either prior to the application of DMI, or after the inhibitory effect of DMI on the response to transmural stimulation had been established, the calcium did not prevent or antagonize the inhibition. Thus, Toda (181) favors an involvement of DMI with α-receptors, though α-blockade cannot explain the inhibitory effect of DMI on the vascular response to nonadrenergic stimulants such as barium and potassium (90). Obviously, the mechanism involved is still uncertain.

C. Hypotensive effects

An undesirable action of the tricyclics both in animals (24, 147) and man (17, 26, 85, 94, 102, 103, 113, 137) is hypotension. The hypotension is mainly postural and particularly severe in patients with cardiovascular disease (94, 137). The incidence of hypotension with imipramine is relatively high, Lund and Kristiansen (113) reporting that 45 to 85 patients with endogenous depression had an average fall of 20-30 mm Hg of systolic blood pressure. Muller et al (137) reported that blood pressure and heart rate were not affected by imipramine in patients in the recumbent position whereas hypotension and tachycardia occurred after assuming an upright position. In patients without cardiac disease, the incidence of postural hypotension was 7.3 per cent whereas 24. 4 per cent of patients with cardiac disease developed severe postural hypotension while receiving imipramine. Blumberg et al (17) have pointed out that changes in blood pressure with imipramine were significantly related to diagnosis, age, and initial levels of pressure. Blood pressure was decreased by imipramine in normal and depressed patients whereas it was increased in schizophrenics.

D. Antagonism of adrenergic neuron blocking agents

The tricyclic antidepressants protriptyline, imipramine, amitriptyline, and their desmethyl derivatives have been demonstrated to be capable of inhibiting catecholamine depletion in hearts of mice induced by α-methyl-*m*-tyrosine, metaraminol, guanethidine, and 6-hydroxydopamine, but not reserpine (177). These antidepressants also antagonized the action of guanethidine in reducing responses of the cat nictitating membrane and dog heart produced by sympathetic nerve stimulation (101, 104, 119, 177) and antagonized or prevented the antihypertensive action of guanethidine in patients (78, 109, 132, 133, 142). These antagonistic effects of the tricyclic antidepressants are apparently directly related to their ability to inhibit the amine uptake pump although they are not actively transported themselves (10, 185). It has been demonstrated that the adrenergic neuron blocking drugs guanethidine, bretylium, bethanidine, and debrisoquin are taken up and selectively concentrated into adrenergic neurons (30, 34, 134) and that this explains the highly selective pharmacologic effects of these drugs on adrenergic neurons (see 8, 19, 34). Although some dispute remains (35, 43), it appears that the competitive inhibition of uptake of the adrenergic neuron blocking agents by the tricyclic antidepressants thus provides an explanation of the antagonism of these former drugs.

The ability of DMI to prevent the antihypertensive activity of adrenergic neuron blocking agents is shown in Figure 3. Bethanidine , 60 mg/kg. P. O., caused a significant decrease in the blood pressure of spontaneously hypertensive rats (SHR's). Re-

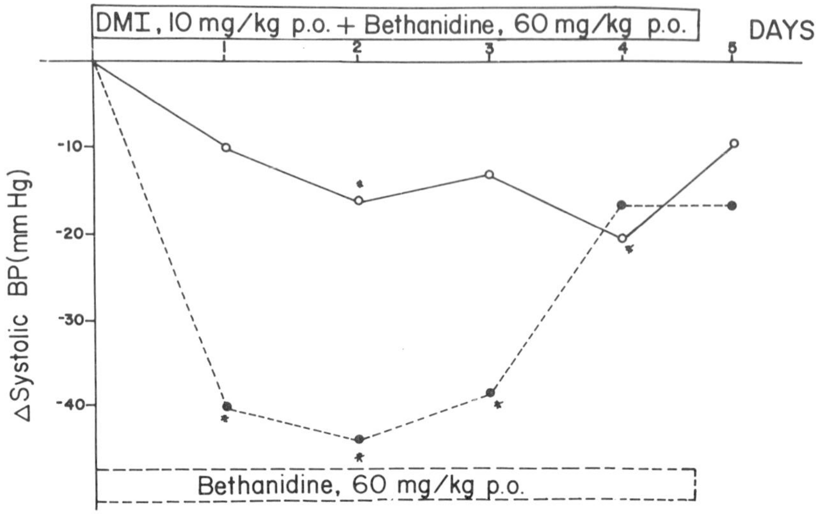

FIGURE 3 Effects of bethanidine alone (●- - - - -●) and after pretreatment with desipramine (DMI) (○———○) on systolic blood pressure of spontaneously hypertensive rats over a 4 day period of treatment. Blood pressure was measured indirectly by sphygmomanometry two hours after bethanidine (n=6 for each group).

sponses to stimulation of the spinal cord of SHR's after pretreatment with bethanidine (using the pithed rat preparation of Gillespie and Muir [71]) were essentially abolished; pressor responses to norepinephrine were potentiated whereas those to tyramine were inhibited (Table II). After a 30 minute pretreatment of SHR's with DMI (10 mg/kg P.O.), both the antihypertensive effect of bethanidine (Figure 3) and the ability of the latter to inhibit responses to sympathetic nerve stimulation were completely prevented (Table II).

An apparent exception to the generalization that tricyclics which inhibit norepinephrine uptake also inhibit effects of adrenergic blocking agents, is doxepin. Although doxepin blocked H^3-norepinephrine uptake to the same extent as guanethidine and amitriptyline and potentiated the norepinephrine pressor response, it did not antagonize the inhibition by guanethidine of the cat nictitating membrane response to sympathetic nerve stimulation (104). This relative lack of effect on responses to nerve stimulation is paralleled by the weak antagonism of the hypotensive effects of guanethidine in man by doxepin (140).

E. Cardiac toxicity

Cardiac side effects following the administration of tricyclic antidepressants were regarded as rare until Coull et al (44), using

TABLE II

Effects of Bethanidine [60 mg/kg p.o. for 1 hr], Desipramine [DMI] [10 mg/kg p.o. for 30 min] and DMI Pretreatment before Bethanidine on Pressor Responses [mm Hg] to Various Procedures in the Pithed Spontaneously Hypertensive Rat

Procedure	Control [n = 9]	DMI 10 mg/kg [n = 6]	Bethanidine 60 mg/kg [ ]	DMI + Bethanidine [n =6]
Sympathetic Stimulation 10 Hz for 20 sec	138 ± 14.5	147 ± 12.7	3 ± 1.2****	103 ± 10.3
NE 1 μg/kg	14 ± 2.0	19 ± 4.3	89 ± 5.4***	98 ± 9.5***
NE 3 μg/kg	36 ± 4.8	49 ± 8.7*	139 ± 5.7***	146 ± 12.5***
Tyramine 300 μg/kg	26.2 ± 3.7	1 ± 1.2***	11 ± 11.1*	10 ± 1.9*
Tyramine 1,000 μg/kg	70.1 ± 12.5	1 ± 1.2****	9 ± 0.8***	14 ± 6.4**

NE = Norepinephrine.
*$p < 0.05$; **$p < 0.02$; ***$p < 0.01$; ****$p < 0.001$.
Shown are mean values ± the standard error of the mean.

a drug-monitoring system, reported that 6 out of 53 patients with cardiac disease died suddenly after receiving amitriptyline, whereas there were no sudden deaths in a control series of patients. These preliminary results were expanded and confirmed by many groups. Moir et al (135) found that there were 13 sudden deaths in a group of 119 amitriptyline patients with cardiac disease but only 3 in a matched control group. After overdosage with the tricyclics, there have been reports of sudden death from cardiac arrest (50, 57, 59, 86, 118, 164) and several editorials have appeared stressing the possible cardiac complications which may occur from tricyclic antidepressant drugs especially in patients with cardiac disease (53-56). A report from the Boston Collaborative Drug Surveillance Program (55) reported that there was no evidence of an association between the tricyclic antidepressant drugs and cardiotoxic effects in 260 patients. However, the lack of positive correlation in that study may have been due to the lack of a diagnosed cardiac disease in the patients tested since cardiac complications with the tricyclics appear to be significant only in patients with a compromised cardiovascular system, or after overdosage (135).

Severe electrocardiographic changes in humans have been reported following the tricyclic antidepressants, mostly after overdosage (1, 2, 33, 57, 70, 81, 157, 158, 186), and also in animals (13, 116). Impaired cardiac conduction of varying degrees, including prolongation of the P-R interval, widening of the QRS complex, right bundle branch block, and complete heart block have been reported following tricyclic overdosage. Many of the EKG changes resemble those of hyperkalemia (81) but potassium levels have been determined to be normal or decreased in many cases (22, 178). Others have variously attributed the cardiotoxic effects to an atropine-like anticholinergic activity (178), adrenergic potentiating effect (41), or a direct myocardial toxic effect resulting in decreased contractility, decreased cardiac output, and hypotension (33, 136, 164).

F. Anticholinergic effects

The tricyclic antidepressants, particularly imipramine and DMI, have both central (179) and peripheral (147) anticholinergic properties which may be responsible for some or all of the tachycardia which is sometimes observed with these drugs (24, 103, 173). The cholinolytic effects are, like the adrenergic potentiating effects, bi-phasic in nature. Thus, vasodepression following peripheral vagal stimulation was enhanced by small doses of imipramine and decreased or abolished by large doses (147). This dual effect was also observed in the urinary bladder and gut preparation as well as in the ciliary beat of the frog's larynx (147). Hypotensive doses of exogenously administered acetylcholine were enhanced by imipramine whereas lower doses of imipramine had no effect on acetylcholine-induced hypotension (147). The dry mouth frequently associated with tricyclic antidepressant therapy may be a consequence of a peripheral anti-acetycholine action, but it may also result from a central action. Enhancement of noradrenergic responsiveness on the CNS, by inhibition of neuronal uptake of transmitter, may result in dry mouth in the same way as clonidine. The antidotal effects of anticholinesterase drugs used in the event of overdosage with the tricyclic drugs, may be achieved by offsetting the noradrenergic dominance in both central and peripheral locations.

G. Iprindole

Iprindole, although a tricyclic antidepressant (47, 58, 83, 99, 129), differs from the imipramine type by being an indole with an eight-membered saturated-ring (Figure 1). Iprindole, in common with the imipramine type tricyclics, shares the ability to potentiate the central effects of amphetamine and cardiovascular effects of directly-acting sympathomimetics (74, 131), although the latter action is considerably weaker than that of imipramine. However, iprindole does not inhibit H^3-norepinephrine uptake either centrally or peripherally (63, 74, 108,111), does not block the cardiovascular actions of indirectly-acting sympathomimetic amines, nor block the sympatholytic effects of guanethidine on the vas deferens preparation (74). Iprindole has been shown to increase levels of amphetamine in tissues by inhibiting *p*-hydroxylation of amphetamine (63). Although this may explain the enhancement of the central effects of amphetamine by iprindole, it does not explain the potentiation of responses to sympathomimetic amines. Furthermore, iprindole has been shown to decrease the peripheral effects of amphetamine (74). Thus, the effects of iprindole on the cardiovascular responses to sympathomimetics are unique and unexplainable at this time.

Iprindole has minimal anticholinergic and antihistamine activity (74). It prolongs A-V conduction at high doses and decreases maximal atrial following frequency in dogs (13). However, atrial and ventricular conduction velocity and ventricular excitability, which were depressed by high doses of imipramine, were unchanged by equal doses of iprindole (13).

II. MONOAMINE OXIDASE INHIBITORS (MAOI)

A. Hypotensive effects

All of the MAOI can produce hypotension (6, 80, 139, 144). The hypotension is usually orthostatic in nature and resembles that produced by sympathetic blockade. There is usually a delay in onset which appears to correlate chronologically with the degree of MAO inhibition (112, 145). The blood pressure lowering effects of pargyline are sufficient to warrant its commercial use as an antihypertensive agent, though other MAOI have also been tried for this indication (72, 80, 120). Oates et al (141) found pargyline to be equal to guanethidine and α-methyldopa as an antihypertensive agent in clinical trials.

B. Possible Mechanisms

The hypotensive action of MAOI appears paradoxical at first glance since they inhibit an enzyme which is important in destroying neurohumoral agents. Since this inhibition results in no change or even an accumulation of norepinephrine in sympathetically-innervated tissues (5, 20, 45, 114, 138, 153, 166, 175), no change or an increase in blood pressure might be expected. However, experimental evidence indicates that responses to adrenergic nerve stimulation are diminished after MAOI (5, 49, 69). Several explanations have been suggested to explain the decreased responses by MAOI to sympathetic activation: 1) Ganglion blockade—MAOI results in the accumulation of norepinephrine at sympathetic ganglionic synapses and it has been suggested that this accumulation impairs transmission thereby leading to a decrease in postganglionic nerve impulses (68, 75). However, it has been demonstrated that MAOI actually increase the number of action potentials in the cat superior cervical ganglion (48) and that responses to postganglionic sympathetic nerve stimulation were also reduced in MAO-inhibited animals (5, 49, 92); 2) False transmitters-MAOI have been shown to alter the nature of the adrenergic transmitter stores by causing the accumulation of false transmitter substances in vesicles that normally contain norepinephrine (28, 105-107).

According to some authors (39, 61, 105-107), octopamine and other similar β-hydroxylated amines which accumulate in the sympathetic nerves after inhibition of MAO, can function as false neurochemical transmitters. After pretreatment with MAOI, there is a marked increase in the synthesis of octopamine from tyramine (5, 107) and accumulation of octopamine in adrenergic nerve endings (29, 61, 100). Kopin et al (107) suggested that the norepinephrine content, whether raised or lowered by MAOI, was not relevant to the adrenergic blockade caused by MAO inhibition. Since only a limited number of amine molecules are released per nerve impulse, replacement with a relatively inactive false transmitter such as octopamine would result in a diminished release of norepinephrine and an apparent adrenergic blockade. Thus, according to this theory, MAO inhibition should always cause a diminished response to adrenergic nerve stimulation regardless of norepinephrine content. However, Smith (174) and Obianwu (143) found that acute administration of pargyline had no effect upon responses to accelerans nerve stimulation in open-chest guinea pigs or isolated left atrial strips to field stimulation or contraction of rat eyelid to cervical nerve stimulation. Also, Antonaccio and Smith (5) found that responses to field stimulation were not altered even after chronic dosage with pargyline alone or in combination with tryamine, a regimen of treatment specifically designed to increase the amount of octopamine in adrenergic nerve endings. Thus, it appears that effective substitution by false transmitters of lesser potency than norepinephrine does not sufficiently account for the adrenergic blocking effects of MAOI; 3) adrenergic neuron blockade—Several studies have indicated that MAOI may prevent release of norepinephrine from adrenergic nerve endings in a manner similar to the adrenergic neuron blocking drugs. Using various MAOI, Gatgounis and Aycock (67) showed that the cardiac contractile and blood pressure responses to the intraortic injection of nicotine or tetramethyl-ammonium were decreased or blocked at a time when the sensitivity of the response to norepinephrine was unchanged. While not ruling out ganglionic blockade as a possible explanation, they suggested that interference with catecholamine release might be a contributing factor. Davey et al (48) suggested that MAOI inhibited the post ganglionic release of norepinephrine since large doses of nialamid or iproniazid had no effect on evoked ganglion potentials. Furthermore, responses to splenic (49) and splanchnic (69) nerve stimulation in the cat were reduced by MAOI, and norepinephrine output to nerve stimulation was similarly reduced. Antonaccio and Smith (5) reported that, unlike responses to field stimulation, responses to accelerans nerve stimulation were inhibited by chronic pretreatment with pargyline and pargyline plus tyramine. This effect of pargyline was noted to be like that of bretylium and β-TM 10 which prevented responses of isolated atria to accelerans nerve stimulation (91) in concentrations which did not alter responses to field stimulation (16).

C. Antianginal effects

Because of their adrenergic blocking actions, the MAOI have been used in the treatment of angina pectoris. However, evaluation of these drugs for angina has yielded conflicting results. Many initial studies showed that, as a class, MAOI were very effective as antianginal drugs (25, 31, 32, 40, 42, 77, 87, 117, 170, 182). Later studies failed to show any greater effectiveness than placebo (11) but it is generally accepted that adequate doses of MAOI are effective in relieving angina. A rationale for the antianginal effect has been suggested on the basis of hemodynamic effects of MAOI; namely, decreased cardiac work, especially in response to exercise (76, 88). However, EKG changes indicative of myocardial hypoxia do not appear to be prevented by MAOI and may actually become more severe during treatment (117, 162). The possibility that pain perception rather than myocardial ischemia could be reduced by MAOI was discounted by Horwitz and Sjoerdsma (88) who found no change in subjective pain caused by forearm claudication whereas anginal pain was significantly reduced by pargyline.

D. Enhancement of responses to indirectly-acting sympathomimetic amines

The effects of indirectly-acting sympathomimetic amines are markedly enhanced after pretreatment with MAOI (5, 64, 143, 174). Both acute (174) and chronic (5) pretreatment with pargyline enhanced responses of cardiac tissues isolated from guinea pigs to tryamine, *d*-amphetamine, and mephentermine. Inhibition of MAO does not alter the sensitivity of cardiac or vascular tissues to norepinephrine (4, 5, 65, 159, 174). The enhancement of responses to tyramine may result in part from decreased oxidative deamination of tyramine. However, this explanation does not account for the enhancement of responses to mephentermine and *d*-amphetamine, since these latter substances are poor substrates for MAO. Furchgott and Garcia (64) attributed this enhancement to the accumulation of increased amounts of norepinephrine within storage sites sensitive to indirectly-acting sympathomimetic amines. However, Antonaccio and Smith (5) found no correlation between atrial norepinephrine content and reponses to indirectly-acting amines. Another explanation of this enhancement is that MAO inhibition prevents the oxidative deamination of norepinephrine released intraneuronally by indirectly-acting sympathomimetic amines (5, 143, 174). Indirectly-acting amines can release norepinephrine intraneuronally where it may be oxidatively deaminated by MAO. Tyramine itself is an excellent substrate for MAO and is also metabolized by intraneuronal MAO whereas *d*-amphetamine and mephentermine are not substrates. Thus, after inhibition of MAO, there is an increased release of norepinephrine not only after tyramine, which is no longer metabolized by MAO, but also after *d*-amphetamine and mephentermine. Since the norepinephrine released by nerve stimulation is not readily available to MAO, responses to nerve stimulation are not enhanced by MAO inhibition (4, 5, 143, 174).

The enhancement of responses to indirectly-acting amines was less after chronic than after acute treatment with pargyline (5). It was suggested that chronic MAO inhibition might allow for a partial substitution of octopamine or some similar substance of lesser potency than norepinephrine in the storage sites sensitive to indirectly-acting amines (5).

E. Hypertensive Crises

Probably directly related to the ability of MAOI to enhance the cardiovascular responses of indirectly-acting amines is the most serious cardiovascular complication produced by MAOI; namely, hypertensive crisis. These attacks occur with a frequency of about 8% (14) and are characterized by sudden throbbing headache, flushing, hyperpyrexia, and high systolic and diastolic pressures (14, 15, 46, 150). In rare instances, cerebrovascular accidents, heart failure, and death have been reported (52). The most common precipitating agent has been tyramine, found in significant concentration in cheeses, wines, beers, chicken livers, and pickled herring (82, 87, 156). However, hypertensive crises have been reported for other substrates of MAO including dopa, dopamine, and tryptophan (52, 84, 120). Hypertension caused by other indirectly-acting amines which are not good substrates for MAO because of their α-methyl group has been reported for amphetamine, tranylcypromine, mephentermine, ephedrine, and phenylpropanolamine in MAO-inhibited patients (21, 37, 46, 115, 130). The hypertension caused by this latter group of drugs is probably due to an increased amount of norepinephrine reaching receptor sites because of decreased intraneuronal metabolism (5, 151, 174). The other major pharmacological mechanism involved in the production of hypertensive crises is inhibition of MAO in the gastrointestinal tract allowing a large percentage of active amine, usually tyramine, to be released into the circulation (149-152).

A further complication arises with MAOI which also act as indirectly-acting releasing agents and/or inhibitors or norepinephrine uptake such as tranylcypromine, phenelzine and pheniprazine since relatively small doses would be expected to result in marked hypertension (38, 64, 151).

III. PSYCHOMOTOR STIMULANTS

A. Methylphenidate as a prototype agent

Drugs included in this class are the amphetamines, pipradrol, deanol, and methylphenidate (51). Because of the large volume of literature already available on the cardiovascular effects of the amphetamines, this review will be concerned mainly with methylphenidate, a prototype agent for the non-amphetamine psychomotor stimulants.

Most of the cardiovascular effects of methylphenidate resemble those of the tricyclic antidepressants. Methylphenidate enhances the pressor and smooth muscle stimulant actions of directly-acting sympathomimetics and antagonizes responses to tyramine and other indirectly-acting amines, both *in vivo* and *in vitro* (121, 125-128, 155). Methylphenidate has also been reported to decrease the uptake of norepinephrine both in peripheral and central adrenergic neurons (60, 122, 168). An interesting difference between the effects of methylphenidate-type compounds and the tricyclic antidepressants on norepinephrine uptake was recently demonstrated by Ferris et al (60). These authors showed that, unlike the periphery or other areas of the brain, the "phenethylamine uptake pump" of the striatum of rats could be easily inhibited by deoxypipradrol and methylphenidate, whereas very high concentrations of DMI were required to inhibit uptake. It was suggested that the receptors of the striatum phenethylamine pump were different from those in other areas and that the molecular configuration of the different molecules could account for the differences observed.

Although the inhibition of norepinephrine uptake in the periphery by methylphenidate might explain the potentiation of the cardiovascular responses to norepinephrine much like the tricyclic antidepressant, Maxwell (121) has offered an alternative suggestion. He suggested that potentiation of the pressor agents on isolated vascular smooth muscle by methyphylphenidate was due to a post-synaptic sensitization of effector cells. This was supported by the observation that the responses to angiotensin were also enhanced by methylphenidate, indicating a non-specific supersensitivity. Like the tricyclic antidepressants, methylphenidate (1) causes moderate and short-lasting reductions in blood pressure (127), (2) inhibits the reflex pressor response to bilateral carotid artery occlusion (126), (3) does not significantly alter the magnitude of responses to sympathetic nerve stimulation although the duration is prolonged (126), (4) has a bi-phasic effect on the contractile responses of vascular smooth muscle to norepinephrine and serotonin, enhancing at low and inhibiting at high concentrations (121), and (5) reverses the circulatory effects of reserpine (154).

Unlike the tricyclic antidepressants, methylphenidate appears to cause no significant clinical incidence of hypotension or cardiotoxicity. However, the drug does cause inhibition of imipramine metabolism (148), and has been reported to cause hypertensive episodes when given to patients taking the tricyclics (62).

REFERENCES

1. Alexander, C. S. and Nino, A.: Cardiovascular complications in young patients taking psychotropic drugs, a preliminary report, *Am. Heart J.*, **78**:757, 1969.
2. Alps, B. J., Harry, T. V. A., and Wilson, A. B.: E.C.G. and tricyclic antidepressant drugs, *Brit. Med. J.*, **3**:743, 1968.
3. Antonaccio, M. J. and Robson, R. D.: Pharmacological alterations of vagally-induced tachycardia, *Europ. J. Pharmacol.*, **3**:19, 1974.
4. Antonaccio, M. J., Robson, R. D., and Burrell, R.: The effects of L-dopa and α-methyldopa on reflexes and sympathetic nerve function, *Europ. J. Pharmacol.*, **25**:9, 1974.
5. Antonaccio, M. J. and Smith, C. B.: Effects of chronic pretreatment with pargyline upon responses of the atrial pacemaker and of left arterial strips of guinea pigs to tyramine, mephentermine, *d*-amphetamine, and adrenergic nerve stimulation, *J. Pharmacol. Exp. Ther.*, **170**:97-107, 1979.
6. Assali, N. S. and Dasgupta, K.: Hypotensive effects of iproniazid and carboxazid, *J. Am. Med. Assoc.*, **173**:1540-1552, 1960.
7. Astrom, A.: Potentiating action of desmethylimipramine on the cardiovascular effects of noradrenaline and some other pressor agents, *Acta. Physiol. Scand.*, **80**:510-518, 1970.
8. Atkinson, R., Watkinson, B., and Weetman, D. F.: The interaction between desmethylimipramine on guanethidine on the rabbit ileum. The importance of the noradrenaline uptake process in the reversal of the guanethidine-induced adrenergic neurone blockade, *Arch. int. Pharmacodyn.*, **198**:385-391, 1972.
9. Axelrod, J., Whitby, L. G., and Hertting, G.: Effect of psychotropic drugs on the uptake of ^{3}-H-norepinephrine by tissues, *Science*, **133**:383-384, 1961.
10. Babulova, A., Bareggi, S. R., Bonaccorsi, A., Garattini, S., Morselli, P. L., and Pantarotto, C.: Correlation between desipramine levels and (-) noradrenaline uptake and chronotropic effect in isolated atria of rats, *Brit. J. Pharmac.*, **48**:464-474, 1973.
11. Barber, J. M., Murphy, F. M., and Cheesman, E. A.: A clinical trial of isocarboxazid (Marplan) in angina pectoris, *Br. Heart. J.*, **24**:192-194, 1962.
12. Barnett, A., Symchowicz, S., and Taber, R. I.: The effects of drugs inhibiting catecholamine uptake on tyramine and noradrenaline-

induced contractions of the isolated vas deferens, *Brit. J. Pharmacol.,* **34**:484-492, 1968.
13. Baum, T., Shropshire, A. T., Rowles, G., and Gluckman, M. I.: Antidepressants and cardiac conduction: iprindole and imipramine, *Europ.J. Pharmacol.,* **13**: 287-291, 1971.
14. Bethune, H. C., Burrell, R. H., Culpan, R. H., and Ogg, G. J.: Vascular crises associated with MAOI, *Amer. J. Psychiat.,* **121**:245-248, 1964.
15. Blackwell, B., Marley, E., Price, J., and Taylor, D.: Hypertensive interactions between monoamine oxidase inhibitors and food stuffs, *Brit.J. Psychiat.,* **113**:349-365, 1967.
16. Blinks, J. R.: Field stimulation as a means of effecting the graded release of autonomic transmitters in isolated heart muscle, *J. Pharmacol. Exp. Ther.,* **151**:221-235, 1966.
17. Blumberg, A. G., Klein, D. F., and Pollack, M.: Effects of chlorpromazine and imipramine on systolic blood pressure in psychiatric patients: relationships to age, diagnosis and initial blood pressure, *J. Psychiat. Res.,* **2**:51-60, 1964.
18. Boakes, A. J., Laurence, D. R., Teoh, P. C., Barar, F. S. K., Benedikter, L. T., and Prichard, B. N. C.: Interactions between sympathomimetic amines and antidepressant agents in man, *Brit. Med. J.,* **1**:311-315, 1973.
19. Boura, A. L. A. and Green, A. F.: Adrenergic neurone blocking agents, *Ann. Rev. Pharmacol.,* **5**:183-212, 1965.
20. Brodie, B. B., Spector, S., and Shore, P. A.: Interaction of monoamine oxidase inhibitors with physiological and biochemical mechanisms in brain, *Ann. N. Y. Acad. Sci.,* **80**:609-614, 1959.
21. Brownlee, G. and Williams, G. W.: Potentiation of amphetamine and pethidine by monoamine oxidase inhibitors, *Lancet,* **1**:669, 1963.
22. Bucher, H. W. and Stuki, P.: Cardiac complications in desipramine intoxication. *Schweiz. Med. Wschr.,* **97**:519-521, 1967.
23. Burn, J. H. and Rand, M. J.: The action of sympathomimetic amines in animals treated with reserpine, *J. Physiol.,* **144**:314-336, 1958.
24. Cairncross, K. D. and Gershon, S.: A pharmacological basis for the cardiovascular complications of imipramine medication, *Med.J.Aust.,* **1**:372-375, 1962.
25. Calatayud, J. B., Orvis, H. H., and Prandoni, A. G.: Double-blind evaluation of an iproniazid analog (Ro 4-1634) in the treatment of angina pectoris, *J. Amer. Geriat. Soc.,* **9**:432-436, 1961.
26. Carlsson, A.: Pharmacological depletion of catecholamine stores, *Pharmacol. Rev.,* **18**:541-549, 1966.
27. Carlsson, A., Corrodi, H., Fuxe, L., and Hokfelt, T.: Effect of some antidepressant drugs on the depletion of intraneuronal brain 5-hydroxytryptamine stores caused by 4-methyl-α-ethyl-meta-tyramine, *Europ. J. Pharmacol.,* **5**:357-366, 1969.
28. Carlsson, A. and Lindquist, M.: *In vivo* decarboxylase of α-methyl-*m*-tyrosine, *Acta Physiol. Scand.,* **54**: 87-94, 1962.
29. Carlsson, A. and Waldeck, B.: β-hydroxylation of tyramine *in vivo, Acta Pharmacol. Toxicol.,* **20**:371-374, 1963.
30. Carlsson, A. and Waldeck, B.: Mechanism of amine transport in the cell membranes of the adrenergic nerves, *Acta Pharmacol. Toxicol.,* **22**:293-300, 1965.
31. Cesarman, T.: Iproniazid in cardiovascular therapy, with specific

reference to its action in angina pectoris and blood pressure, *Ann. N.Y. Acad. Sci.*, **80**:988-1008, 1959.
32. Cesarman, T.: Marsilid in the treatment of angina pectoris, *Exptl. Psychopathol.*, **19**:169-174, 1959.
33. Chahine, R. A. and Castellanos, A. J.: Myocardial toxicity produced by desipramine over-dosage, *Chest*, **59**:566-568, 1971.
34. Chang, C. C., Chen, T. F., and Cheng, H. C.: On the mechanism of neuromuscular blocking action of bretylium and guanethidine, *J. Pharmacol. Exptl. Ther.*, **158**:89-98, 1967.
35. Chang, C. C., Costa, E., and Brodie, B. B.: Interaction of guanethidine with adrenergic neurons, *J. Pharmacol. Exptl. Ther.*, **147**:303-312, 1965.
36. Chang, C. C. and Lee, M. C.: Studies of the effect of phenoxybenzamine on the uptake of noradrenaline and on the response to sympathetic stimulation of rat hearts, *Arch. Int. Pharmacodyn.*, **201**:400-414, 1973.
37. Clark, J. A.: Side effects of tranylcypromine, *Lancet*, **1**:618-619, 1961.
38. Clineschmidt, V. and Horita, A.: Auto-potentiation and potentiation by inhibition of monoamine oxidase of the sympathomimetic action of phenelzine and pheniprazine, *Brit.J. Pharmacol.*, **30**:67-77, 1967.
39. Cohen, R. A., Kopin, I. J., Creveling, C. R., Mussacchio, J. M., Fischer, J. E., Crout, J. R., and Gill, J. R., Jr.: False neurochemical transmitters, *Ann. Int. Med.*, **65**:347-362, 1966.
40. Cole, S. L., Kaye, H., and Griffith, G. C.: Assay of anti-anginal agents: a long-acting nitrate, psychic energizers and a tranquilizer, *Ann.J. Cardiol.*, **11**:639-645, 1963.
41. Colvard, C.: Overdosage of desipramine hydrochloride with marked EKG abnormalities, *Southern Med.J.*, **61**:1218, 1968.
42. Cossio, P.: The treatment of angina pectoris and other muscular pain due to ischemia with iproniazid and isoniazid, *Am. HeartJ.*, **56**:113-118, 1959.
43. Costa, E., Boullin, D. J., Hammer, W., Vogel, W., and Brodie, B. B.: Interactions of drugs with adrenergic neurons, *Pharmacol. Rev.*, **18**:577-597, 1966.
44. Coull, D. C., Crooks, J., Dingwall-Fordyce, I., Scott, A. M., and Weir, R. D.: Amitriptyline and cardiac disease, *Lancet*, **2**:590-591, 1970.
45. Crout, J. R., Creveling, C. R., and Udenfriend, S.: Norepinephrine metabolism in rat and heart, *J. Pharmacol. Exptl. Ther.*, **132**:269-277, 1961.
46. Cuthbert, M. F., Greenberg, M. P., and Morley, S. W.: Cough and cold remedies: A potential danger to patients on monoamine oxidase inhibitors, *Brit. Med.J.*, **1**:404-406, 1969.
47. Daneman, E. A.: Treatment of depressed patients with iprindole, *Psychosomatics*, **8**:216-221, 1967.
48. Davey, M. J., Farmer, J. B., and Reinert, H.: Hypotension and monoamine oxidase inhibitors, *Chemotherapia*, **4**:314-328, 1962.
49. Davey, M. J., Farmer, J. B., and Reinert, H.: The effects of nialamide on adrenergic function, *Brit.J. Pharmacol.*, **20**:121-134, 1963.
50. Davies, D. M. and Allaye, R.: Amitriptyline poisoning, *Lancet*, **2**:543, 1963.
51. Davis, J. M., Klerman, G. L., and Schildkraut, J. J.: Drugs used in the treatment of depression, *in* Efron, D. H., editor: *Psychopharma-*

cology– review of progress, Public Health Service Publication, Washington, D. C. 1968, pp. 719-748.
52. Ebert, M. H. and Shader, R. I.: Cardiovascular effects, *in* Shader, R. I. and DiMascio, A., editors: *Psychotropic drug side effects,* The Williams & Wilkins Co., Baltimore. 1970, pp. 149-163.
53. Editorial: Amitriptyline and cardiac diseases, *Med.J. Aust.,* **2**:940-941, 1970.
54. Editorial: Cardiovascular complications from psychotropic drugs, *Brit. Med.J.,* **1**:3, 1971.
55. Editorial: Cardiovascular implications of tricyclic antidepressants, *New Zeal. Med.J.,* **74**:390-391, 1971.
56. Editorial: Adverse reactions to the tricyclic-antidepressant drugs. Report from Boston Collaborative Drug Surveillance Program, *Lancet,* **1**:529-531, 1972.
57. Edwards, J.: Fatal imipramine overdosage, *Med. J. Aust.,* **1**: 839-840, 1966.
58. El-Deiry, N. K., Forrest, A. D., and Littman, S. K.: Clinical trial of a new antidepressant (Wy-3263), *Brit. J. Psychiat.,* **113**:999-1004, 1967.
59. Fatteh, A., Blanke, R., and Mann, G.: Death from imipramine poisoning, *J. Forensic Sci.,* **13**:124-128, 1968.
60. Ferris, R. M., Tang, F. L. M., and Maxwell, R. A.: A comparison of the capacities of isomers of amphetamine, deoxypipradrol and methylphenidate to inhibit the uptake of tritiated catecholamines into rat cerebral cortex slices, synaptosomal preparations of rat cerebral cortex, hypothalamus and striatum and into adrenergic nerves of rabbit aorta, *J. Pharmacol. Exptl. Ther.,* **181**:407-416, 1972.
61. Fischer, J. E. Horst, W. D., and Kopin, I. J.: β-hydroxylated amines as false neurotransmitters, *Brit.J. Pharmacol.,* **24**:477-484, 1965.
62. Flemenbaum, A.: Hypertensive episodes after adding methylphenidate (Ritalin) to tricyclic antidepressants, *Psychosomatics,* **13**:265-268, 1972.
63. Freeman, J. J. and Sulser, F.: Iprindole - amphetamine interactions in the rat: the role of aromatic hydroxylation of amphetamine in its mode of action, *J. Pharmacol. Exptl. Ther.,* **183**:307-315, 1972.
64. Furchgott, R. F. and Garcia, P. S.: Effects of inhibition of monoamine oxidase on the actions and interactions of norepinephrine, tyramine and other drugs on guinea pig left atrium, *J. Pharmacol. Exptl. Ther.,* **163**:98-122, 1968.
65. Furchgott, R. F., Kirpekar, S. M., Riecker, M., and Schwab, A.: Actions and interactions of norepinephrine, tyramine and cocaine on aortic strips of rabbit and left atria of guinea pig and cat, *J. Pharmacol. Exptl. Ther.,* **142**:39-58, 1963.
66. Garcia, A. G., Martin, A. V., Sierra, R. M., and Garcia, P. S.: Evidence for a different site of action of phenoxybenzamine and desmethylimipramine on the catecholamine uptake system, *Experientia,* **28**:671-673, 1972.
67. Gatgounis, J. and Aycock, J.: Effects of monoamine oxidase inhibitors on adrenal medullary responses to nicotine and tetramethylammonium, *J. Pharmacol. Exptl. Ther.,* **141**:50-57, 1963.
68. Gertner, S. D.: The effects of monoamine oxidase inhibitors on ganglionic transmission, *J. Pharmacol. Exptl. Ther.,* **131**:223-230, 1961.

69. Gessa, G. L., Cuenca, E., and Costa, E.: On the mechanism of hypotensive effects of monoamine oxidase inhibitors, *Ann. N.Y. Acad. Sci.*, **107**:935-944, 1963.
70. Giles, H.: Imipramine poisoning in childhood, *Brit. Med.J.*, **2**:844-846, 1963.
71. Gillespie, J. S. and Muir, T. C.: A method of stimulating the complete sympathetic outflow from the spinal cord to blood vessels in the pithed rat, *Brit.J. Pharmac.*, **30**:78-87, 1967.
72. Gillespie, L., Terry, L. L., and Sjoerdsma, A.: The application of a MAOI 1-phenyl-2-hydrazino-propane (JB-516) to the treatment of primary hypertension, *Amer. HeartJ.*, **58**:1-12, 1959.
73. Glowinski, J. and Axelrod, J.: Inhibition of uptake of tritiated noradrenaline in the intact rat brain by impramine and structurally related compounds, *Nature*, **204**:1318-1319, 1964.
74. Gluckman, M. I. and Baum, T.: The pharmacology of iprindole, a new antidepressant, *Psychopharm.*, **15**:169-185, 1969.
75. Goldberg, L. I. and DaCosta, F. M.: Selective depression of sympathetic transmission by intravenous administration of iproniazid and harmine, *Proc. Soc. Exp. Biol.*, **105**:223-227, 1961.
76. Goldberg, L. I., Horowitz, D., and Sjoerdsma, A.: Attenuation of cardiovascular responses to exercise as a possible basis for effectiveness of monoamine oxidase inhibitors in angina pectoris, *J. Pharmacol. Exptl. Ther.*, **137**:39-46, 1962.
77. Grant, A. P.: Sequential trial of isocarboxazid in angina pectoris, *Brit. Med.J.*, **1**:513-515, 1962.
78. Gulati, O. D., Dave, B. T., Gokhale, S. D., and Shah, K. M.: Antagonism of adrenergic neuron blockade in hypertensive subjects, *Clin. Pharmacol. Ther.*, **7**:510-514, 1966.
79. Haefely, W., Hürlimann, A., and Thoenen, H.: Scheinbar paradoxe beeinflussung von peripheren noradrenalinwirkungen durch einige thymoleptica, *Helv. Physiol. Pharmacol. Acta.*, **22**:15-33, 1964..
80. Harnes, J.: Effect of marsilid on blood pressure in hypertensive patients, *J. Clin. Exp. Psychopath.*, Suppl. 1, **19**:152-154, 1958.
81. Harthorne, J. W., Marcus, A. M., and Kaye, M.: Management of massive imipramine overdosage with manittol and artificial dialyses, *New Eng.J. Med.*, **268**:33-36, 1963.
82. Hedberg, D. L., Gordon, M. W., and Glueck, B. C.: Six cases of hypertensive crisis in patients on tranylcypromine after eating chicken livers, *Amer.J. Psychiat.*, **122**:933-937, 1966.
83. Hicks, J. T.: Iprindole, a new antidepressant for use in general office practice. A double-blind, placebo-controlled study, *Illinois Med.J.*, **128**:622-626, 1965.
84. Hodge, J. V. and Nye, E. R.: Monoamine oxidase inhibitors, broad beans and hypertension, *Lancet*, **1**:1108, 1964.
85. Honigfeld, G. and Newhall, P. N.: Hemodynamic effects of imipramine, acetophenazine and trifluoperazine in geriatric psychiatry, *Dis. Nerv. Syst.*, **26**:427-429, 1965.
86. Horn, A. S., Coyle, J. T., and Snyder, S. H.: Structure activity relationships of drugs with differential effects on dopamine and norepinephrine neurons, *Mol. Pharmacol.*, **7**:66-80, 1970.
87. Horwitz, D., Lovenberg, W., Engelman, K., and Sjoerdsma, A.: Monoamine oxidase inhibitors, tyramine and cheese, *J. Amer. Med. Assoc.*, **188**:1108-1110, 1964.

88. Horwitz, D. and Sjoerdsma, A.: A basis for the use of monoamine oxidase inhibitors in angina pectoris, *Ann. N.Y. Acad. Sci.*, **107**:1033-1042, 1963.
89. Hrdina, P., Bonaccorsi, A., and Garattini, S.: Pharmacological studies on isolated and perfused rat renal arteries, *Europ.J. Pharmacol.*, **1**:99-108, 1967.
90. Hrdina, P. D. and Ling, C. M.: Studies on the mechanism of the inhibitory effect of desmethylimipramine (DMI) on vascular smooth muscle contraction, *J. Pharmacol. Exptl. Ther.*, **173**:407-415, 1970.
91. Hukovic, S.: The action of sympathetic blocking agents on isolated and innervated atria and vessels, *Brit.J. Pharmacol.*, **15**:117-121, 1960.
92. Hukovic, S. and Muscholl, E.: Die noradrenalin-freisetzung aus dem isolierten herzen durch sympathische nervenreizung, *Arch. exp. Path. Pharmak.*, **243**:348, 1962.
93. Hurlimann, A., Thoenen, H. and Haefely, W.: The action of tricyclic antidepressant drugs and related compounds on the α-adrenergic receptors and re-uptake of neurally released norepinephrine, *in* Garratini, S. and Dukes, M. N. G., editors: *Proceedings of the first international symposium on antidepressant drugs*, Excerpta Medica Foundation, Amsterdam, 1967, pp. 168-171.
94. Idestrom, C. M. and Cadenius, B.: Imipramine-desmethylimipramine. A pharmacological study on human beings, *Psychopharm.*, **5**:431-439, 1964.
95. Costa, E. and Garratini, S., editors: *International symposium on amphetamines and related compounds*, Raven Press, New York, 1970.
96. Iversen, L. L.: Inhibition of noradrenaline uptake by drugs, *J. Pharm. Pharmacol.*, **17**:42-64, 1965a.
97. Iversen, L. L.: The uptake of catecholamines at high perfusion concentrations in the rat isolated heart: A novel catecholamine uptake process, *Brit.J. Pharmacol.*, **25**:18-33, 1965b.
98. Jacquot, C., Bralet, J., Cohen, Y., and Valette, G.: Effet de la stimulation de la chaine sympathique sur la liberation de la noradrenaline-^{3}H dans la circulation du rat: influence de la guanethidine, de la phenoxybenzamine, de la cocaine et de la desipramine, *in vivo*, *Arch. int. Pharmacodyn.*, **187**:245-264, 1970.
99. Johnson, J. and Maden, J. G.: A new antidepressant pramindole (WY-3263). A double-blind controlled trial, *J. Clin. Trials*, **4**:787-791, 1967.
100. Kakimoto, Y. and Armstrong, M.D.: On the identification of octopamine in mammals, *J. Biol. Chem.*, **237**:422-427, 1962.
101. Kaumann, A., Basso, N., and Aramendia, P.: The cardiovascular effects of N-(α-methylamino-propyl-imino-dibenzyl)-HCl (desmethylimipramine) and guanethidine, *J. Pharmacol. Exp. Ther.*, **147**:54-64, 1965.
102. Klerman, G. L.: *In* discussion of the paper by Sulser and Dingell. *In* Effron, D. H. and Kety, S. S., editors: *Antidepressant drugs of non-MAO inhibitor type*, Department of Health, Education and Welfare, Washington, D. C., 1966, p. 36.
103. Klerman, G. L. and Cole, J. D.: Clinical pharmacology of imipramine and related antidepressant compounds, *Pharmacol. Rev.*, **17**:101-141, 1965.

104. Koe, B. K. and Constantine, J. W.: Blocking H^3-norepinephrine uptake and some guanethidine-induced effects with tricyclic psychotherapeutic drugs, *Arch. int. Pharmacodyn.,* **195**:71-80, 1972.
105. Kopin, I. J.: False adrenergic transmitters, *Ann. Rev. Pharmacol.,* **8**:377-394, 1968.
106. Kopin, I. J., Fischer, J. E., Musacchio, J., and Horst, W. D.: Evidence for a false neurochemical transmitter as mechanism for the hypotensive effect of monoamine oxidase inhibitors, *Proc. Nat. Acad. Soc.,* **52**:716-721, 1964.
107. Kopin, I. J., Fischer, J. E., Musacchio, J. M., Horst, W. D., and Weise, V. K.: "False neurochemical transmitters" and the mechanism of sympathetic blockade by monoamine oxidase inhibition, *J. Pharmacol. Exp. Ther.,* **147**:186-193, 1965.
108. Lahti, R. A. and Maickel, R. P.: The tricyclic antidepressants - Inhibition of norepinephrine uptake as related to potentiation of norepinephrine and clinical efficacy, *Biochem. Pharmacol.,* **20**:482-486, 1971.
109. Leishman, A. W. D., Mathews, H. L., and Smith, A. J.: Antagonism of guanethidine by imipramine, *Lancet,* **1**:112, 1963.
110. Leitz, F. H. and Stefano, F. J. E.: Effect of ouabain and desipramine on the uptake and storage of norepinephrine and metaraminol, *Europ. J. Pharmacol.,* **11**:278-285, 1970.
111. Lemberger, L., Sernatinger, E., and Kuntzman, R.: Effect of desmethylimipramine, iprindole and DL-erythro-α-(3,4-dichlorophenyl)-β-(t-butylamino) propanol HCl on the metabolism of of amphetamine, *Biochem. Pharmacol.,* **19**:3021-3028, 1970.
112. Levine, R. J. and Sjoerdsma, A.: Direct measurement of monoamine oxidase inhibition in humans, *Clin. Pharmacol. Therap.,* **4**:22-27, 1963.
113. Lunn, V. and Kristiansen, E. S.: Cardiac complications in the course of treatment with Tofranil, *Wien. Med. Wschr.,* **110**:754, 1960.
114. Malmfors, T.: Studies on adrenergic nerves, *Acta. Physiol. Scand.* (Supple. 248), **64**:1-93, 1965.
115. Mark, L. C., Marx, G. F., Arkins, R. E., Kepres, E. K., Radnay, P. A., Schapira, M., Stein, S. N., and Waldbauer, M.: Hypotension following use of monoamine oxidase inhibitors, *N.Y. State J. Med.,* Feb. 15, 1967, pp. 570-572.
116. Marmo, E., Coscia, L., and Cataldi, S.: Cardiac effects of antidepressants, *Japan J. Pharmacol.,* **22**:283-292, 1971.
117. Master, A. M.: Iproniazid (Marsilid) in angina pectoris, *Am. Heart J.,* **56**:570-582, 1958.
118. Masters, A. B.: Delayed death in imipramine poisoning, *Brit. Med. J.,* **3**:866-867, 1967.
119. Matsumoto, C. and Horita, A.: Antagonism of bretylium by sympathomimetic amines, *Nature,* **195**:1212-1213, 1962.
120. Maxwell, M. H., Bernstein, H., Roth, S., and Kleeman, C.: Monoamine-oxidase inhibitors in hypertension, *Amer. J. Cardiol.,* **6**:1146-1151, 1960.
121. Maxwell, R. A.: Concerning the mechanism of action of methylphenidate on the responses of rabbit vascular tissue to norepinephrine, *J. Pharmacol. Exp. Ther.,* **147**:289-297, 1965.

122. Maxwell, R. A., Chaplin, E., Eckhardt, S. B., Soares, J. R., and Hite, G.: Conformational similarities between molecular models of phenethylamine and of potent inhibitors of the uptake of tritiated norepinephrine by adrenergic nerves in rabbit aorta, *J. Pharmacol. Exp. Ther.*, **173**:158-165, 1970b.
123. Maxwell, R. A., Eckhardt, S. B., and Hite, G.: Kinetic and thermodynamic considerations regarding the inhibition of tricyclic antidepressants of the uptake of tritiated norepinephrine by the adrenergic nerves in rabbit aortic strips, *J. Pharmacol. Expt. Ther.*, **171**:62-69, 1970a.
124. Maxwell, R. A., Plummer, A. J., Povalski, H., and Schneider, F.: Concerning a possible action of guanethidine (Su-5864) in smooth muscle, *J. Pharmacol. Expt. Ther.*, **129**:24-30, 1960.
125. Maxwell, R. A., Plummer, A. J., Povalski, H., Schneider, F., and Coombs, H.: A comparison of some of the cardiovascular actions of methylphenidate and cocaine, *J. Pharmacol. Exp. Ther.*, **126**:250-257, 1959.
126. Maxwell, R. A., Plummer, A. J., Ross, S. D., and Daniel, A. I.: Studies concerning the cardiovascular actions of the central nervous stimulant methylphenidate, *J. Pharmacol. Exp. Ther.*, **123**:22-27, 1958.
127. Maxwell, R. A., Plummer, A. J., Ross, S. D., Paytas, J. J., and Dennis, A. D.: Antihypertensive effects of the central nervous stimulant methylphenidate, *Arch. int. Pharmacodyn.*, **112**:26-35, 1957.
128. Maxwell, R. A., Sylwestrowicz, H. D., Holland, R., Schneider, F., and Daniel, A. I.: Some actions of methylphenidate on the vascular system, arterial tissue and the nictitating membrane, *J. Pharmacol. Exp. Ther.*, **131**:355-365, 1961.
129. McClatchey, W. T., Moffat, J., and Irvine, G. M.: A double-blind study of WY-3263, imipramine and placebo, *J. Ther. Clin. Res.*, **5**:13-15, 1967.
130. McClure, J. L.: Reactions associated with tranylcypromine, *Lancet*, **1**:1351, 1962.
131. Miller, K. W., Freeman, J. J., Dingell, J. G., and Sulser, F.: On the mechanism of amphetamine potentiation by iprindole, *Experientia*, **26**:863-864, 1970.
132. Mitchell, J. R., Arias, L., and Oates, J. A.: Antagonism of the antihypertensive action of guanethidine sulfate by desipramine hydrochloride, *J. Amer. Med. Assoc.*, **202**:973-976, 1967.
133. Mitchell, J. R., Cavanaugh, J. H., Arias, L., and Oates, J. A.: III Antagonism by drugs which inhibit the norepinephrine pump in man, *J. Clin. Invest.*, **49**:1596-1604, 1970.
134. Mitchell, J. R. and Oates, J. A.: Guanethidine and related agents. I. Mechanism of the selective blockade of adrenergic neurons and its antagonism by drugs, *J. Pharmacol. Exp. Ther.*, **172**:100-107, 1970.
135. Moir, D. C., Cornwell, W. B., Dingwall-Fordyce, I. Crooles, J., O'Malley, K., Turnbull, M. J., and Weir, R.: Cardiotoxicity of amitriptyline, *Lancet*, **2**:561-564, 1972.
136. Motin, J., Evreux, J. C., and Vedrinne, J.: Toxicite cardiovasculaire de l'imipramine, *Rev. Lyon Med.*, **16**:309-310, 1967.
137. Muller, O. F., Goodman, N., and Bellet, S.: The hypotensive effect of imipramine hydrochloride in patients with cardiovascular disease, *Clin. Pharmacol. Therap.*, **2**:300-307, 1961.
138. Muscholl, E.: Die wirkung von harmalin auf die konzentration von

noradrenalin und adrenalin in herzen, *Experientia,* **15**:428-429, 1959.

139. Nussbaum, H. E., Leff, W., Mattia, V. D., Jr., and Hillman, E.: Effects of iproniazid phosphate (Marsilid) on hypertension, *Angiology,* **8**:198-200, 1957.
140. Oates, J. A., Fann, W. E., and Cavanaugh, J. A.: Effect of doxepin on the norepinephrine pump. A preliminary report, *Psychosomatics,* Sec. II, **10**:12-13, 1969.
141. Oates, J. A., Seligmann, A. W., Clarke, M. A., Rouseau, P., and Lee, R. E.: The relative efficacy of guanethidine, methyldopa and pargyline as antihypertensive agents, *New Eng. J. Med.,* **273**:729-734, 1965.
142. Ober, K. F. and Wang, R. I. H.: Drug interactions with guanethidine, *Clin. Pharmacol. Therap.,* **14**:190-195, 1973.
143. Obianwu, A. O.: Possible functional differentiation between the stores from which adrenergic nerve stimulation, tyramine and amphetamine release noradrenaline, *Acta. Physiol. Scand.,* **75**:92-101, 1969.
144. O'Connor, J. B., Howlett, K. S., Jr., and Wagner, R. R.: Side effects accompanying use of iproniazid, *Am. Rev. Tuberc.,* **68**:270-272, 1953.
145. Orvis, H. H., Tamagna, I. G., Horwitz, D., and Thomas, R.: Correlation of hypotensive effects and urinary tryptamine levels during paragyline therapy, *Ann. N.Y. Acad. Sci.,* **107**:958-965, 1963.
146. Osborne, M.: Interaction of imipramine with sympathicomimetic amines and reserpine, *Arch. int. Pharmacodyn.,* **138**:492-504, 1962.
147. Osborne, M. and Sigg, E. B.: Effects of imipramine on the peripheral autonomic system, *Arch. int. Pharmacodyn.,* **129**:273-289, 1960.
148. Perel, J. M., Black, N., Wharton, R. N., and Malitz, S.: Inhibition of imipramine metabolism by methylphenidate (Ritalin), *Fed. Proc.,* **28**:418, 1969.
149. Pettinger, W. A., Mitchell, J. R., and Oates, J. A.: Cardiovascular effects and toxicity of psychotropic agents in man, *in* Efron, S. H., editor: *Psychopharmacology. A review of progress,* Public Health Service Publication, Washington, D.C., 1968, pp. 589-605.
150. Pettinger, W. A. and Oates, J. A.: Supersensitivity to tyramine during monoamine oxidase inhibition in man, *Clin. Pharmacol. Therp.,* **9**:341-344, 1968a.
151. Pettinger, W. A. and Oates, J. A.: Supersensitivity to tyramine during monoamine oxidase inhibition in man. Mechanism at the level of the adrenergic neuron, *Clin. Pharmacol. Therap.,* **9**:341-344, 1968b.
152. Pettinger, W. A., Soyangco, F. G., and Oates, J. A.: Inhibition of monoamine oxidase in man by furazolidone, *Clin. Pharmacol. Therap.,* **9**:442-447, 1968.
153. Pletscher, A., Gey, K. F., and Zeller, P.: Monoamine oxidasehemmer. Biochemie, Chemie, Pharmacologie, Klinik, *Prog. Drug. Res.,* **2**:417-459, 1960.
154. Plummer, A. J., Maxwell, R. A., and Earl, A. E.: The influence of ritalin (methylphenidate) on the behavioral and circulatory effects of reserpine, *Schweiz. Acad. Wochem.,* **14**:39-51, 1957.
155. Povalski, H. J. and Goldsmith, E. D.: Effect of methylphenidate on cardiovascular actions of pressor amines, *Proc. Soc. Exp. Biol. Med.,* **101**:717-721, 1959.

156. Price, K. and Smith, S. E.: Cheese reaction and tyramine, *Lancet,* **1**:130-131, 1971.
157. Rao, A. V.: Imipramine-induced auricular fibrillation, *J. Indian Med. Assoc.,* **47**:36, 1966.
158. Rasmussen, J.: Amitriptyline and imipramine poisoning, *Lancet,* **2**:850-851, 1965.
159. Robson, R. D.: Modification of the cardiovascular effects of L-dopa in anesthetized dogs by inhibition of enzymes involved in catecholamine metabolism, *Circ. Res.,* **28**:662-669, 1971.
160. Robson, R. D., Antonaccio, M. J., and Fehn, P.: The cardiovascular pharmacology of neuroleptics, in Fielding, S. and Lal, H. (eds.) *Industrial Pharmacology. Neuroleptics,* Futura Publishing Company, New York, 1974.
161. Ross, S. B., Renzi, A. L., and Ogren, S. O.: Inhibition of the uptake of noradrenaline and 5-hydroxytryptamine by chlorphentermine and chlorimipramine, *Europ. J. Pharmacol.,* **17**:107-112, 1972.
162. Russek, H. I.: Monoamine oxidase inhibitors in the treatment of angina pectoris, *Angiology,* **11**:76-80, 1960.
163. Ryall, R. W.: Effects of cocaine and antidepressant drugs on the nictitating membrane of the cat, *Brit. J. Pharmacol.,* **17**:331-357, 1961.
164. Sacks, M. H., Bonforte, R., Lasser, R., and Dimick, I.: Cardiovascular complications of imipramine intoxication, *J. Amer. Med. Assoc.,* **205**:580-590, 1968.
165. Schaeppi, U.: Die beinflüssung der reizübertragung in peripheren sympathicus durch tofranil, *Helv. Physiol. Pharmacol. Acta.,* **18**:545-562, 1960.
166. Schaepke, H. G. and Wiegand, R. G.: Relation between norepinephrine accumulation or depletion and blood pressure responses in the cat and rat following pargyline administration, *Ann. N.Y. Acad. Sci.,* **107**:924-934, 1963.
167. Scriabine, A.: Some observations on the adrenergic blocking activity of desipramine and amitriptyline on aortic strips of rabbits, *Experientia,* **25**:164-165, 1969.
168. Shafi'ee, A. and Hite, G.: The absolute configuration of the pheniramines, methylphenidates and pipradols, *J. Med. Chem.,* **12**:260-270, 1969.
169. Shaskan, E. G. and Snyder, S. H.: Kinetics of serotonin accumulation into slices from rat brain: relationship to catecholamine uptake, *J. Pharmacol. Exp. Ther.,* **175**:404-418, 1970.
170. Shoshkes, M., Rothfeld, E. L., Becker, M. C., Finkelstein, A., Smith, C. C., and Wachtel, F. W.: Iproniazid in angina pectoris. A double-blind study, *Circulation,* **20**:17-24, 1959.
171. Sigg, E. B.: Pharmacological studies with Tofranil, *Am. Psychiat. Assoc., J.,* **4**:575-583, 1959.
172. Sigg, E. B., Osborne, M., and Koral, B.: Cardiovascular effects of imipramine, *J. Pharmacol. Exp. Ther.,* **141**:237-243, 1963.
173. Sigg, E. B., Soffer, L., and Gyermek, L.: Influence of imipramine and related psychoactive agents on the effect of 5-hydroxytryptamine and catecholamines on the cat nictitating membrane, *J. Pharmacol. Expt. Ther.,* **142**:13-20, 1963.
174. Smith, C. B.: The role of monoamine oxidase in the intraneuronal metabolism of norepinephrine released by indirectly acting sym-

pathomimetic amines or by adrenergic nerve stimulation, *J. Pharmacol. Exp. Ther.,* **51**:207-220, 1966.

175. Spector, S., Shore, P. A., and Brodie, B. B.: Biochemical and pharmacological effects of the monoamine oxidase inhibitors, iproniazid, 1-phenyl-2-hydroazinopropane (JB-516) and 1-phenyl-3-hydrazino butane (JB-835), *J. Pharmacol. Expt. Ther.,* **128**:15-21, 1960.
176. Steinberg, M. and Smith, C. B.: Uptake, retention and metabolism of H^3-tyramine in rat atria, *J. Pharmacol. Exp. Ther.,* **176**:139-148, 1971.
177. Stone, C. A., Porter, C. C., and Vernier, V. G.: Some autonomic properties of aminethylene, a new antidepressant, *Fed. Proc.,* **22**:627, 1963.
178. Sueblinvong, V. and Wilson, J. F.: Myocardial damage due to imipramine intoxication, *J. Pediat.,* **74**:475-478, 1969.
179. Sulser, F., Bickel, M. H., and Brodie, B. B.: An action of desmethylimipramine in counteracting sedation and cholinergic effects of reserpine, *J. Pharmacol. Expt. Ther.,* **144**:321-330, 1964.
180. Svihovecova, P. and Svihovec, J.: Mechanism of catecholamine potentiation by dibenzazepines and cocaine. *Proc. Can. Fed. Bio. Soc.,* **10**:159, 1967.
181. Toda, N.: Influence of cocaine and desipramine on the contractile response of isolated rabbit pulmonary arteries and aortae to transmural stimulation, *J. Pharmacol. Exp. Ther.,* **179**:198-206, 1971.
182. Towers, M. D. and Wood, P.: Use of iproniazid in ischaemic angina pectoris, *Brit. Med. J.,* **2**:1067-1068, 1958.
183. Turker, R. K. and Khairallah, P. A.: Desmethylimipramine (desipramine), an adrenergic blocking agent, *Experientia,* **23**:252, 1967.
184. Ursillo, R. C. and Jacobson, J.: Potentiation of norepinephrine in the isolated vas deferens of the rat by some CNS stimulants and antidepressants, *J. Pharmacol. Exp. Ther.,* **148**:247-251, 1965.
185. Wilbraudt, W. and Rosenberg, T.: The concept of cardiac transport and its corollaries in pharmacology, *Pharmacol. Rev.,* **13**:109-183, 1961.
186. Williams, R. B., Jr. and Sherter, C.: Cardiac complications of tricyclic antidepressant therapy, *Am. Int. Med.,* **74**:395-398, 1971.

9

Toxicology of the Antidepressant Agents

STEVEN L. MALISH, PH.D. and
THEODORE O. KING, PH.D.

I. INTRODUCTION

The preclinical safety assessment of all new drugs in animals is designed to detect toxic hazards which may define the risk of administering such agents to man. The toxicological evaluation of these new drugs must follow general Food and Drug Administration (FDA) guidelines for preclinical testing (Table I). Safety testing must be consistent with the length of drug administration in man (12) and therefore must include acute, subacute, and chronic toxicity studies. In addition, since 1966, the FDA has required teratological studies for all drugs which may be administered to women of child bearing age. Carcinogenicity testing in rodents has also become important in evaluating chronic use drugs and, in many laboratories, mutagenicity testing is receiving considerable attention.

Since 1958 two distinct classes of drugs have become available for the treatment of mental depression. These classes are the monoamine oxidase inhibitors (MAOIs) and the tricyclic compounds. The MAOIs have declined in use partly because of many drug and food interactions which are frequently encountered. The tricyclic antidepressant agents have, on the other hand, increased in popularity and in 1972 accounted for 14% of the leading 200 drugs, equivalent to 20.3 million prescription (3) (Table II).

II. HISTORY OF ANTIDEPRESSANT AGENTS

In 1951 iproniazid was introduced for the treatment of tuberculosis and was found to have a pronounced euphoric effect in some patients. This phenomenon was subsequently related to monoamine oxidase inhibition and to excitation in animals. In

TABLE I
General FDA Guidelines for Animal Toxicity Studies*

Category	Duration of Human Administration	Phase[1]	Subacute or Chronic Toxicity[2]	Observations	Special Studies
Oral or Parenteral	Several days	I, II, III, NDA	2 species, 2 weeks	Body weights, food consumption, behavior, hemogram, coagulation tests, liver and kidney function tests, fasting blood sugar, ophthalmological examination, metabolic studies, gross and microscopic examination, others as appropriate.	For parenterally administered drugs; irritation studies, compatibility with blood where applicable.
	Up to 2 weeks	I	2 species, 2 weeks		
		II	2 species, up to 4 weeks		
		III, NDA	2 species, up to 3 months		
	Up to 3 months	I, II	2 species, 4 weeks		
		III	2 species, 3 months		
		NDA	2 species, up to 6 months		
	6 months to unlimited	I, II	2 species, 3 months		
		III	2 species, 6 months or longer		
		NDA	2 species, 12 months (nonrodent), 18 months (rodent)		

* Adapted from Goldenthal, E. I.: current views on safety evaluation of drugs, *FDA Papers,* **2**:13-18 (May) 1968.
[1] Phases I, II, and III are defined in § 130.0 of the New Drug Regulations.
[2] Acute toxicity should be determined in 3 to 4 species; subacute or chronic studies should be by route to be used clinically.

TABLE II
Tricyclic Antidepressant Drugs Most Frequently
Prescribed in 1972* +

Rank Use of All Drugs	Drug: Generic Name	Drug: Brand Name	Total No. of Prescriptions (Millions)
39	Amitriptyline hydrochloride	Elavil hydrochloride®	6.4
53	Amitriptyline hydrochloride and Perphenazine	Triavil®	5.7
198		Etrafon®	1.6
88	Imipramine hydrochloride	Tofranil®	3.8
127	Doxepin hydrochloride	Sinequan®	2.8

* Adapted from Blackwell, B.: Psychotropic drugs in use today, *JAMA*, **225**:1638, 1973.
\+ Based on figures for first 6 months.

Table 3
Monoamine Oxidase Inhibitors

Generic Name[47] Tradename (Manufacturer)	Structural Formula[47] (chemical name)	Oral Clinical Dose (mg/day)
Isocarboxazid Marplan Tablets (Roche Laboratories)	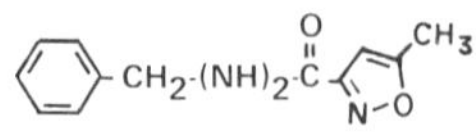 *1-Benzyl-2-(5-methyl-3-isoxazolyl-carbonyl)hydrazine*	Adults: 30 mg, as soon as clinical improvement is observed reduce to 10-20 mg daily (or less)(10)
Nialamide Niamid* (Pfizer Laboratories Division)[48]	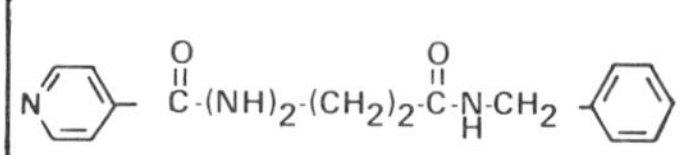 *Isonicotinic acid 2-[2-(Benzyl-carbamoyl)ethyl]hydrazide*	Adults: 75 to 100 mg; increase if necessary to 200 mg. (47)
Pargyline hydrochloride Eutonyl Tablets (Abbott Laboratories)	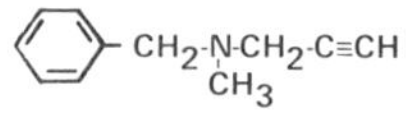 · HCl *N-Methyl-N-2-propynylbenzylamine hydrochloride*	Recommended as an antihypertensive, not as an antidepressant (10)
Phenelzine Sulfate Nardil Tablets (Warner-Chilcott)	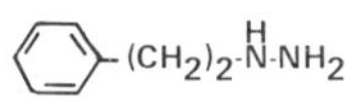 · H_2SO_4 *Phenethylhydrazine sulfate*	Adults: 45 mg; increase if necessary to 75 mg. When satisfactory response is obtained reduce to maintenance dose (10)
Tranylcypromine Sulfate Parnate Tablets (Smith Kline & French Laboratories)	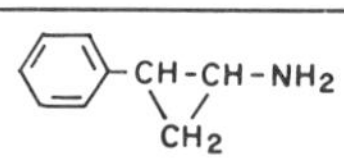 · 1/2 H_2SO_4 *trans-D,L-2-phenylcyclopropyl-amine sulfate*	Adults: 20 mg; increase if necessary to 30 mg. When satisfactory response is obtained reduce to maintenance dose (10)

1957, iproniazid, was introduced into psychiatry for the treatment of mental depression (18).

The MAOIs now available for use in the United States, are divided into the hydrazine or nonhydrazine class according to their chemical structure. The hydrazines are exemplified by isocarboxazid (Marplan®) and nialamide (Niamid®)* while the nonhydrazine MAOIs are illustrated by phenelzine sulfate (Nardil®), tranylcypromine (Parnate®) and pargyline hydrochloride (Eutonyl®) (Table III). The latter compound, while having marked MAOI properties, is not recommended as an antidepressant but rather as an antihypertensive agent (32).

In 1948, Geigy S. A. of Switzerland became interested in iminodibenzyl derivatives as possible therapeutic agents (15). Some of these compounds aroused further interest when it was shown that a structurally similar analog, chlorpromazine, was useful in psychiatry. One derivative, G-22355, later to be known as imipramine, was investigated by Kuhn in 1954. Although no

*Withdrawn from the market

chlorpromazine-like activity was found, the compound appeared to be useful in the treatment of mental depression (21). After further clinical trials, the first tricyclic antidepressant agent, imipramine hydrochloride, was introduced in Europe in 1958 (15).

III. ACUTE TOXICITY

Acute toxicity refers to the toxic effects produced by a single dose of a compound. The lethal dose of a substance is normally expressed as the LD_{50}—a calculated dose level that will kill 50% of a group of animals. Table III shows the name, manufacturer, chemical structure and the clinical dose of the monoamine oxidase inhibitors. Table IV lists the acute toxicities expressed as the LD_{50}'s in 4 species of animals. Tables V and VI present similar information concerning the tricyclic antidepressant compounds. The large variation noted in the LD_{50} in a particular species when the drug is administered by a specific route may be attributable to different experimental conditions e.g. a difference in the strain of rat, maturity of the animal, sex, concentration of drug used, etc.

A. Factors Modifying Acute Toxicity

1. Species

Differences in metabolism, in part, may account for some of the LD_{50} differences seen among species with the antidepressant compounds (Tables IV, VI). The finding that the antidepressant action of imipramine hydrochloride could be evoked in the rat, but was nct as apparent in mice and rabbits, points out the need for acute toxicity testing in more than a single species. Rats rapidly demethylate imipramine to desmethylimipramine—the active metabolite—which is then only slowly oxidized. Rabbits and mice, however, rapidly metabolize both imipramine and desmethylimpramine at about the same rate (9).

2. Strain

The LD_{50} of imipramine hydrochloride in the adult male Holtzmann rat is 682 mg/kg although it is 355 mg/kg in the adult male Charles River CD rat (13). (Table VII). This phenomenon has been seen with other drugs in several different strains and suggests that genetic constitution is an important factor in drug toxicity.

3. Sex

Orally administered imipramine hydrochloride or imipramine pamoate appear to be more toxic in female rats than in male rats.

TABLE IV
Acute Toxicities-LD_{50}-(mg/kg) of Monamine Oxidase Inhibitors

Generic Name (Route of Administration)	Species: Mouse	Rat	Monkey	Dog
Isocarboxazid (47)				
Oral	193	280	160	
Intravenous				>40
Intraperitoneal	49	199		
	190			
Subcutaneous	150			
Nialamide*				
Oral	1000 (10)	1700 (10)		≈500+
	590 (10)			
Intravenous	120 (10)			200+
Intraperitoneal	742 (10)	760 (10)		
	435 (10)			
	580 (10)			
Parglyine hydrochloride (47)				
Oral	680	250		175
Intravenous	175	175		
Intraperitoneal	370	175	150	
Phenelzine Sulfate				
Oral	156	210		
	166			
Intravenous	157			
Intraperitoneal	168			
Subcutaneous	150			
Tranylcypromine Sulfate (47)				
Oral	38			
Intravenous	37			
Intraperitoneal	130			
	91			
	41			

*Withdrawn from the market
+ Unpublished data

This effect appears to be due to differences in metabolism of the compound by the liver microsomal enzyme system (9, 38). The LD_{50} of the hydrochloride salt in the female is 305 mg/kg, versus 355 mg/kg in the male (Table VI). A more pronounced difference is noted with the pamoate salt which has an LD_{50} of 1142 mg/kg in the female compared to 1807 mg/kg in the male (Table VI). At least in rats, these facts underscore the need for acute toxicity studies in both sexes. Other common laboratory animals e.g. guinea pig and mouse that also metabolize these compounds by the microsomal enzyme system do not show this sex difference (9, 38).

TABLE V

TRICYCLIC ANTIDEPRESSANTS

Generic Name Tradename (Manufacturer)	Structural Formula (chemical name)	Usual Clinical Dose (mg/day) (Oral unless stated)
Amitriptyline hydrochloride Elavil HCl (Merck Sharpe & Dohme)[48]	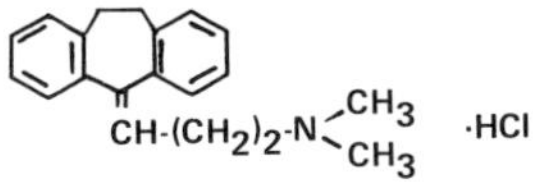 *10,11-Dihydro-N,N-dimethyl-5H-dibenzo[a,d]cycloheptent-* Δ^{5}*,gamma propylamine hydrochloride*[48]	Adults: 75 mg, increase if necessary to (→) 150 mg; Adults (hospitalized): 100 mg → 200-300; Adults (intramuscular): 80-120 mg; Adolescent/Geriatric: 30 mg plus 20 mg at bedtime[11]
Desipramine hydrochloride Pertofrane (USV Pharmaceutical Corp.) Norpramine (Lakeside Laboratories, Inc.)[48]	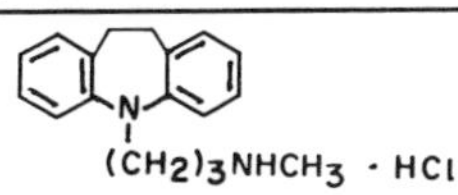 *10,11-Dihydro-5-[3-(methylamino)-propyl]-5H-dibenz[b,f]azepine hydrochloride*[48]	Adults: 150 mg → after 7-10 days to maximum of 200 mg; Adolescent/ Geriatric: 25-50 mg → 100 mg[11]
Doxepin hydrochloride Sinequan (Pfizer Laboratories Division)[11] Adapin (Pennwalt Corp.)[11]	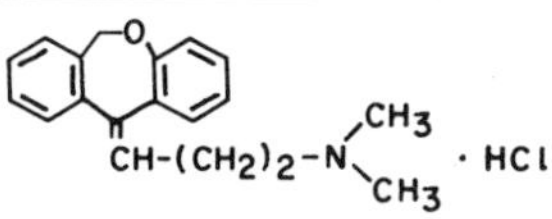 *N,N-Dimethyldibenz[b,e]oxepin-* $\Delta^{11(6H)}$*,gamma-propylamine hydrochloride*[48]	Adults: 75-150 mg – usual optimum range → to maximum of 300 mg[11]
Imipramine hydrochloride Tofranil (Geigy Pharmaceuticals) Presamine (USV Pharmaceutical Corp.)[48]	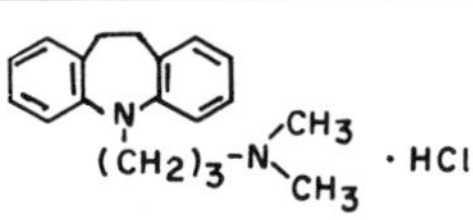 *5-[3-(Dimethylamino)propyl]-10,11-dihydro-5H-dibenz[b,f]-azepine hydrochloride*[48]	Adults (hospitalized): 100 mg → 200-300 mg; Adults (intramuscular): 100 mg; Adults (outpatients): 75 mg → 150-200 mg[11]

4. *Isolation*

Lal and Brown (23) noted a 35% increase in the LD_{50} of the hydrochloride salt of imipramine or desipramine in isolated mice compared to aggregated mice. Furthermore, clonic convulsions or death occured sooner in the aggregated group than in isolated animals. These authors speculate that aggregation provides excessive sensory stimulation to the peripheral and central nervous systems causing a large increase in the quantity of catecholamines released. Since these drugs block the normal reuptake mechanism which inactivates the catecholamines, toxicity was increased in aggregated animals.

5. *Age*

As can be seen from examination of Table VII, the tricyclic agents, like many other drugs, are more toxic to the neonate than to adult rats, the most striking example being the acute toxicity of imipramine pamoate in the Sprague-Dawley rat. While this compound has an oral LD_{50} of 251 mg/kg in 2 day old rats, the LD_{50} is

TABLE V
TRICYCLIC ANTIDEPRESSANTS (continued)

Generic Name Trademark (Manufacturer)	Structural Formula (chemical name)	Usual Clinical Dose (mg/day) (Oral unless stated)
Imipramine pamoate Tofranil-PM (Geigy Pharmaceuticals)[46]	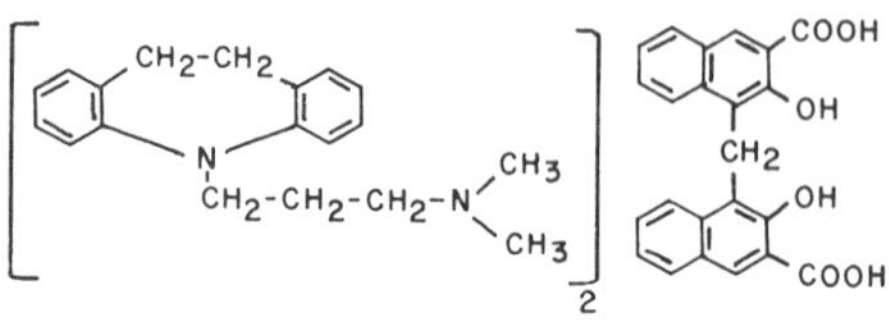 *5-[3-(Dimethylamino)propyl]-10,11-dihydro-5H-dibenz[b,f]-azepine compounds (2:1) with 4,4-methylene-bis-[3-hydroxy-2-naphthoic acid]* [46]	Same dosage as Imipramine hydrochloride [46]
Nortriptyline hydrochloride Aventyl HCl (Eli Lilly and Company)[48]	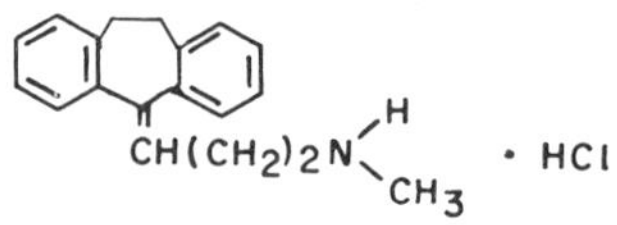 *5-[3-(Methylamino)propyl]-10,11-dihydro(5H)-dibenzo [a,d] cycloheptene hydrochloride* [48]	Adults: 75-100 mg Adolescent/Geriatric: 30-50 mg[11]
Protriptyline hydrochloride Vivactil (Merck Sharpe & Dohme)[48]	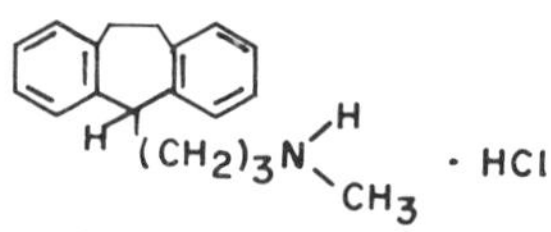 *N-Methyl-5H-dibenzo[a,d]-cycloheptene-5-propylamine hydrochloride* [48]	Adults: 15 to 40 mg → 60 mg Adolescent/Geriatric: 15 mg [11]

7500 mg/kg in the adult. The large difference in acute toxicity in the neonate versus the adult animal is probably related to the state of maturation of the enzyme systems needed to metabolize these substances.

6. Different Salt Forms

In the mouse, rat, and dog, imipramine pamoate appears to be less toxic than imipramine hydrochloride when the base equivalents of the two salts are compared (Table VI). Part of the decreased toxicity may be due to the slow and sustained release of the pamoate salt which produces a relatively constant blood level for long periods of time. This constant blood level decreases the possibility that the detoxification mechanisms will be stressed.

B. Symptomatology

Although the LD_{50} determination is useful as a basis of comparison with other compounds, an equally important finding is the acute symptomatology observed at the various dose levels together with the onset and duration of these effects.

When the hydrazine-type of MAO inhibitors, nialamide or isocarboxazid, were administered by the oral or the intraperitoneal routes to rodents, the most commonly observed signs were excitation, loss of weight, decreased respiration and depression. In dogs, both compounds produced an increase in heart and respiratory rates, an elevation of body temperature, stiffness and extension of the hind limbs, hyperesthesia, ataxia, convulsions, and death (8).

These signs may be compared with the symptomatology produced by the tricyclic compounds. Imipramine hydrochloride, depending on the dose, produced signs which progressed from depression, irregular respiration, ataxia to convulsions and death in both dogs and rats (33).

Severe ataxia and sedation were prominent in both dogs and cats given nortriptyline hydrochloride at doses of 25 mg/kg or greater. This compound, administered in doses greater than 50 mg/kg, produced signs of central nervous system (CNS) stimulation in the rat, mouse, dog and cat. Dogs given 50 or 75 mg/kg of nortriptyline hydrochloride (LD_{50} >75 mg/kg) experienced prolonged periods of tremors and short episodes of clonic convulsions. Cats administered 50 mg/kg of nortriptyline hydrochloride were noted to have tremors, emesis, and marked hyperpnea before clonic convulsions ensued (24). Mice and rats given lethal doses of nortriptyline hydrochloride showed signs of hyperexcitability and experienced convulsive seizures. This stimulation, however, was also accompanied by signs of profound CNS depression which were seen shortly after administration of a toxic dose. Rodents lost their righting reflex prior to or during convulsions and became completely prostrate before death. Narcosis was frequently seen in nonconvulsive animals and death appeared to be due to respiratory depression. Following intravenous administration of nortriptyline hydrochloride nearly all deaths occurred within the first hour. Death from subcutaneous administration were scattered throughout a 48 hour period. Most of the animals that failed to survive oral administration died within 48 hours; a few latent deaths occurred up to 5 days after the drug was given (24).

Examination of Table VIII shows the symptomatology produced when a lethal dose of either doxepin hydrochloride or amitriptyline hydrochloride was administered to mice (ICR strain), rats (Sprague-Dawley strain) or dogs (mongrel) by oral and parenteral routes. Signs of toxicity were characterized by muscle relaxation, prostration, ataxia, clonic convulsions and dyspnea. Frequently death was preceded by lacrimation, salivation and cyanosis. Emesis was observed in dogs. Local dermal changes were produced by subcutaneous administration in all species (26).

TABLE VI
Acute Toxicities-LD_{50}-(mg/kg) of Tricyclic Antidepressants

Generic Name (Route of Administration)	Species			
	Mouse	Rat	Rabbit	Dog
Amitriptyline hydrochloride				
Oral (48)	140	530		
	27			
	289			
	196			
Intravenous (48)	21	14	9.9	
	38			
Intraperitoneal (48)	76	72		
	73			
	94			
Subcutaneous (48)	328	1290		
Desipramine hydrochloride				
Oral	935 (48)	320 (13)		
	315 (48)	625 (48)		
		55		
Intravenous (48)	22	29	12	25
Intraperitoneal (48)	42	19		
	88	55		
	97			
Subcutaneous (48)	180	250		
Doxepin hydrochloride				
Oral	135 (48)	147 (48)		≈200 (9)
	148-178 (34)	346-460 (34)		

Intravenous	26 (48)	16 (47)	11 (9)	≈16 (9)
	14.6 to 19.6 (34)	12.7 to 18.8 (36)		
Intraperitoneal (48)	79	182		
Subcutaneous	720 (48)			
Imipramine hydrochloride				
Oral	666 (48)	682 (13)	400 (48)	100 to 215 (48)
		305 ♀, 355 ♂ (13)		
Intravenous (48)	35	22	18	
Intraperitoneal (48)	115	79		
Subcutaneous (48)	189	250		
Imipramine pamoate				
Oral	2185 (46)	1142 ♀ (46)	1016 (46)	693* (46)
		1807 ♂ (46)		
		7500 ♂ (13)		
Nortriptyline hydrochloride				
Oral (48)	329	503		
	275			
Intravenous (48)	28.7	22.3		
Intraperitoneal (48)				
Subcutaneous (48)	145	666		
Intramuscular (48)				>75
Protriptyline hydrochloride				
Oral	211 (13)	299 (13)	310 (48)	400 (48)
	269 (48)	480 (48)		
		720 (48)		
Intravenous (48)	37		8.2	
Intraperitoneal (48)		44		
Subcutaneous (48)	192			

*Emesis effective dose 50

TABLE VII

LD_{50} Values in Newborn and Adult Animals of some Tricyclic Antidepressants*[b]

Drug Name	Species	Strain	Age (days)	Sex	LD_{50} (mg/kg)	Route	Adult/newborn Ratio
Desipramine HCl	Rat	Charles River	1-3	-	128±10	Oral	2.5
			Adult	-	320±18		
Imipramine HCl	Rat	Charles River-CD	1-2	-	98	Oral	3.4
			Adult	M	355 (304-413)		
			Adult	F	305 (239-388)		
		Holtzman	Adult	M	682 (403-1150)		7.0
Imipramine pamoate	Rat	Sprague-Dawley	2	-	251 (199-318)	Oral	29.9
			Adult	M	7500		
Protriptyline	Rat [c]	Charles River COBS	3	-	111	Oral	2.7
			90	-	299 (256-349)		
	Mouse	Charles River COBS	3	-	86	Oral	2.5
			49	-	211 (195-228)		

* Adapted from Goldenthal, E. I. (1971). A compilation of LD_{50} values in newborn and adult animals, *Toxicol. Appl. Pharamcol.*, **18**:185-207, 1968.

b The species, strain and route of administration are the same for adult and newborn animals for each drug unless otherwise indicated.

c LD_{50}'s performed concurrently.

TABLE VIII
Main Symptoms Observed Following Administration of a Lethal Dose of Doxepin Hydrochloride or Amitriptyline Hydrochloride in the Mouse, Rat and Dog.*

			Time Post Dose			
Compound	Route	Species	Onset	Duration	Maximum Death	Main Symptoms
Doxepin hydrochloride	Oral	Mouse	5 min	within 16 hr	15-30 min	Depression, Ataxia, Muscular Relaxation, Clonic Convulsion, Loss of Righting Reflex, Dyspnea, Emesis (Dog), Vomiting (Dog), Lacrimation (Mouse, Rat), Salivation (Mouse, Rat)
		Rat	5 min	24-48 hr	15-30 min	
		Dog	10-20 min	48 hr	6 hr	
	Intravenous	Mouse	immediately after dosing	within 16 hr	1-3 min	Ataxia, Straub Tail, Clonic Convulsion, Opisthotonos, Prostration
		Rat	immediately after dosing	within 16 hr	2-5 min	
	Intraperitoneal	Mouse	1-2 min	within 16 hr	10-15 min	Ataxia, Muscular Relaxation, Clonic Convulsion, Prostration
		Rat	1-2 min	within 16 hr	10-15 min	
	Subcutaneous	Mouse	10 min	16-24 hr	5-16 hr	Depression, Ataxia, Muscular Relaxation, Clonic Convulsion, Salivation, Prostration, Cyanosis, Loss of Righting Reflex, Lacrimation, Local Dermal Change
		Rat	10 min	48-72 hr	24-48 hr	
Amitriptyline hydrochloride	Oral	Mouse	3-5 min	within 20 hr	30 min.-1 hr	Depression, Ataxia, Muscular Relaxation, Clonic Convulsion, Loss of Righting Reflex, Dyspnea, Emesis (Dog), Vomiting (Dog), Lacrimation (Mouse, Rat), Salivation (Mouse, Rat)
		Rat	2-3 min	24-48 hr	18-20 hr	
		Dog	2-5 min	48 hr	8 hr	
	Intravenous	Mouse	immediately after dosing	within 16 hr	1-3 min	Ataxia, Straub Tail, Clonic Convulsion, Opisthotonos, Prostration
	Subcutaneous	Mouse	10 min	24-48 hr	5-16 hr	Depression, Ataxia, Muscular Relaxation, Clonic Convulsion, Salivation, Prostration, Cyanosis, Loss of Righting Reflex, Lacrimation, Local Dermal Change

* from Noguchi, Y., Sakai, T., Ishiko, J., and Suginoto, S.: Acute toxicity of doxepin hydrochloride, *Pharmacometrics*, **6**:889-897, 1972.

C. Cardiovascular Effects

In animals and in man the tricyclic agents have been associated with various cardiac abnormalities.

In dogs, low doses of imipramine hydrochloride have an anticholinergic and/or direct sympathetic action which produces an increased heart rate (5, 44). Higher dose levels (2-5 mg/kg, i.v.), however, decrease myocardial contractility, heart rate and coronary blood flow. Imipramine hydrochloride (1-8 mg/kg) injected intravenously into anesthetized dogs also lowers the blood pressure (44).

Desipramine hydrochloride was infused at a dose of 0.5 mg/kg/min for a total of 25 mg/kg in anesthetized mongrel dogs (22). An initial sympathomimetic effect was observed which was followed by a depression of contractile force with a lowering of blood pressure. A prolongation of the P-R interval and QRS complex was also noted. Ventricular ectopic beats and multifocal ventricular tachycardia were observed in some experiments. The drug was withdrawn when the contractile force was depressed by 66% of control values, but the myocardial depression was not reversed and proceeded to complete cardiac arrest (22). Scharer (41) noted varying degrees of conduction defects which were characterized as atrioventricular or bundle branch blocks or both. These changes, however, appeared reversible. The same cardiac changes were noted in experimental amitriptyline poisoning in guinea pigs (4). Nymark and Rassmussen (29) observed electrocardiographic changes in rabbits administered 50 mg/kg of amitriptyline intraperitoneally. The time interval between the injection and the first changes varied between 3 and 10 minutes and the duration of these effects was never less than one hour. The electrocardiographic changes may have resulted from a shift in the autonomic balance toward adrenergic dominance.

In humans, cardiac effects have been associated with imipramine, desipramine and amitriptyline after excessive doses were given. Congestive heart failure has been produced or aggravated and acute myocardial infarction has occurred. Electrocardiographic abnormalities, congestive heart failure and myocardial infarction seem to occur more frequently with imipramine hydrochloride, while sinus tachycardia, rather than arrhythmias, are more commonly associated with amitriptyline (6, 20. 45).

IV. LONG TERM TOXICITY

Two main goals are important in long term toxicity testing—the observation of toxicity, and the determination of the highest dose that will produce minimal or no toxic effects. This "*no effect level*" allows an estimation of the *safety margin* of the drug—that being the ratio of the maximum chronically tolerated dose to the therapeutic dose as determined during the pharmacological evaluation.

The results of the toxicology testing serve as a guide to the physician involved in clinical studies of a new drug. The toxic signs and altered clinical parameters observed in animals, hopefully, will alert the investigator to make appropriate observations.

A. Tricyclic Agents

1. *Subacute Toxicity*

Doxepin hydrochloride was administered orally to SPF Sprague-Dawley rats of both sexes at dose levels of 25, 50, 100 and 200 mg/kg/day for 33 days. All males and 10 of 12 females died at the 200 mg/kg/day dose level, while 2 of 11 males and 5 of 11 females died at the 100 mg/kg/day level. At the 50 mg/kg/day level 1 of 9 males also died. A decrease in body weight gain was observed in the two higher dose level groups. However, there were no adverse changes in food consumption, urinalysis, hematology, clinical chemistry or in gross or histopathology at any dose level (27).

In a similar study, amitriptyline hydrochloride administered orally to SPF Sprague-Dawley rats at a dose level of 100 mg/kg/day produced death in 3 of 7 animals within one month. At necropsy the livers of these animals showed hydropic degeneration or focal cytoplasmic degeneration associated with nuclear pyknosis (29).

2. *Chronic Toxicity*

Sprague-Dawley (SPF) rats were administered doxepin hydrochloride by oral intubation for 180 days at dose levels of 5, 10, 20, 40 or 80 mg/kg//day. No adverse effects were found at the three lowest dosage levels. The higher dosage levels (80 mg/kg/day both sexes, 40 mg/kg/day in males) caused decreases in weight gain but no deaths. There were no adverse effects on hematology, urinalysis, clinical chemistry or food consumption and no abnormalities were noticed in the gross or microscopic pathology (25).

Other long term studies were conducted with Charles River CD rats. These animals received doxepin hydrochloride in the feed at dose levels of 5, 25, 50 and 100 mg/kg/day for 12-18 months. At the two highest dose levels males developed fatty metamorphosis of the liver, a condition that did not occur in the female (1, 36). Similar changes have also been seen in rats given amitriptyline hydrochloride at a dose level of 100 mg/kg/day (unpublished data).

Doxepin hydrochloride was also administered to dogs at dose levels of 5, 25 and 50 mg/kg/day for 1 year. At the 5 mg/kg/day level dogs were practically asymptomatic, but slight emesis, tremors, ptosis, sedation and twitching occurred at the higher dose levels. There were no abnormal laboratory values or histopathological changes attributable to the drug (1, 34).

Meyers et al (24) administered nortriptyline hydrochloride subcutaneously to Wistar rats at dose levels of 2, 5, 10 and 20 mg/kg/day for 246 days. The 246-day mean body weight curves showed a slight growth retardation in the males that received 20 mg/kg/day of the drug, but in all groups weight gains were within normal limits. Dose related declines in hematocrits, hemoglobins and red blood cell counts were also noted, although these values remained within accepted physiologic limits. Tissue changes, except for ulceration at the injection site, were not observed.

Rats of the Harlan strain were administered nortriptyline hydrochloride in medicated feed at dose levels of 0.015, 0.03, 0.075 and 0.15% of diet for approximately 54 weeks. A dose related retardation in weight gain was noted at the 0.075 and 0.15% levels and the efficiency of food utilization was markedly lowered in both sexes at the highest dose level. Hematology parameters were considered to be within the normal range. The only changes in organ weights were apparent increases in the relative weights of the adrenals, thyroids and ovaries of the female rats receiving the diet containing the highest dose level. Very slight to moderate fatty degenerative changes were seen in some of the liver and kidney sections of both control and treated rats (24).

Dogs were given daily oral doses of 5, 10, 20 or 40 mg/kg of nortriptyline hydrochloride by capsule for 1 year. Three of the 4 dogs at the 40 mg/kg/day level died during the first week of study, and the fourth animal died on the 27th day, following a series of convulsive seizures. The animals that died during the first week showed vomiting, mydriasis, ataxia, and occasional clonic convulsions prior to death. One of the animals that died during the first week showed slight metamorphosis of the liver, mild pyelonephritis, pulmonary vascular congestion and edema. Generally abnormalities were not evident in animals receiving 20 mg/day or less of the drug (24).

Imipramine pamoate administered orally to dogs at 90 mg/kg/day (10 times the maximum human dose) for 3 months produced histological changes in the testes. These findings ranged from degeneration to complete atrophy of the seminiferous tubules with cessation of spermatogenesis. Imipramine paomate, however, administered to rats at the same dose level, was noted to be free of deleterious effects on the testes (46). No effects on the testes has been reported in man.

3. Anticholinergic Effects

The anticholinergic actions of the tricylic compounds in human medicine are frequently the cause of side effects such as urinary retention, constipation, and paralytic ileus, and has also been associated with blurred vision and glaucoma (2, 40).

In patients known to be predisposed to acute narrow angle glaucoma, anticholinergic drugs constitute a risk that is proportional to their effect in dilating the pupil (14). In this regard, mydriasis has been observed in reserpine-treated mice given the hydrochloride salts of imipramine, desmethylimipramine or amitriptyline (16). Amitriptyline was found to be the most potent agent producing pupillary dilatation while desmethylimipramine was the least potent (16). Mydriatic effects were also noted with doxepin hydrochloride in mice (43).

4. Withdrawal Syndrome

Abrupt cessation of imipramine hydrochloride treatment (and possibly other tricyclic agents) in man has produced a withdrawal syndrome characterized by mild to marked symptoms such as nausea, headache, fatigue, cramps, restlessness, insomnia and irritability (42). This symptomatology has not been reproduced in animals with the hydrochloride salts of doxepin or amitriptyline. Administration of the hydrochloride salts of doxepin or amitriptyline to beagle dogs at doses of 6, 25 and 50 mg/kg/day and 25 and 50 mg/kg/day, respectively, did not produce evidence of withdrawal after 120 to 132 days of treatment (28). Furthermore, no withdrawal symptoms occurred in either mice or rats forced to drink a doxepin hydrochloride solution for 30 days (19).

5. Reproductive Studies

Imipramine hydrochloride was found capable of inducing abnormal fetal development in rabbits when administered subcutaneously at 30 mg/kg. However, this result was attributed to a maternal toxicity. Lower parenteral doses (5 and 15 mg/kg) did not produce a teratogenic effect although embryotoxicity (reduced litter size, etc.) was noted. Oral doses of 5 and 15 mg/kg were without any significant effect (17).

In the mouse, repeated oral and parenteral doses of 150 and 40 mg/kg, respectively, were without significant effect (17).

When rats were fed imipramine hydrochloride in medicated feed at 5 and 15 mg/kg a small reduction in litter size and an increased loss of young during rearing were observed. The latter response was probably due to a drug effect on the dam (17).

Imipramine pamoate when fed to albino rats of both sexes for 28 weeks at dose levels of 15 and 40 mg/kg through two breeding cycles produced no teratogenic effects. The only changes noted were a decrease in the mean litter size and growth suppression in the nursing pups of both sexes at the high dose level and in the females at the low dose level. Furthermore, the lactation index (ratio of the number of pups weaned divided by the number left to nurse) was lower in the second litter of the high dose group (46).

Nortriptyline hydrochloride was administered to rats of both sexes in medicated feed at dose levels of 0.015% and 0.03% for 61 days. The animals were followed through two breeding cycles. The only changes seen were at the high dose level where a depressed viability index (percentage of young surviving 4 or more days) was evident in the first litter (25).

Doxepin hydrochloride administered orally to Sprague-Dawley—JCL rats at 10, 30, 90 or 270 mg/kg/day from 9 to day 14 of gestation was without teratogenic effect. Maternal and fetal toxicity were noted at the two higher dose levels (15 and 45 times the maximum human dose) (30). Other reports indicate that doxepin hydrochloride, administered orally to Japanese white rabbits at dose levels of 5, 25 or 100 mg/kg/day from day 8 to day 16 of gestation produced no maternal toxicity or teratogenic effects. However, at the highest dose level a significantly increased fetal mortality was observed, and at all dose levels the drug produced delayed ossification of the fifth sternebrae together with an increased likelihood of the absence of the 13th rib (31). These effects are evidence of delayed development rather than of teratogenesis.

B. Monoamine Oxidase Inhibitors

1. Subacute Toxicity

Daily intraperitoneal injections of pargyline hydrochloride administered at 75 mg/kg to Sprague-Dawley rats for 7 days produced necrosis and myopathic changes in skeletal muscle. These changes were characterized by grouped lesions, excess connective tissue, and a sarcoplasmic fluorescence indicative of monoamine accumulation. Histopathologically, the lesions were similar to those seen in Duchenne muscular dystrophy (49). No evidence was presented concerning recovery or reversibility of this lesion.

Further studies will be required to elucidate the significance of these findings.

2. Chronic Toxicity

Male and female weanling rats were fed diets containing 3, 10, 30, 100 and 300 mg/kg/day of nialamide for 26 weeks. Except for a severe growth depression seen in both sexes at the 300 mg/kg/day dose level no other changes were noted (8).

Mongrel dogs were administered nialamide orally at dose levels of 3, 10, 30 and 60 mg/kg 6 days a week for 6 months. The only toxic effect observed was a non-progressive mild hypochromic anemia characterized by a reduction in the red cell count and hemoglobin levels (8).

Monkeys, orally treated with nialamide at 10, 25 and 50 mg/kg/day for 3 months, also showed a slight reduction in hemoglobin and red cell counts at the highest dose level (8).

The hydrazine-type MAOIs have been reported to produce liver damage in man in the form of drug-induced hepatitis. Iproniazid was frequently implicated in this regard (1 in 5000 patients) and has since been withdrawn from the market. Other reports, however, have indicated a lower incidence of this condition (7).

Drug-induced hepatitis cannot in most cases be reproduced in animals. This fact, together with the relatively low incidence in man indicates that these agents are not intrinsic hepatotoxins but may exert their toxic effects through either a metabolic defect or an allergic response (39, 50).

When iproniazid was administered orally at a dose level of 50 mg/kg/day to dogs, a drug-induced acute toxic hepatitis developed in about one week in 18/20 animals (8). In another study, Popper noted that pretreatment of the rat with iproniazid will not produce hepatic changes, but will enhance liver necrosis induced by the hepatotoxin, carbon tetrachloride (35).

3. Reproductive Studies

The effects of a number of MAOIs were investigated with respect to their ability to prevent pregnancy in mice. All compounds were given a non-toxic dose, subcutaneously on either days 1 to 3, 1 to 6, 4 to 7, 7 to 11, or 11 to 16 of gestation. Iproniazid, at a dose of 5 mg/kg/day interrupted some of the pregnancies or prevented nidation when administered on days 1 to 6, 4 to 7 and 6 to 11, the most marked effect being on days 6 to 11 where no pregnancies were found (36). Nialamide given at 4 mg/kg/day on days 1 to 6, 6 to 11 and 11 to 16 produced a depression of litter size during the first two time periods. Phenelzine given at 25 mg/kg on days 1 to 6 also reduced litter size (36, 37). In contrast, the non-hydrazine MAOI, tranylcypromine administered at dose level of 38.5 mg/kg produced no effect on pregnancy during any time period (36).

CONCLUSIONS

The toxicological evaluation of both the MAOIs and the tricyclic agents have shown that these compounds have a relatively low order of toxicity. Moreover, clinically, these drugs have also proved to be relatively safe when used in the recommended quantities.

It should be noted, howver, that with any drug, a small percentage of individuals may have an allergic response or a metabolic defect that will result in toxic effects. These problems usually cannot be predicted from the standard toxicological tests.

REFERENCES

1. Avery, G. S.: Doxepin: A review, *Drugs,* **1**:194-227, 1971.
2. Belfer, M. L. and Shader, R. I.: Autonomic effects (Chapter 13), *in* Shader, R. I. and DiMuscio, A. editors: *Psychotropic Drug Side Effects,* The Williams & Wilkins Co., Baltimore, 1970, pp. 116-123.
3. Blackwell, B.: Psychotropic drugs in use today, *JAMA,* **225**:1637-1641, 1973.
4. Boissier, J. R., Simon, P., and Witchitz, S.: Étude chez le cobaye de la toxicité cardiaque de l' imipramine, de l' amitriptyline et de leurs dérivés monodesyméthylés, *Thérapie,* **20**:67-75, 1965.
5. Cairncross, K. E. and Gershon, S.: A pharmacological basis for the cardiovascular complications of imipramine intoxication, *Med. J. Aust.,* **49**:373, 1962.
6. Crocker, J. and Morton, B.: Tricyclic (antidepressant) drug toxicity, *Clin. Toxicol.,* **2**:397-401, 1969.
7. D'Arcy, P. F. and Griffin, J. P.: *Iatrogenic Diseases,* Oxford University Press, London, 1972, p. 81.
8. Delahunt, C. S. and Pepin, J. M.: Toxicology of nialamide, a new psychotherapeutic agent, *Toxicol. Appl. Pharmacol.,* **1**:524-533, 1959.
9. Dingell, J. V., Sulser, F., and Gillette, J. P.: Species differences in the metabolism of imipramine and desmethylimipramine (DMI), *J. Pharmacol. Exp. Ther.,* **143**:14-22, 1964.
10. *Facts and Comparisons,* Facts and Comparisons, Inc., St. Louis, Missouri, 1972, Isocarboxazid, p. 260, Pargyline hydrochloride, p. 170, Phenelzine Sulfate p. 170b, Tranylcypromine p. 260 h.
11. *Facts and Comparisons,* Facts and Comparisons, Inc., St. Louis, Missouri, 1972, Amitriptyline hydrochloride p. 260a, Nortriptyline hydrochloride p. 260, Protriptyline hydrochloride p. 260c, Desipramine hydrochloride p. 260c, Doxepin hydrochloride pp. 260, 523.
12. Goldenthal, E. I.: Current views on safety evaluation of drugs, *FDA Papers,* **2**:14-18, 1968.

13. Goldenthal, E. I.: A compilation of LD_{50} values in newborn and adult animals, *Toxicol. Appl. Pharmacol.*, **18**:185-207, 1968.
14. Grant, W. M.: Ocular complications of drugs, *JAMA*, **207**:2089-2091, 1969.
15. Hafliger, F.: Chemistry of tofranil, *Canad. Psychiatr. Assoc. J.*, **4**:S-69-S-74, 1959.
16. Halliwell, G., Quinton, R. M., and Williams, F. E.: A comparison of imipramine, chlorpromazine and related drugs in various tests involving autonomic functions and antagonism of reserpine, *Brit. J. Pharmacol.*, **23**:330-350, 1964.
17. Harper, K. H., Palmer, A. K., and Davies, R. E.: Effect of imipramine upon the pregnancy of laboratory animals, *Arzneim. Forsch.*, **15**:1218-1221, 1965.
18. Jarvik, M. E.: Drugs used in the treatment of psychiatric disorders (Chapter 12), *in* Goodman, L. S. and Gilman, A., editors: *The Pharmacological Basis of Therapeutics*, 3d ed. The Macmillan Co., New York, 1965, pp. 191-198.
19. Kaneto, H., Masao, K., and Tsuchie, F.: Studies on tolerance and physical dependence liability of doxepin, *Folia. Pharmacol. Jap.*, **68**:704-715, 1972.
20. Kristiansen, E. S.: Cardiac complications during treatment with imipramine (tofranil), *Acta Psychiatr. Neurol. Scand.*, **36**:427-441, 1961.
21. Kuhn, R.: The treatment of depressive states with G-22355 (imipramine hydrochloride), *Am. J. Psychiatry*, **115**:459-464, 1958.
22. Laddu, A. R. and Somani, P.: Desipramine toxicity and its treatment, *Toxicol. Appl. Pharmacol.*, **15**:287-294, 1969.
23. Lal, H. and Brown, R. M.: Enhanced toxicity of imipramine and desipramine in aggregated mice, *J. Pharm. Pharmacol.*, **20**:581-582, 1968.
24. Meyers, D. B., Small, R. M., and Anderson, R. C.: Toxicology of nortriptyline hydrochloride, *Toxicol. Appl. Pharmacol.*, **9**:152-159, 1966.
25. Noguchi, Y., Sakai, T., Ishiko, J., and Suginoto, S.: Acute toxicity of doxepin hydrochloride, *Pharmacometrics*, **6**:889-897, 1972.
26. Noguchi, Y., Sakai, J., Arakawa, M., and Nabata, H.: Subacute toxicity of doxepin hydrochloride in rats, *Pharmacometrics*, **6**:899-928, 1972.
27. Noguchi, Y., Sakai, J., Arakawa, M., and Nabata, H.: Chronic toxicity of doxepin hydrochloride in rats, *Pharmacometrics*, **6**:929-954, 1972.
28. Noguchi, Y., Sugmimot, S., and Sawada, Y.: Physical dependence test of doxepin hydrochloride in beagle dogs, *Pharmacometrics*, **6**:1243-1254, 1972.
29. Nymark, M. and Rasmussen, J.: Effect of certain drugs upon amitriptyline induced electrocardiographic changes, *Acta Pharmacol. Toxicol.*, **24**:148-156, 1966.
30. Owaki, Y., Momiyama, H., and Onodera, N.: Effects of doxepin hydrochloride administered to pregnant rats upon the fetus and their postnatal development, *Pharmacometrics*, **5**:913-924, 1971.
31. Owaki, Y., Momiyana, H., and Onodera, N.: Effects of doxepin hydrochloride administered to pregnant rabbits upon the fetuses, *Pharmacometrics*, **5**:905-912, 1971.
32. *Physicians' Desk Reference*, 27th ed., Medical Economics Co., Oradell, N. J., 1973, p. 513.

33. *Physicians' Desk References,* 27th ed. Medical Economics Co., Oradell, N. J., 1973, p. 765-766.
34. *Physicians' Desk Reference,* 27th ed. Medical Economics Co., Oradell, N. J., 1973, p. 1106.
35. Popper, H.: Hepatic injury in patients who had received iproniazid, *Ann. N.Y. Acad. Sci.,* **80**:551-1045, 1959.
36. Poulson, E. and Robson, J. M.: The effect of amine oxidase inhibitors on pregnancy, *J. Endocrincol.,* **27**:147-152, 1963.
37. Poulson, E. and Robson, J. M.: Effect of phenelzine and some related compounds on pregnancy and on sexual development, *J. Endocrincol.,* **30**:205-215, 1964.
38. Quinn, G. P., Axelrod, J., and Brodie, B. B.: Species, strain and sex differences in metabolism of hexobarbitone, aminopyrine, antipyrine and aniline, *Biochem. Pharmacol.,* **1**:152-159, 1958.
39. Randolph, H. and Joseph, S.: Toxic hepatitis with jaundice occurring in a patient treated with isoniazid, *JAMA,* **152**:38-40, 1953.
40. Rosselet, E.: Misuse of psychotropics blamed for increase in eye disorders, *Psychiatr. News.,* **3**:3, 1968.
41. Scharer, K.: Toxizitätsstudie mit amitriptylin, *Schweiz. Med. Wochschr.,* **95**:173-176, 1965.
42. Shaton, C.: Withdrawal symptoms after abrupt termination of imipramine *Canad. Psychiatr. Assoc.,* **11**:S150-S158, 1966.
43. Schaumann, W. and Ribbentrop, A.: Interference of central anticholinergic action in animal experiments testing of potential antidepressive drugs, *Arzneim. Forsch.,* **16**:646-649, 1966.
44. Sigg, E. B., Osborne, M., and Koed, B.: Cardiovascular effects of imipramine, *J. Pharmacol. Exp. Ther.,* **141**:237-243, 1963.
45. Sloman, L.: Myocardial infarction during imipramine treatment of depression, *Canad. Med. Assoc. J.,* **82**:20-22, 1960.
46. Tofranil PM (Package insert), Geigy Pharmaceuticals, Division of Ciba-Geigy Corp., Ardsley, New York, 1973.
47. Usdin, E. and Efron, D. H.: *Psychotropic Drugs and Related Compounds,* 2nd ed., DHEW Publication, No(HSM), 72-9074, 1972, Isocarboxazid p. 240, Nialamide p. 269, Pargyline hydrochloride p. 401, Tranylcypromine sulfate p. 359.
48. Usdin, E. and Efron, D. H.: *Psychotropic Drugs and Related Compounds,* 2nd ed., DHEW Publication, No(HSM), 72-9074, 1972. Amitriptyline hydrochloride p. 60, Nortriptyline hydrochloride p. 83, Protriptyline hydrochloride p. 83, Imipramine hydrochloride p. 78, Desipramine hydrochloride p. 70.
49. Yu, M. K., Wright, T. L., Dettbarn, W. D., and Olson, W. H.: Pargyline-induced myopathy with histochemical characteristics of duchenne muscular dystrophy, *Neurology,* **24**:237-244, 1974.
50. Zimmerman, H. J.: Drug-induced hepatic injury, *in* Salinter M., editor: *Hypersensitivity to Drugs,* Pergamon Press, Oxford and New York, 1972.

10

Absorption, Distribution, Excretion, and Metabolism of Antidepressants

CLAUDE I. JUDD, PH.D. and
RICHARD C. URSILLO, PH.D.

I. METHODOLOGICAL CONSIDERATIONS

Studies concerned with the absorption, metabolism, and excretion of investigational drugs play an important role in the new drug development process. The initial concern should be the elaboration of the proper information for the safe and rational use of the drug in man. To this end it is obviously ideal, though not always possible, to gain a thorough knowledge of the metabolic disposition of a therapeutic agent in a species in which the compound is handled in a manner similar to the human. Since this cannot be predicted, metabolism data during preclinical studies are usually gathered in the rat, dog, and often in the primate as well. These studies also serve to complement the preclinical toxicological studies which are traditionally done in these species. The data collected in the initial studies consist of absorption, tissue distribution, excretion, plasma level, and some estimate of plasma elimination curves. With the development of some similar data in man during Phase I clinical studies the investigators are in a more secure position to relate animal pharmacological and toxicological data to plasma levels and to make some reasonable estimates of safe human doses and frequency of administration. These data also serve as the basis for selection of animal species for chronic toxicological study.

The ever increasing availability of radioactive intermediates makes possible the economic synthesis of carbon-14 or tritium labelled compound of high specific activity. Thus the initial information generated is most conveniently done with radio-labelled compound administered usually at a level below 100 μc. The dose of total compound should, in the first studies, relate to the pharmacological dose. Collection of 24-hour urine and fecal output over a period of 5 days and frequent blood samples from the large animals on the first day following oral administration of drug constitutes the usual balance study and additionally gives estimates of the rate of plasma clearance and rate and major route of excretion of parent compound and metabolites. A similar study by a parenteral route of administration coupled with a study in bile-fistula animals serves to identify the source of tracer appearing in feces and gives an estimate of the degree of absorption. These studies should include animals of either sex for apparent reasons. The balance study can then be followed by one using several animals of each species in which animals are sacrificed at an appropriate interval following oral administration of tracer and the tissues analyzed for tracer content thus giving some indication of the organs which concentrate the drug or metabolites. The foregoing are usually carried on concurrently with the acute and sub-acute toxicological studies.

At this stage, investigation proceeds to the human at the earliest opportunity in Phase I studies. Here again, using radioactively labelled compound, tracer plasma kinetics and balance study can be carried out. It is useful if these subjects are then included in the multiple dose portion of Phase I studies and the tracer study repeated at the conclusion of multiple dosing in order to detect any change in tracer kinetics due to multiple doses of cold compound.

It is obvious that the foregoing represents the simplest line of pursuit of information concerning metabolic disposition of the new compound. There may be compelling reasons, such as species variability in pharmacological response, species specific toxicity, or suspicion of formation of an active or toxic metabolite, that would demand a much more elaborate study design in the initial investigative stages. In any event, methods for the quantitation of parent compound and for the identification of major metabolites should also proceed at the earliest possible time and usually include inquiry by means of chemical and physical methodology, such as thin-layer chromatography, high-pressure liquid chromatography, gas-liquid chromatography, and its combination with mass spectometry, densitometry, or radioimmunoassay.

Finally, attention should be given to such special areas as placental transfer of drug and metabolites, pediatric metabolism, drug interaction, and methods of influencing absorption or excretion in the treatment of toxic overdose.

The following discussion of the metabolism of known antidepressants illustrates the application of these principles in varying degrees of complexity among the various agents and a study of the cited literature will point out the quality of information derived as result of the progressive development of newer methodology.

II. METABOLIC DISPOSITION

A. Absorption

The time within which tricyclic antidepressants or their metabolites appear in detectable amounts in plasma after single doses indicates that they are absorbed at a moderate rate following most routes of administration in man and animals. Significant plasma levels of imipramine in man are achieved within 2 hr and peak in less than 4 hr after an oral dose (79). Substantial amounts are absorbed by the buccal route within 5 min (28). Similar absorption is indicated following intraperitoneal, subcutaneous, or oral administration in rats (28, 26, 107, 21, 83), oral administration to rabbits and mice (83), and intraperitoneal injection in guinea pigs (28). Peak plasma levels in man were obtained within approximately 4 hr after oral administration of amitriptyline (57). The two N-monomethyl congeners of these two agents, i. e., desipramine and nortriptyline, show similar times to peak plasma levels in man (1, 2, 5, 4, 69) and the rat (96). Significant plasma levels of protriptyline were seen in man in 2 hr following an oral dose, but peak plasma concentrations were not achieved until the 10th hr (43). Peak plasma levels were reached in 1 to 3 hr in the dog with doxepin (85), in approximately 1 hr in the rat with noxiptilin (56); in less than 1 hr in the rat with dimetacrine (89), and with trimeprimine, in about 1 hr in the rabbit and within 2 to 4 hr in the dog (102).

The data obtained principally by balance studies in animals and man indicate that the antidepressants are well absorbed. The difficulty with most such studies in assessing accurately the quantity absorbed lies in the fact that of the amounts excreted in feces a portion represents material derived from biliary excretion. This is substantial in the rat and dog and much less so in man. This problem has been surmounted by several investigators by comparison of excretory patterns after oral and parenteral administration. Such comparisons have been made with nortriptyline in man (5) and the rat (96); with clomipramine in man, dog, and rat (19); in the rat with noxiptilin (56), doxepin (85), and dimetacrine (106); and in the rabbit with imipramine (83). Fecal excretion in man has been measured with imipramine (50) and protriptyline (43). These data show that the antidepressants are absorbed nearly completely following oral administration in all species studied.

B. Plasma Levels

Peak plasma levels achieved with all of the antidepressants on oral administration in man and animals are rather low, indicating a large apparent volume of distribution. This has been shown to be due to rapid redistribution from blood to tissues. On intravenous administration plasma concentration falls rapidly and within minutes appreciable tissue levels are seen (42, 41, 39, 63, 60). Rapid sequestration has been clearly demonstrated in isolated perfused rat lung (90) and liver (25, 16, 14, 105). Table I gives the plasma levels observed in various species following oral single doses or multiple daily doses. It is obvious from the single dose data that the total amount of drug circulating in plasma represents only a very small fraction of the dose even at these peak plasma levels.

Within a group of subjects mean plasma levels have been shown to be linearly related to the dose (99, 74, 117). However, inter-individual levels may vary widely. In six subjects receiving 150 mg of desipramine daily, Yates et al (117) reported steady state levels of 0.69 to 1.51 mcg/ml. Hammer et al (74) and Moody et al (99) also emphasized the differences in plasma levels among subjects. These three studies also point out that the plasma level is characteristic for a particular individual since the values are consistent within individuals when measured weeks apart. This is clearly demonstrated in Figure 1, where both the time to steady state level and the steady state levels are in good agreement between the first and second drug administration periods irrespective of the actual plasma level achieved. That the concomitant administration of other medication can be one factor responsible for large differences in plasma levels of antidepressants among individuals was demonstrated by Hammer et al (74). These authors showed that treatment with phenobarbital, presumably stimulating liver microsomal enzyme systems, reduced desipramine steady state plasma levels from 100 ng/ml to 60 ng/ml. Examples of drugs which tend to increase plasma levels of antidepressants are aspirin and chloramphenicol (104), methylphenidate (118), haloperidol, perphenazine, and chlorpromazine (69), hydrocortisone and testosterone (18). Alexanderson et al (6) also found differences in plasma levels attributable to concomitant drug therapy in a study of nortriptyline plasma concentrations in twins.

However, in the absence of treatment with other drugs, the large inter-individual differences in plasma levels of antidepressants (Figs. 2, 3) appear to be due to genetic factors (6, 76). The role of genetics in the response to antidepressants was first suggested by the observation by Angst (8, 9), of the resistance of certain families

TABLE I
Plasma Levels of Antidepressants
after Oral Doses in Various Species

Drug	Species	N	Dose	Dose Frequency	Peak or Steady State Level* ng/ml	Ref.
Imipramine	man	5	50 mg.	s.d.	30 (I) 20 (DMI)	99
Imipramine	rat	5	50 mg/kg	s.d.	720 (DMI)	27
Clomipramine-C^{14}	man	2	25 mg.	s.d.	20	63
Desipramine	man	10	25 mg.	t.i.d.	39.6	74
Desipramine	man	8	1 mg/kg	s.d.	26.7	2
Desipramine	man	8	0.4 mg/kg	t.i.d.	42.7	2
Amitriptyline	man	15	50 mg.	t.i.d.	70 (AT) 66 (NT)	35
Amitriptyline-C^{14}	man	4	25 mg.	s.d.	185.8 (AT+NT)	57
Nortriptyline-C^{14}	rat	4	5 mg/kg	s.d.	600	96
Nortriptyline	man	8	1 mg/kg	s.d.	42.3	2
Nortriptyline	man	6	0.4 mg/kg	t.i.d.	84.3	2
Nortriptyline	man	49	25 mg.	t.i.d.	101.9	12
Nortriptyline	man	10	25 mg.	t.i.d.	79	74
Protriptyline-C^{14}	man	2	47.5 mg.	s.d.	238	43
Doxepin-C^{14}	dog	2	10 mg/kg	s.d.	26.5	85
Doxepin-C^{14}	dog	3	10 mg/kg	q.d.	52.8	85
Doxepin-C^{14}	rat	4	10 mgPkg	s.d.	600	85
Dimetacrine-H^3	rat	15	20 mg/kg	s.d.	3500	89

* Given or calculated from author's graphs or tables
I = Imipramine DMI = Desipramine A = Amitriptyline NT = Nortriptyline s.d. = single dose

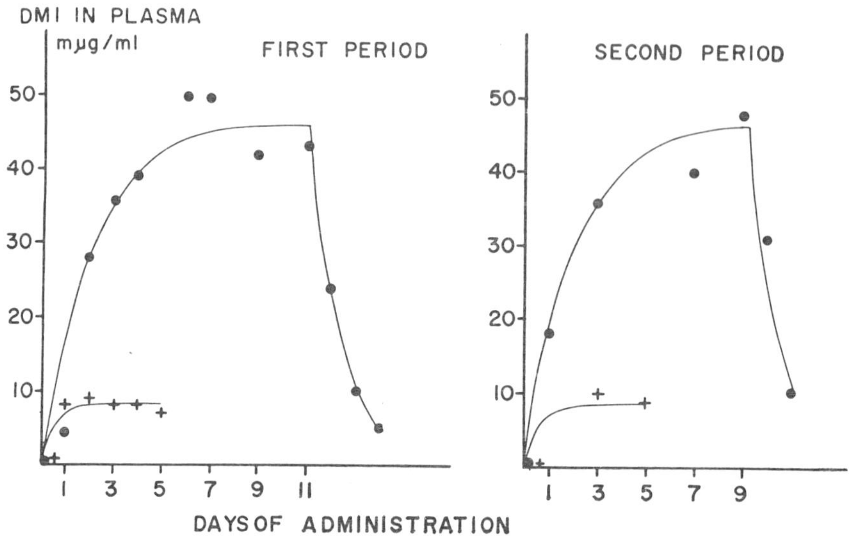

FIGURE 1 Plasma concentrations of desipramine (DMI) in 2 patients at two time periods five weeks (patient K. A. ●●) and seven weeks (patient K. E. ++) apart. 25 mg, p.o., at 6 a.m., 2 p.m. and 10 p.m. Blood samples taken at 1 p.m. (Reprinted with permission of Hammer et al. (74), Proceeding of the first international symposium on antidepressant drugs, 1967, Excerpta Medica Foundation.)

to the antidepressant effects of imipramine. Moody et al (99), and Hammer and Sjöqvist (76) suggested that this resistance might be due to the genetic control of rates of metabolism. This view is consistent with the data from two studies showing 1) similar patterns of desipramine or nortriptyline plasma levels in 5 individuals after they received either of these two compounds or after administration of imipramine or amitriptyline (Fig. 4); and 2) a correspondence between the plasma half-life of oxyphenbutazone in the same individual (Fig. 5). The inferences from these two studies are necessarily limited due to the small subject number; however, the correspondence between desipramine and nortriptyline plasma levels has been confirmed in a crossover study in a larger population (vide infra).

C. Plasma Kinetics

In rats following a 50 mg/kg intraperitoneal dose of imipramine no detectable plasma level of parent compound was seen. However, substantial levels of the metabolite, desipramine, were found which peak in 30 min. This was followed by a rapid redistribution phase during the next 30 min and an exponetial decline thereafter

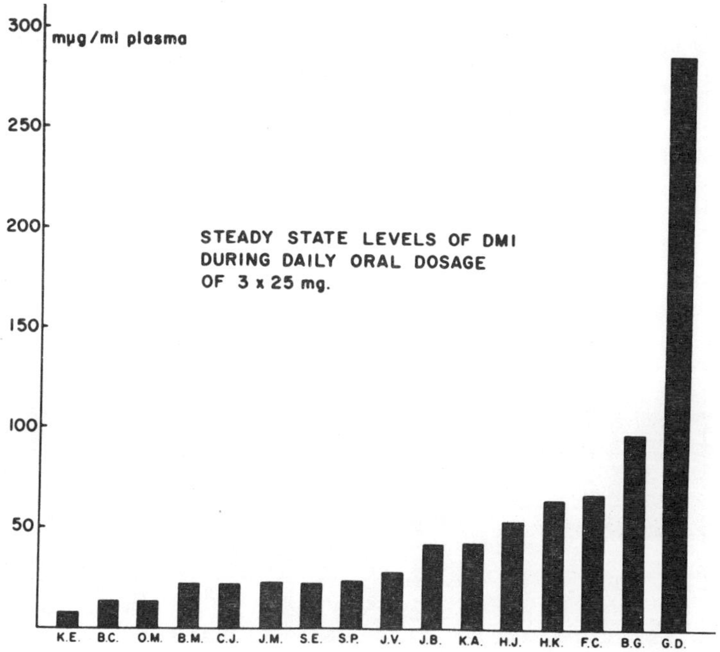

FIGURE 2 Interindividual variability in steady-state plasma levels of desipramine. (Reprinted with permission from Hammer and Sjöqvist (76), *Life Sciences,* 1967, Pergamon Press).

with a half-life of about 20 hr (99). In man, low but very variable levels of imipramine were seen with doses of 75 and 150 mg/day. Substantial levels of desipramine which reached a steady state within 10 to 20 days were measured (99). After intravenous administration of amitriptyline to rats a mean half-life of about 195 min was found (57). In man, the t ½ after intravenous administration was compared with that obtained on oral administration (57); these ranged from 16.9 to 35.1 hr (i.v.) and from 44 to 76.6 hr (p.o.). A study of protriptyline in two individuals (43) indicates a half-life of approximately 4 days after a single oral dose. In rats a plasma half-life of about 7 hr for doxepine (14) and 24 hr for dimetacrine (89) was found.

By far the most extensive and careful investigation of plasma kinetics with antidepressants has been carried out in humans with desipramine and nortriptyline by Alexanderson (1, 2) and Alexanderson et al (5). The basic data obtained in these studies are shown in Tables II and III. In general the peak plasma levels after single dose and the steady state levels during multiple dosing were higher with nortriptyline than with desipramine. The plasma half-life of desipramine was shorter both after a single dose and

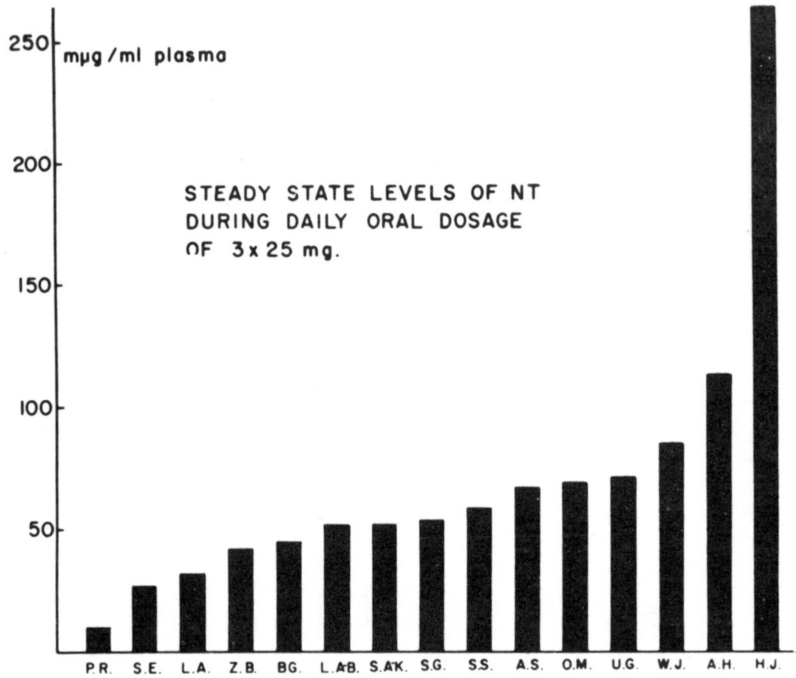

FIGURE 3 Interindividual variability in steady-state plasma levels of nortriptyline. (Reprinted with permission from Hammer and Sjöqvist (76), *Life Sciences,* 1967, Pergamon Press).

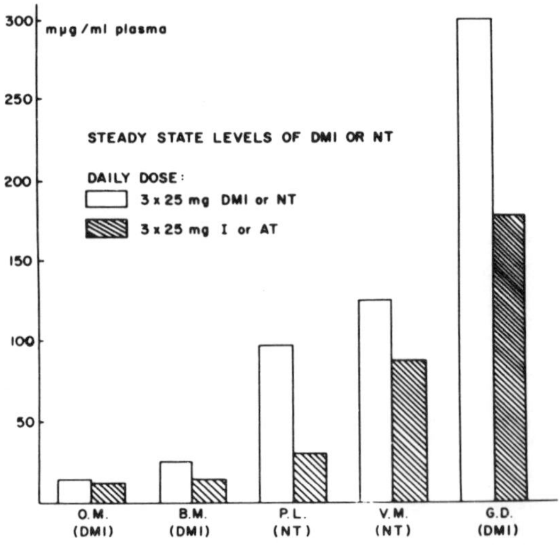

FIGURE 4 Steady-state plasma levels of desipramine (DMI) or nortriptyline (NT) during administration of these compounds or their N-dimethyl analogues, imipramine (I) or amitriptyline (AT). (Reprinted with permission from Hammer and Sjöqvist (76), *Life Sciences,* 1967, Pergamon Press).

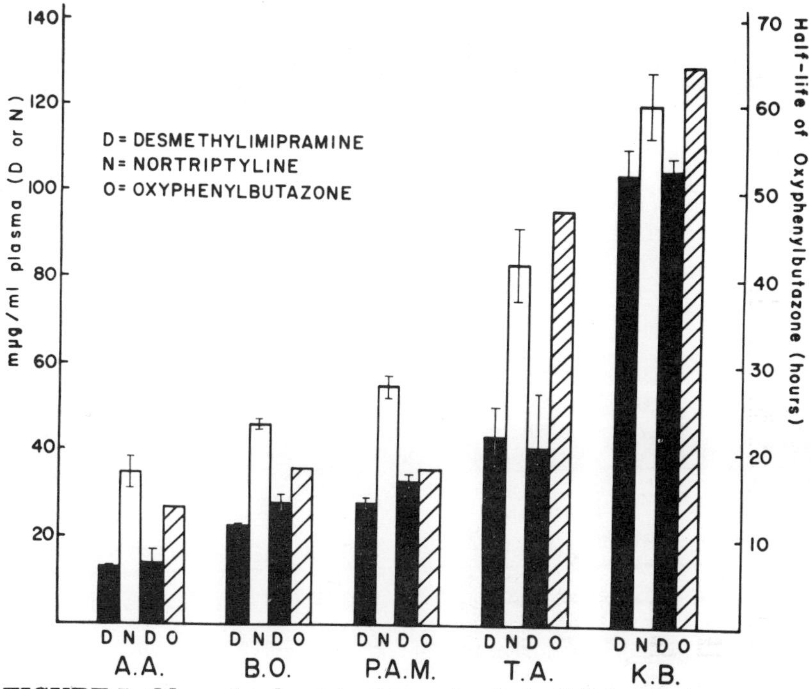

FIGURE 5 Mean steady-state plasma levels (± S. D.) of desipramine or nortriptyline (25 mg, t. i. d.) and oxyphenbutazone plasma half-life in 5 hospitalized psychiatric female patients. Drugs given separately in order shown in figure. (Reprinted with permission from Hammer et al. (75), *Clin. Pharmacol. Therap.*, 1969, C. V. Mosby Co.)

after multiple dosing in comparison with nortriptyline. The data also indicate that steady state plasma levels can be predicted from single dose kinetics. Numerous correlations of the various kinetic parameters both within drugs and between drugs were carried out by the authors. Significant correlations were found between drugs for peak single dose plasma levels, single dose half-lives, and single dose plasma clearance rates. The steady state plasma levels of both drugs correlated well with their respective single dose plasma half-lives, and with the post steady state plasma half-life with desipramine but not with nortriptyline.

D. Plasma Protein Binding

The antidepressants are highly bound to plasma proteins (32), the binding apparently involving mainly the albumin fraction (29). Considerable species difference in binding has been reported (33). In this latter study the percentages of unbound desipramine

TABLE II
Plasma Concentration and Pharmacokinetic Parameters Calculated for Single Oral Doses of Desipramine (DMI) and Nortriptyline (NT) (1 mg/kg)

Subject	Peak Plasma Level ng/ml		t ½ hr.		Vd 1/kg	
	DMI	NT	DMI	NT	DMI	NT
B. A.	39.0	61.2	21.2	34.2	31.9	21.1
G. A.	29.1	47.1	21.2	18.2	32.3	24.6
I. B.	18.0	30.5	12.5	20.2	52.1	41.6
O. B.	18.1	29.9	14.3	19.0	54.7	29.1
M. G.	29.9	37.6	17.8	24.7	27.7	22.9
M. L.	23.6	40.7	14.7	30.4	41.3	29.2
A. R.	36.7	49.8	24.7	35.0	35.6	21.2
M. A,	19.1	43.1	22.3	32.5	59.8	25.1
Mean	26.7	42.5	18.6	26.8	41.9	26.9
± S. D.	±8.3	±10.4	±4.4	±7.1	±12.1	±6.7

(Data from Alexanderson (2))

TABLE III
Plasma Concentrations and Pharmacokinetic Parameters for Multiple Oral Doses of Desipramine (DMI) and Nortriptyline (NT) (0.4 mg/kg every 8 hours for 15 (DMT) and 14 (NT) Days Respectively

Subject	Css ± SE ng/ml		(t ½) ss hrs.		(Vd) ss 1/kg	
	DMI	NT	DMI	NT	DMI	NT
B. A.	64.3±2.3	111.0±4.9	21.3	25.1	23.9	16.3
G. A.	21.1±2.3	60.5±1.3	12.1	18.1	41.4	21.6
I. B.	28.8±1.0	—	17.3	—	43.3	—
O. B.	20.7±4.6	51.7±3.1	10.6	27.4	37.1	38.2
M. G.	61.1±4.0	92.3±3.0	19.5	29.8	23.1	23.3
M. L.	35.3±1.1	76.7±3.4	18.0	29.5	36.8	27.8
A. R.	61.3±2.9	113.8±5.8	21.9	31.7	25.8	20.1
M. A.	48.6±1.5	—	26.4	—	39.1	—
Mean	42.7	84	18.4	26.9	33.8	24.5
± S. D	±18.5	±25.8	±5.2	±4.9	±8.2	±7.7

(Data from Alexanderson (2))

were found to be 8.6 to 10.8 in plasma from man, 6.0 to 10.6 in the rat, 13.8 to 16.4 in the rabbit, 0.7 to 4.0 in the dog, and 1.5 to 3.2 in the cat. Investigation of plasma from 41 blood donors showed that the amount of unbound desipramine varied approximately two-fold over the total samples with the majority of samples showing an unbound fraction of 8 to 11% (112). The degree of binding changes little over the therapeutic concentration range (32). Of a variety of drugs tested acetylsalicylic acid, aminopyrine, phenacetin, meprobamate, and diphenylhydantoin in therapeutic concentrations were capable of displacing desipramine from plasma proteins *in vitro*. The latter agent was the most potent causing an additional 3.3% of the total to appear in the unbound fraction (32). In an investigation of nortriptyline binding in plasma from twins receiving daily doses, Alexanderson and Borga (3) concluded that the degree of binding could be influenced by both genetic and environmental factors. Additionally, these authors could find no correlation between steady state plasma levels and the degree of binding which agrees with the *in vitro* observations with desipramine cited above.

E. Tissue Distribution

Tissue content of antidepressants in various sub-human species has been investigated for imipramine (26, 21, 60, 59), amitriptyline (57, 41), nortriptyline (96), clomipramine (63), doxepin (85), dimetacrine (89, 106), and noxiptyline (56). Distribution data in man has been presented in cases of fatal intoxication with imipramine (109, 80, 64) and amitriptyline and nortriptyline (31).

In general, all of the antidepressants are widely distributed in all animal species and the human with the highest concentrations found in the liver, lungs, spleen, kidney, and adrenals; the content of the remaining tissues is relatively low. The relative amount found in the brain depends upon the route of administration. Significant brain levels can be developed after intramuscular, intraperitoneal, or intravenous administration but not after oral administration (107, 27, 108). There are also species differences in the absolute levels developed. In the rabbit and mouse, which metabolize imipramine rapidly (54), lower peak levels were found after oral administration and tissue levels decreased rapidly in contrast to the rat whose tissue levels gradually increased over a period of 8 hours. However, in spite of the differences in tissue kinetics in these three species, the highest amounts were found in the liver, kidney, and lungs in all three.

In mice, rats, and humans, the antidepressants have been shown to enter the fetal circulation rapidly and become distributed in fetal tissue in a manner similar to the adult (39, 3, 40, 55, 110). In rats, for example, an equilibrium between maternal and fetal plasma was reached in 1 minute after an intramuscular injection of desipramine (88) though the fetal plasma levels were lower at all time points up to 20 minutes after the injection. Lower newborn than maternal plasma levels were also seen in an infant delivered 20 hr after the ingestion of a toxic dose of nortriptyline by the mother (110). Since fetal microsomes are capable of hydoxylating desipramine (and presumably nortriptyline) this difference in maternal-fetal plasma level might be due to a lower ability of a newborn's plasma to bind the drug (110).

F. Excretion

1. Urinary, Fecal, and Biliary Excretion

Studies on the excretory pattern in rats after imipramine given orally or intraperitoneally have shown that the major portion of the administered dose is excreted within 24 hr and within 5 to 7 days the excretion is essentially completed (26, 50). Approximately 50% of the administered dose appears in the urine, 50% in feces. This pattern is not changed in animals pretreated with imipramine for several days prior to the balance study (50). Analysis for intact drug in the urine shows that only 0.7-5% of the total dose is excreted in the urine unchanged, the remainder of the urinary total consisting mainly of polar metabolites. Fecal excretion also contains little unchanged drug (105). Since the antidepressants are absorbed nearly completely on oral administration and since the excretory patterns following parenteral or oral administration are quite similar, it is evident that a major portion of the fecal excretion represents material arriving via bile and not reabsorbed. This is substantiated by the fact that in bile-fistula rats given imipramine intraperitoneally, nearly 70% of the administered dose appears in the bile within 5 hr (25). Obviously in the rat there is considerable enterohepatic circulation of imipramine metabolites (5% unchanged drug, 80% glucuronides) (25). In man, urinary excretion of imipramine plus metabolites is somewhat higher than in rats with about 60 to 80% of the administered dose appearing in the urine, the majority being excreted in the first 72 hr (50, 45). Biliary excretion thus seems to be less in man than in rats since only up to 22% appeared in feces. As in the rat, intact drug in urine was found to be approximately 1% of the total excreted. Three per cent of total urinary excretion was accounted for by desipramine (45).

The excretion of amitriptyline is similar to that of imipramine.

In mice given the drug intravenously, 50 to 60% of the dose appears in the urine in the first 24 hr (41) and thus is more rapidly excreted than in the rat and man. In female rats, after oral administration, 32% was excreted in urine and 38% in feces in 11 days. In males, 44% in urine and 17% in feces was found (57). Thus total recovery in this study was rather low. A study in 4 humans given an oral dose indicated excretion of 68.5 to 83.8% of the dose in urine and 6.9 to 9.7% in feces after 11 days (57). About 30% of the dose appears in the urine in the first 24 hr (52). Again this difference in fecal excretion between rat and man may be due to differences in biliary excretion since in the rat 50% of an injected dose of amitriptyline can be recovered in bile within 6 hr (41).

The excretion of nortriptyline is essentially quantitatively similar in respect to both quantity and rate to amitriptyline. In the first 24 hr, man excretes approximately 58% of an oral dose in the urine (7). Total urinary excretion after either a single dose or daily doses amounts to an average of 62% of the administered oral dose (4). Excretion of unchanged nortriptyline amounts to only 1 to 3% of the total urinary recovery.

A comparison in the rat of the excretory pattern following oral or intraperitoneal excretion has been carried out with dimetacrine (89). After oral administration 21% of the dose appeared in urine and 48% in feces in 48 hr. With intraperitoneal administration 16% was found in urine and 42% in feces. Biliary excretion is not as marked as with the above compounds since only 24% of the administered dose was excreted in bile in 24 hours after oral administration in bile-fistula rats.

A study of the excretion of protriptyline in two human subjects (43) indicates that this compound and its metabolites are very slowly eliminated in comparison to the compounds discussed above. Only 6.1 and 11% of the administered dose was recovered in urine in 24 hr. A mean of 50% of the dose was excreted by the 16th day. Fecal excretion amounted to 2% of the dose after 10 days.

Although closely related in structure to imipramine, clomimpramine shows a markedly different pattern of excretion in rats and dogs than in man (63). In the former, about 80% of the dose was eliminated in feces and 10 to 20% in urine after three days following either oral or intravenous application. Conversely, in man, about 50% of an oral dose appeared in urine and 20 to 30% in feces during a 14-day collection. The majority of excretion occurred within 72 hr.

Noxiptilin and doxepin are eliminated more rapidly than other antidepressants. With the former, after either intravenous or oral administration in rats, 75% of the total renal elimination had occurred in 8 hr and was essentially complete in 16 hr (56). The pattern of excretion was apparently dose dependent with greater urinary excretion the higher the dose. At 3 mg/kg, 59% of the total dose was collected in urine and 40% in feces after an intravenous injection. Urinary excretion after the same dose, orally, was approximately 41% compared to 58% in feces. Excretion of doxepin was similarly rapid in the rat where nearly all of the material excreted could be accounted for in 24 hr (85). Approximately 60% of the dose was excreted via urine and 30% via feces following either intraperitoneal or oral dosing.

2. Excretion and Urinary pH

The effect of alkalinization or acidification of urine on the excretion of unchanged imipramine, desipramine, and nortriptyline and, in some cases, their metabolites has been examined in the rat, dog, and human (28, 50, 111, 68). In general, alkalinization of urine decreases and acidification increases excretion of unchanged drug; phenolic or conjugated metabolite excretion does not change significantly. However, since the total amount of unchanged drug in urine at normal pH is a small proportion of the administered dose, the increased excretion (1 to 5% of the total dose) in acid urine is still insignificant in relation to the proportion metabolized and would be of no importance in the treatment of toxic overdose with these agents (111).

3. Gastric Secretion

The antidepressants are secreted in gastric juice in minor amounts (57, 111) commensurate with their weakly basic properties. In rats, approximately 0.1% of an administered dose of amitriptyline reaches the stomach contents by this route. In the dog, elimination of desipramine and nortriptyline is similarly insignificant by this route even during betazole-induced gastric secretion. Thus treatment of toxic overdose by continuous gastric lavage would be expected to be of little use in promotion excretion of the antidepressants (111).

G. Relationship of Plasma Levels to Clinical Effects

Early studies which attempted to relate clinical effect with the plasma levels of tricyclic antidepressants are difficult to interpret due to either insufficient diagnostic criteria or inadequate methods used for the plasma level determinations. More recent studies, however, have yielded interesting relationships. Hammer et al (74) treated seven patients with endogenous depression, three with desipramine, and four with nortriptyline. All four responded favorably to nortriptyline yielding plasma levels ranging from 48 to 80 ng/ml. One responder to desipramine had a plasma level of 14 ng/ml while two nonresponders had levels of 8 and 14 ng/ml. The plasma levels of the responders to nortriptyline are interesting in view of two subsequent studies of nortriptyline, one of 2 weeks' and one of 4 weeks' duration (11, 93), which suggested that plasma levels of at least 50 ng/ml were necessary for a beneficial response. These authors also suggested a poor clinical response at levels above 175 ng/ml. This biphasic response, however, was not confirmed by Braithwaite et al (35) in a study of amitriptyline over a six-week period. A positive correlation between response and the levels of both parent compound and nortriptyline was found at the end of six weeks. The highest level of nortriptyline achieved was 206 ng/ml and the highest combined level was 313 ng/ml. A correlation was achieved also at four weeks but not at two weeks. This biphasic response was also not seen with nortriptyline in a 6-week study by Burrows et al (37). These authors also found no relationship between plasma level and clinical effect although several of their non-responders did respond at higher doses and such a relationship was stated to have been established in a subsequent unpublished study using various doses. Interesting discussion of these studies appears in recently published comments (93, 70, 36, 38). Two studies relating plasma drug levels after imipramine administration and clinical response have been reported. Walter (114), measuring the total imipramine-desipramine plasma levels, found a significant correlation between levels and response at the end of four weeks; responders had a mean total level of 46.1 ng/ml and non-responders, a level of 13.3 ng/ml. Zeidenberg et al (118) also found a correlation between imipramine + desipramine plasma levels and amelioration of depression; however, all patients were given high doses of imipramine and the range of maximum plasma levels achieved was 170-750 ng/ml. Thus, it is not possible from this study to judge the clinical response at low plasma levels. In three patients where plasma levels and depression ratings are given over the course of treatment (50-70 days), the authors show continuous improvement in the course of the disease in spite of widely fluctuating plasma levels. It is important to note, though, that with the exception of a few days in one patient, plasma levels remained well above 40 ng/ml throughout the study.

A relationship between side effects and plasma levels of antidepressants has been found by some workers, but significance to the relationship was established only early during treatment (2 weeks) but not at later times (35, 12, 10). Those subjects with the highest levels exhibit the most severe side effects (74, 10). Burrows et al (37) found no correlation of plasma levels and side effects at 2, 4 or 6 weeks.

III. METABOLIC ALTERATION

A. Imipramine and Related Drugs

1. Imipramine and Desipramine

Imipramine has been widely studied and shown to be extensively metabolized in man and laboratory animals. There are four principal metabolic pathways involved in imipramine metabolism: 1) hydroxylation at the 2- and 10-positions with aromatic hydroxylation in the 2-position heavily dominating bridge hydroxylation in the 10-position, 2) side chain demethylation, 3) side chain cleavage, and 4) N-oxide formation. Most of the metabolite combinations resulting from these pathways have been isolated and are shown on the flow chart (Fig. 6).

Hermann and co-workers first described the isolation and characterization of the major urinary metabolites from rabbits, rats, mice, and humans (83, 84). Hydroxylation in the 2-position with partial glucuronide conjugation (metabolite, II) and side chain demethylation with 2-position hydroxylation and partial glucuronide formation (metabolites III and IV) were recognized in these early studies as the dominant metabolic pathways. The primary amine (metabolite, V) resulting from the loss of two methyl groups was also described.

Subsequently additional metabolites, although formed in small quantities, were reported which define other metabolic pathways. Fishman and Goldenberg isolated and characterized imipramine N-oxide (metabolite, VI) from human urine (66). Obersteg and Baümler showed the occurrence of metabolites resulting from complete loss of the amino-alkyl side chain with the characterization of iminodibenzyl (metabolite, VII) from an overdosed human (101). Iminodibenzyl, as well as 2-hydroxyiminodibenzyl (metabolite, VIII), were confirmed by Crammer et al as being present in both rat tissues and human urine (47, 49). Hydroxylation at the 10-position occurs as a minor but distinct metabolic pathway leading to 10-hydroxyimipramine (metabolite, IX), 10-hydroxydesipramine (metabolite, X), 10-hydroxydidismethylimipramine (metabolite, XI) and possibly 10-hydroxyiminodibenzyl (metabolite, XII), which are present in both human urine and plasma (48).

Numerous investigators attempted quantitation of urinary metabolites using colorimetric, fluorometric, and paper

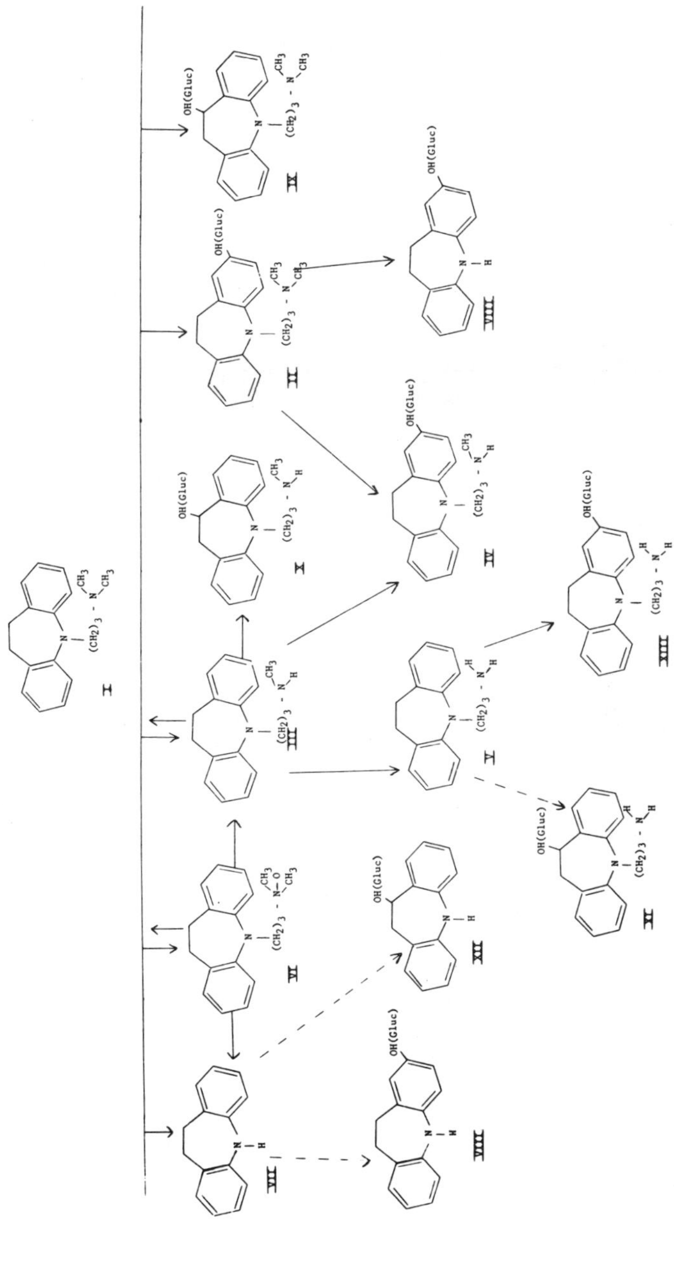

FIGURE 6 Metabolites of imipramine and desipramine

chromatographic procedures (83, 71, 78, 94). Christiansen et al first reported on the use of radioactive imipramine tagged in the 10- and 11-position with C^{14} for quantitation of human urinary metabolites (45). The results of these studies indicated that 43% of the administered dose was excreted in the urine in the first 24 hr and 72% was excreted in 72 hr. Approximately 15% of the radioactivity was recovered as non-conjugated metabolites, 35% as conjugated metabolites and 23% remained as nonextractable. Desipramine, 2-hydroxyimipramine, 2-hydroxydesipramine, and imipramine N-oxide were isolated and identified by thin layer chromatography.

Later a more comprehensive study was reported by Crammer et al (49). Employing a special solvent extraction system of equal parts of tetrahydrofuran and isoamyl alcohol on salt saturated urine at both basic and acidic pHs, they were able to recover 95% of the radioactivity from the urine of subjects dosed with 5 uc of C^{14} imipramine. Using both one way and two way thin layer chromatography, autoradiography, and various color tests, twenty metabolites were provisionally identified. Monitoring both urine and feces it was shown that metabolites retaining the basic side chain with 2-position hydroxylation and side chain demethylation accounted for 70 to 85% of the dose and of this 60 to 70% was excreted in the urine in the form of free phenols and conjugates and 10 to 15% in the feces in the form of free phenols. Side chain cleavage, leading to iminodibenzyl and 2-hydroxyiminodibenzyl, accounted for possibly 10 to 15% of the metabolites, suggesting this to be a more important metabolic pathway than previously realized. The conjugated metabolites were mostly glucuronides but new acid labile conjugates of unknown structure were found. The excretion of imipramine N-oxide was minor, accounting for only 1 to 3% of the dose. Complete demethylation to desmethyldesipramine and 10-position hydroxylation were not shown to be quantitatively significant pathways. Similar results were obtained from subjects treated with desipramine instead of imipramine except that 2-hydroxyimipramine in either conjugated or free form and imipramine N-oxide were not present.

In studies reported on rats, rabbits, mice, and humans no qualitative difference in the formation of metabolites has been observed. One possible exception is the recent report that *in vitro* metabolism of imipramine and desipramine in liver fractions from rabbits and guinea pigs yields N-hydroxylated desipramine (20). This metabolite has not been reported as a urinary metabolite from any species studied to date. However, Dingell et al (54) have observed that kinetic differences do exist as evidenced by the conversion of imipramine to desipramine in rats and man with further metabolism of desipramine being slower, thus resulting in the accumulation of desipramine. In contrast, mice and rabbits rapidly metabolize desipramine and at a rate approximately equal to the rate of metabolism of imipramine.

Imipramine and desipramine are metabolized principally by liver microsomal enzymes to demethylated and hydroxylated metabolites as demonstrated by experiments with isolated liver perfusion preparations, liver microsomal enzyme preparations, and hepatectomized rats (25, 54, 47, 24, 98, 15). Extrahepatic tissues, e.g. lung, kidney, heart, gut, and brain, have been reported to cause some imipramine metabolism, but the conversions are low and, indeed, investigators are not in agreement as to whether all are metabolizing tissues (54, 47, 98). In any case, it seems unlikely that tissues other than liver are of quantitative significance in imipramine metabolism.

Imipramine-N-oxide presents a special case since it is reported to be a potentially useful antidepressant drug (19, 65). Oxidation of imipramine to form this metabolite occurs in the liver (98). In contrast to imipramine, the N-oxide is metabolized in many extrahepatic tissues by reduction to imipramine and demethylation to desipramine (98). However, the metabolic conversion of imipramine-N-oxide to desipramine is a different metabolic pathway from the direct demethylation of imipramine (30, 23).

As stated above the formation of desipramine from imipramine is largely a hepatic process. However, Minder et al (98) have shown that the gastrointestinal contents of rats and humans also cause this conversion and to a degree that could be significant in the accumulation of desipramine in plasma. The mechanism for this demethylation is unknown. To a small degree methylation of desipramine to imipramine has been shown to occur in rat liver and in rabbit liver and lung (25, 53).

Numerous analytical methods for the determination of imipramine and its metabolites in urine and biological tissues have been described. Thin layer and paper chromatographic methods have been used extensively for studies concerned with the broad spectrum of metabolites (83, 80, 84, 44) and, coupled with the use of radioactive drugs, provide the best quantitative estimates of the amounts of the various metabolites formed (45, 47, 49).

Mechanisms to study the possibility that the antidepressant activity of imipramine is mediated through the metabolite desipramine required that highly sensitive and selective analytical methods be developed for plasma determinations. Early fluorometric methods suffered from low sensitivity and were not selective (117, 54). The method of Moody et al described the fluorometric estimation of both imipramine and desipramine in plasma through the separation of desipramine by acetylation with a sensitivity down to 20 ng/ml (99). Hammer and Brodie, using an isotope-derivative method based on acetylation of desipramine with tritiated acetic anhydride and scintillation counting, were able to determine desipramine levels with a lower limit of sensitivity of 5 ng/ml (73). A modification of this procedure described by Harris et al additionally provides for the determination of imipramine by the conversion to the C^{14} methyl iodide quaternary salt with a resulting lower limit of sensitivity to either desipramine or imipramine of 15 to 20 ng/ml (77). Gillette et al (67) and Viala et al (113) have described the use of gas chromatography for the determination of imipramine and desipramine in plasma. Weder and Bickel reported on a gas chromatographic method for the determination of imipramine and seven of its major metabolites in biological samples using selective extraction and derivation techniques and flame ionization detection (115). Recently a highly sensitive gas chromatographic method for the determination of desipramine has been described by Ervik et al (58). This involves the treatment of desipramine with trifluoroacetic anhydride resulting in the formation of a bis-trifluoroacetyl derivative in which one trifluoroacetyl group is attached to the secondary amine and the second is inserted in the side chain as a trifluoroacetyl enamine. This allows the use of electron capture detection with resulting sensitivity down to 1 ng/ml. Nagy and Trieber have reported the use of direct densitometry on thin layer chromatograms which provides a method for the estimation of both imipramine and desipramine in the 20 ng/ml sensitivity range. The procedure is specific, relatively simple, and rapid (100).

2. 10-Keto-Imipramine

This derivative of imipramine, containing a ketone carbonyl group in the 10-position, (compound I, Fig. 7) has been reported to be a clinically effective antidepressant (82). In the rabbit it is reduced to 10-hydroxy imipramine, the tertiary amino group is demethylated, and possibly the side chain is cleaved to 10-hydroxy iminodibenzyl. In the rat the compound is rapidly metabolized with an apparent half-life of only 15 min (imipramine, t ½ in rats = 2½ hr).

3. Clomipramine

Clomipramine, a clinically active antidepressant, is 3-chloroimipramine (compound II, Fig. 7). The major metabolic

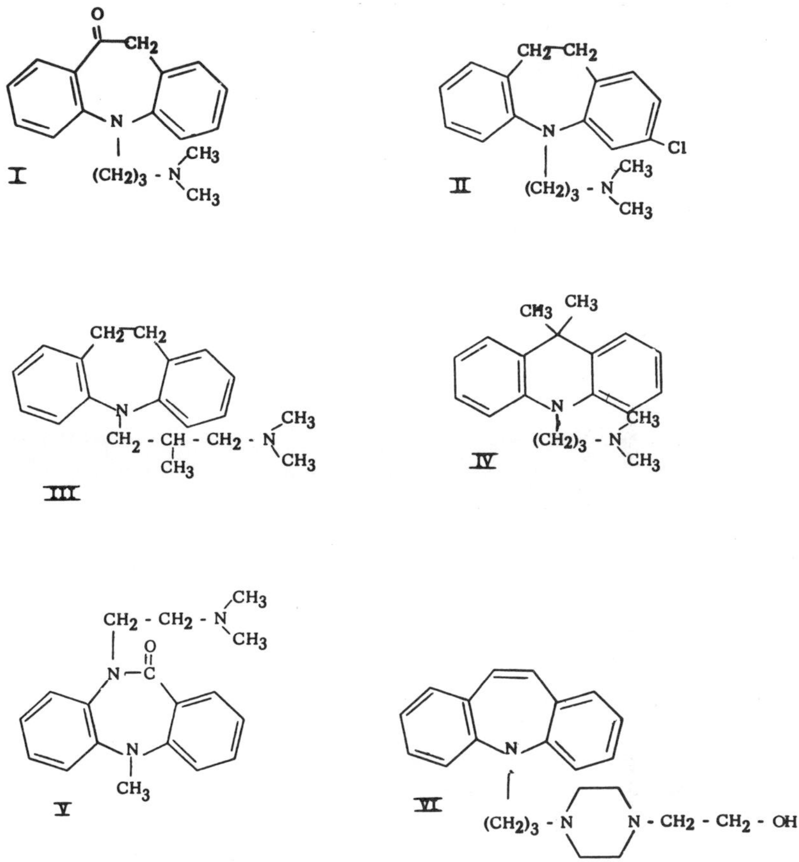

FIGURE 7 Imipramine-related structures

routes are apparently similar to imipramine in rats, rabbits, and man (102, 82). Side chain demethylation, aromatic hydroxylation, and N-oxide formation have been characterized as metabolic pathways.

4. Trimeprimine

Trimeprimine contains a branched methyl group, β to the terminal amine in the imipramine structure, (compound III, Fig. 7). Its metabolism in the rabbit, dog, and man has been studied by Populaire et al (102). As might be anticipated from the similarity in structures, the metabolism closely parallels that of imipramine, with side chain demethylation, aromatic hydroxylation, side chain cleavage, and bridge hydroxylation identified as major metabolic pathways.

5. Dimetacrine

Unlike imipramine which contains a seven membered central ring, dimetacrine is an acridine derivative, with a six membered central ring (compound IV, Fig. 7). Schatz et al have studied its metabolism in dogs and rats and shown that the drug is rapidly metabolized. The major metabolic routes are strikingly similar to imipramine (106). Metabolites corresponding to 2-position hydroxylation, side chain monodemethylation, side chain cleavage, and N-oxide formation have been identified in dog urine.

6. Dibenzepine

Dibenzepine (compound V, Fig. 7) differs significantly from imipramine in the chemistry of the central ring in that it contains two nitrogen atoms (a diazepine ring) with the amino alkyl chain attached to the amide bridge nitrogen. The compound is extensively metabolized in man and laboratory animals. Tissue distribution studies have shown that mouse brain contains both intact drug and the 5-demethylated metabolite (97). Lehner et al studied urinary metabolites in man, dog, and rabbit (95). In dog and man all five possible demethylated metabolites have been identified. In the rabbit a metabolite corresponding to side chain monodemethylation and a metabolite corresponding to 5-position demethylation were the only demethylated metabolites found. All three species excreted phenolic metabolites that were mostly conjugated with glucuronic acid.

7. Opipramol

Opipramol (compound VI, Fig. 7) differs structurally from imipramine and its other derivatives in two important aspects: the central ring is unsaturated and the basic side chain is a hydroxethylpiperazinylpropyl group. Thus demethylation, so important in the metabolism of other members of the imipramine series which contain dimethylamino side chains, is not possible. Herrmann has conducted limited metabolism studies in rats and rabbits and shown that the drug is extensively metabolized with several metabolic products appearing in rabbit urine (81).

B. Amitriptyline and Related Drugs

1. Amitriptyline and Nortriptyline

Like other tricyclic antidepressants, amitriptyline is rapidly and extensively metabolized in man and laboratory animals. In all species studied the major metabolic pathways are side chain demethylation and bridge hydroxylation. The position for hydroxylation of amitriptyline contrasts with imipramine in which bridge hydroxylation is a very minor pathway and hydroxylation in the aromatic portion of the molecule extensive. The known metabolites of amitriptyline and nortriptyline are shown in Figure 8.

Hucker and Porter first reported on the metabolism of amitriptyline in man, rabbits, and rat liver microsomal preparations (87, 86). They identified the demethylated metabolite II, and 10-hydroxylated metabolites III and IV and the 10, 11-hydroxylated metabolite VII. Their studies also suggested that metabolites resulting from oxidative deamination, aromatic hydroxylation, and oxidative rupture of the ethylene bridge were formed. Other investigators have reported on the metabolic conversion of amitriptyline and nortriptyline in man, rats, and rabbits confirming demethylation and bridge hydroxylation as the major metabolic pathways (4, 96, 41, 46, 51, 72). The hydroxylated metabolites are largely excreted as glucuronide conjugates in man and laboratory animals (87, 46).

Introduction of the hydroxyl group at the 10-position in the amitriptyline structure destroys the symmetry around the exocyclic double bond and produces *cis* and *trans* isomers. The stereochemistry of 10-hydroxynortriptyline (IV), the major metabolite of both amitriptyline and nortriptyline, has been extensively studied. Bertilsson and Alexanderson separated both isomers from the urine of subjects treated with nortriptyline and these accounted for about 80% (in conjugated and unconjugated form) of the total metabolites recovered (22). Each of the isomers was shown to be optically active and of different configurations at the asymmetric carbons. The ratio of the two geometric isomers was constant at 1:4-5. Remy et al have reported the synthesis and configuration assignments of the pure *cis* and *trans* isomers of 10-hydroxynortriptyline based on an N.M.R. study using tris (dipivalomethanato) europium as a shift reagent (103). It should therefore now be possible to determine which of the isomers predominates in the metabolic mixture.

The carboxylic acid metabolite VIII, resulting from oxidative deamination of the amitriptyline side chain in the rabbit has been reported by Facino et al (62). Since the acid is present in only trace quantities in urine, it represents a minor metabolic pathway. Beckett and Al-Sarraj have recently described the N-hydroxylation of amitriptyline and nortriptyline by rabbit and guinea pig liver fractions to N-hydroxynortriptyline (20). This

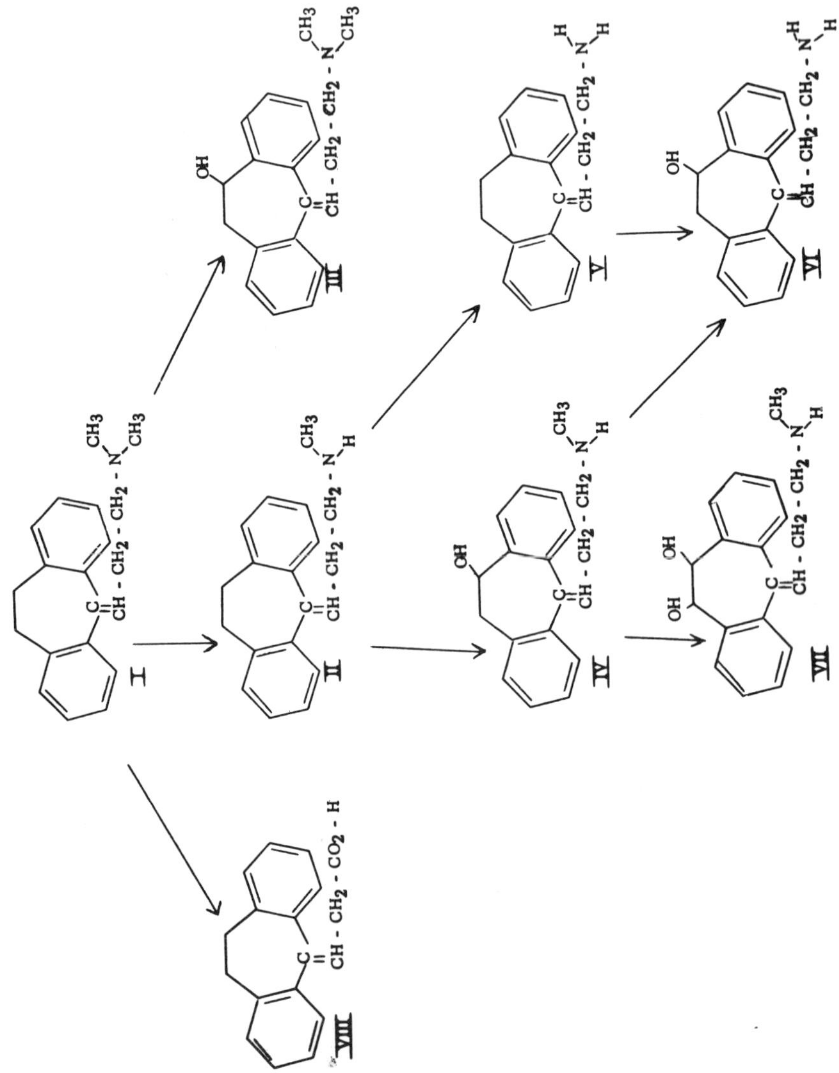

FIGURE 8 Metabolites of amitriptyline and nortriptyline

metabolite in free or conjugated form has not been reported as a urinary metabolite in any species studied to date.

Rat liver microsomal enzyme preparations and rabbit liver slices rapidly metabolize amitriptyline (87, 86). In metabolic rat studies using rat liver microsomes, von Bahr has shown that the rate of demethylation of amitriptyline to nortriptyline was more rapid than either the 10-hydroxylation of amitriptyline or the demethylation of 10-hydroxyamitriptyline which in turn were more rapid than the demethylation of nortriptyline, the formation of 10, 11-dihydroxynortriptyline, or the 10-hydroxylation of nortriptyline (13). Human liver fractions are reported to hydroxylate nortriptyline more slowly than rats' (17).

Whitnach et al have shown that the dog lung is capable of demethylating nortriptyline while the heart does not metabolize the drug (116).

Numerous analytical methods for the determination of amitriptyline, nortriptyline, and their metabolites in urine and biological tissues have been described. These include thin layer chromatography (46, 13, 61), thin layer and column chromatography with radioisotope tagging (96, 41, 52), calorimetric (87), and U.V. spectrophotometric procedures (7). Gas chromatographic methods have been employed for nortriptyline (4, 51). An especially sensitive gas chromatography method, developed by Borga and Carli, measures heptafluorobutyryl derivatives of nortriptyline and its demethylated and hydroxylated metabolites by electron capture detection in concentrations down to 10 ng/ml in human plasma and urine (34).

Hammar et al have applied gas chromatography, mass spectometry, and mass fragmentography to the study of nortriptyline and its metabolites in human biological fluids (72). A special application of these techniques has been described by Knapp et al (92) and Whitnach et al (116) employing nortriptyline labeled with the stable isotopes, deuterium and nitrogen-15.

2. Doxepin .

Doxepin (structure I, Fig. 9) is structurally related to amitriptyline differing only by the replacement of carbon by oxygen on one of the bridge positions. It is a mixture of *cis* and *trans* isomers. Hobbs has studied its metabolism in rats and dogs using drug labeled with C^{14} in the central ring and demonstrated that the major routes of metabolism are similar to imipramine and amitriptyline (85). Metabolites corresponding to demethylation and N-oxide formation have been identified. Hydroxylation with glucuronide conjugation occurs but the structures of the hydroxylated metabolites have not been established.

3. Noxiptilin

Noxiptilin (structure II, Fig. 9), although structurally similar to amitriptyline in the central ring system, differs substantially in the nature of the amino alkyl side chain. Attachment of these two structural moieties is through an oximino bond with the dimethylamino group separated by a two carbon chain. Duhn et al have studied the metabolism of noxiptilin in rats and dogs using C^{14} tagging and shown that the drug is extensively metabolized in both species (56). The profile of metabolites indicates that the metabolic pathways are similar to those found with amitriptyline. Demethylation, bridge hydroxylation with conjugation, and N-oxide formation are the principle metabolic pathways. Both the rat and the dog excrete a significant amount of the drug as the N-oxide (rat 25%, dog 15%), the 10-hydroxy N-oxide (rat 5%, dog 17%), and the 10, 11-dihydroxy N-oxide (rat 4%, dog 3%). Hydroxylation occurs at the 10-position and dihydroxylation at the 10, 11-positions. This metabolic hydroxylation is associated with side chain monodemethylation and N-oxide formation. The non-demethylated metabolite of the parent compound is excreted in only small amounts in both species and the loss of both methyl groups is observed only in the dog and in trace quantities. Possible side chain cleavage at the point of attachment of the oximino group is evidenced by the isolation of a small amount of parent ring ketone. Some acidic metabolic products were also isolated.

4. Protriptyline

Protriptyline (structure III, Fig. 9) differs from amitriptyline in two important aspects. The center ring of the tricyclic structure is unsaturated on the bridge and the side chain is attached through a saturated carbon-carbon bond. Little information is available on the metabolism of protriptyline. Human studies using C^{14} tagged drug show a very slow excretion rate indicating that the drug is not rapidly converted to readily excreted metabolites (43). It is reported that the rat metabolizes the drug to a glucuronide which is excreted in high concentrations in the bile (43).

5. Maprotiline

Maprotiline (structure IV, Fig. 9) is structurally different from other tricyclic antidepressants in the center ring portion of the molecule. It is a bicyclic structure with the center ring rigidly fixed

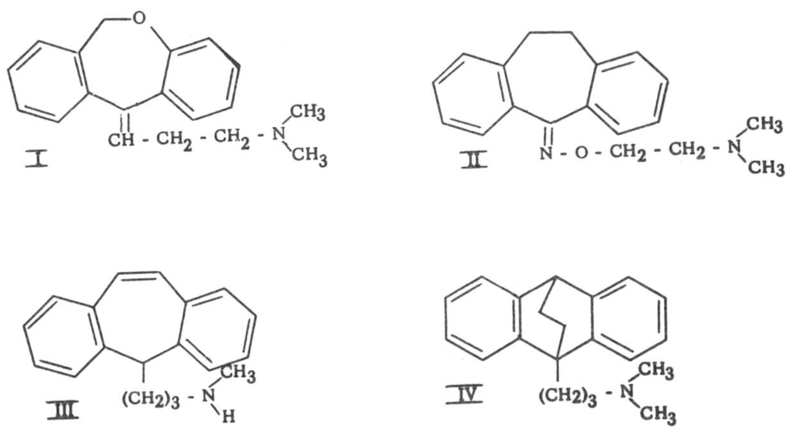

FIGURE 9 Amitriptyline-related structures

by an ethylene bridge. Keberle et al have studied its metabolism in rat, rabbit, dog, and man using tritium labeled drug and identified metabolites in man and dog corresponding to both mono- and di-demethylation, hydroxylation with glucuronide conjugation, and oxidative deamination to a propionic acid side chain (91). The structure of the hydroxylated metabolites has not been determined.

IV. SUMMARY

The study of the metabolism of a new drug can yield a better understanding of its pharmacological and toxicological activity and contribute greatly to its safe and rational use especially during early clinical trials. Such studies on the known antidepressants have demonstrated that they are readily absorbed on oral administration and extensively metabolized. Blood concentrations are never very great and the material present in blood is highly bound to plasma proteins. Plasma half lives are long and tend to be variable between individuals. The main excretory route is renal. Metabolism occurs by three main mechanisms which can be defined as N-alkyl cleavage (mostly demethylation), hydroxylation (either aromatic or activated carbon), and N-oxide formation. Metabolites arising from combination of these mechanisms have been found with all compounds studied. Investigations concerned with the relationship between plasma levels and clinical effects have not been conclusive. More carefully designed studies, with consideration for the definition of clinical change and type of clinical population, are needed.

REFERENCES

1. Alexanderson, B.: Pharmacokinetics of nortriptyline in man after single and multiple oral doses: the predictability of steady-state plasma concentrations from single-dose plasma level data, *Eur. J. Clin. Pharmacol.*, **4**:82-91, 1972.
2. Alexanderson, B.: Pharmacokinetics of desmethylimipramine and nortriptyline in man after single and multiple oral doses—a cross-over study, *Eur. J. Clin. Phcrmacol.*, **5**:1-10, 1972.
3. Alexanderson, B. and Borgå, O.: Interindividual differences in plasma protein binding of nortriptyline in man—a twin study, *Eur. J. Clin. Pharmacol.*, **4**:196-200, 1972.
4. Alexanderson, B. and Borgå, O.: Urinary excretion of nortriptyline and five of its metabolites in man after single and multiple oral doses, *Eur. J. Clin., Pharmacol.*, **5**:174-180, 1973.
5. Alexanderson, B., Borgå, O., and Alván, G.: The availability of orally administered nortriptyline, *Eur. J. Clin. Pharmacol.*, **5**:181-185, 1973.
6. Alexanderson, B., Evans, D. A. P., and Sjöqvist, F.: Steady-state plasma levels of nortriptyline in twins: influence of genetic factors and drug therapy, *Br. Med. J.*, **4**:764-768, 1969.
7. Amundson, M. E. and Manthey, J. A.: Excretion of nortriptyline in man I. Detection and determination of urinary nortriptyline, *J. Pharm. Sci.*, **55**:277-280, 1966.
8. Angst, J.: A clinical analysis of the effects of tofranil in depression, *Psychopharmacologia*, **2**:381-407, 1961.
9. Angst, J.: Antidepressiver effekt und genetische faktoren, *Arzneim. Forsch.*, **14**:496-500, 1964.
10. Asberg, M., Crönholm, B., Sjöqvist, F., and Tuck, D.: The correlation of subjective side-effects with plasma concentrations of nortriptyline, *Br. Med. J.*, **4**:18-21, 1970.
11. Åsberg, M., Crönholm, B., Sjöqvist, F., and Tuck, D.: Relationship between plasma level and therapeutic effect of nortriptyline, *Br. Med. J.*, **3**:331-334, 1971.
12. Asberg, M., Evans, D. A. P., and Sjöqvist, F.: Genetic control of nortriptyline kinetics in man. A study of relatives of propositi with high plasma concentrations, *J. Med. Genet.*, **8**:129-135, 1971.
13. von Bahr, C.: Binding and oxidation of amitriptyline and a series of its oxidized metabolites in liver microsomes from untreated and phenobarbital treated rats, *Xenobiotica*, **2**:293-306, 1972.
14. von Bahr, C., Alexanderson, B., Azarnoff, D. L., Sjöqvist, F., and Orrenius, S.: A comparative study of drug metabolism in the isolated perfused liver and *in vivo* in rats, *Eur. J. Pharmacol.*, **9**:99-105, 1970.
15. von Bahr, C. and Bertilsson, L.: Hydroxylation and subsequent glucuronide conjugation of desmethylimipramine in rat liver microsomes, *Xenobiotica*, **1**:205-212, 1971.
16. von Bahr, C. and Borgå, O.:Uptake, metabolism and excretion of desmethylimipramine and its metabolites in the isolated perfused rat liver, *Acta Pharmacol. Toxicol.*, **29**:359-374, 1971.
17. von Bahr, C., Orrenius, S., and Sjöqvist, F.: Interaction of imipramine, desmethylimipramine, nortriptyline and 1-naphthal with microsomal preparations, *Chem.-Biol. Interact.*, **3**:243-244, 1971.
18. von Bahr, C., Sjöqvist, F., and Orrenius, S.: The inhibitory effect of

hydrocortisone and testosterone on the plasma disappearance of nortriptyline in the dog and the perfused rat liver, *Eur. J. Pharmacol.,* **9**:106-110, 1970.
19. Ban, T. A.: *Psychopharmacology,* The Williams and Wilkins Co., Baltimore, Md., 1969.
20. Beckett, A. H. and Al-Sarraj, S.: Metabolism of amitriptyline, nortriptyline, imipramine and desipramine to yield hydroxylamines, *J. Pharm. Pharmacol.,* **25**:335-336, 1973.
21. Bernhard, L. and Beer, H.: Aktivitäten der expirationskohlensäure, des ZNS und anderer organe nach gaben von[14] C-signiertem N-(γ-dimethyl-aminopropyl)-iminodibenzyl (Psychopharmakon Tofranil) an ratten und hunde, *Helv. Physiol. Acta,* **20**:114-121, 1962.
22. Bertilsson, L. and Alexanderson, B.: Stereospecific hydroxylation of nortriptyline in man in relation to interindividual differences in its steady-state plasma level, *Eur. J. Clin. Pharmacol.,* **4**:201-205, 1972.
23. Bickel, M. H.: Liver metabolic reactions: Tertiary amine N-dealkylation, tertiary amine N-oxidation, N-oxide reduction, and N-oxide dealkylation: 1, Tricyclic tertiary amine drugs, *Arch. Biochem. Biophys.,* **148**:54-62, 1972.
24. Bickel, M. H. and Gigon, P. L.: Intracellular binding and metabolism of imipramine and imipramine-N-Oxide, *Chem.-Biol. Interact.,* **3**:245-246, 1971.
25. Bickel, M. H. and Minder, R.: Metabolism and biliary excretion of the lipophilic drug molecules, imipramine and desmethylimipramine in the rat. I. Experiments in vivo and with isolated perfused livers, *Biochem. Pharmacol.,* **19**:2425-2435, 1970.
26. Bickel, M. H. and Weder, H. J.: The total fate of a drug: kinetics of distribution, excretion and formation of 14 metabolites in rats treated with imipramine, *Arch. Int. Pharmacodyn. Ther.,* **173**:433-463, 1968.
27. Bickel, M. H. and Weder, H. J.: Demethylation if imipramine in the rat as influenced by SKF 525-A and by different routes of administration, *Life Sci.,* **7**(I):1223-1230, 1968.
28. Bickel, M. H. and Weder, H. J.: Buccal absorption and other properties of pharmacokinetic importance of imipramine and its metabolites, *J. Pharm. Pharmacol.,* **21**:160-168, 1969.
29. Bickel, M. H. and Weder, H. J.: Interaction of drugs with proteins I. Binding of tricyclic thymoleptics to human and bovine plasma proteins, *J. Pharm. Sci.,* **59**:1505-1507, 1970.
30. Bickel, M. H., Weder, H. J., and Aebi, H.: Metabolic interconversions between imipramine, its N-oxide and its desmethyl derivative in rat tissues in vitro, *Biochem. Biophys. Res. Commun.,* **33**:1012-1018, 1968.
31. Bonnichsen, R., Maehly, A. C., and Sköld, G.: A report on autopsy cases involving amitriptyline and nortriptyline, *Z. Rechtsmed.,* **67**:190-200, 1970.
32. Borgå, O. Azarnoff, D. L., Forshell, G. P., and Sjöqvist, F.: Plasma protein binding of tricyclic antidepressants in man, *Biochem. Pharmacol.,* **18**:2135-2143, 1969.
33. Borgå, O., Azarnoff, D. L., and Sjöqvist, F.: Species differences in the plasma protien binding of desipramine, *J. Pharm. Pharmacol.,* **20**:571-573, 1968.

34. Borgå, O. and Carle, M.: A gas chromatographic method for the quantitative determination of nortriptyline and some of its metabolites in human plasma and urine, *J. Chromatogr.*, **68**:77-88, 1972.
35. Braithwaite, R. A., Goulding, R., Theano, G., Bailey, J., and Coppen, A.: Plasma concentration of amitriptyline and clinical response, *Lancet*, **1**:1297-1300, 1972.
36. Braithwaite, R. A., Goulding, R., Theano, G., Bailey, J., and Coppen, A.: Clinical significance of plasma levels of antidepressant drugs in the treatment of depression, *Lancet*, **1**:556-557, 1973.
37. Burrows, G. D., Davies, B., and Scoggins, B. A.: Plasma concentration of nortriptyline and clinical response in depressive illness, *Lancet*, **2**:619-623, 1972.
38. Burrows, G. D., Davies, B., and Scoggins, B. A.: Clinical significance of plasma levels of antidepressant drugs in the treatment of depression, *Lancet*, **1**:557-558, 1973.
39. Cassano, G. B.: An autoradiographic study of the distribution of drugs acting on the central nervous system in the whole body and brain, *J. Nucl. Biol. Med.*, **12**:13-25, 1968.
40. Cassano, G. B., Placidi, G. F., and Ghetti, B.: Studio comparativo della distribuzione fetale di alcuni farmaci psicotropi ed ipnotici, *Riv. Neurobiol.*, **13**:105-114, 1967.
41. Cassano, G. B., Sjöstrand, S. E., and Hansson, E.: Distribution and fate of C^{14}-amitriptyline in mice and rats, *Psychopharmacologia*, **8**:1-11, 1965.
42. Cassano, G. B., Sjöstrand, S. E., and Hansson, E.: Distribution of C^{14}-labelled amitriptyline in the cat brain, *Psychopharmacologia*, **8**:12-22, 1965
43. Charalampous, K. D. and Johnson, P. C.: Studies of C^{14}-protriptyline in man: plasma levels and excretion, *J. Clin. Pharmacol.*, **7**:93-96, 1967.
44. Christiansen, J. and Gram, L. F.: Imipramine and its metabolites in human brain, *J. Pharm. Pharmacol.*, **25**:604-608, 1973.
45. Christiansen, J., Gram, L. F., Kofod, B., and Rafaelsen, O. J.: Imipramine metabolism in man. A study of urinary metabolites after administration of radioactive imipramine, *Psychopharmacologia*, **11**:255-264, 1967.
46. Corona, G. L. and Facino, R. M.: Identification and evaluation of amytriptyline and its basic metabolites in rabbit's urine, *Biochem. Pharmacol.*, **17**:2045-2050, 1968.
47. Crammer, J. L. and Rolfe, B.: Metabolism of ^{14}C-Imipramine III. Conversion by rat tissues, *Psychopharmacologia*, **18**:26-37, 1970.
48. Crammer, J. L., and Scott B.: New metabolites of imipramine, *Psychopharmacologia*, **8**:461-468, 1966.
49. Crammer, J. L., Scott, B., and Rolfe, B.: Metabolism of ^{14}C-Imipramine II. Urinary metabolites in man, *Psychopharmacoligia*, **15**:207-225, 1969.
50. Crammer, J. L., Scott, B., Woods, H., and Rolfe, B.: Metabolism of ^{14}C-Imipramine. I. Excretion in the rat and in man, *Psychopharmacologia*, **12**:263-277, 1968.
51. De Leenheer, A. and Heyndrickx, A.: Identification of a major metabolite of nortriptyline in human urine, *J. Pharm. Sci.*, **60**:1403-1405, 1971.

52. Diamond, S.: Human metabolization of amitriptyline tagged with carbon 14, *Curr. Ther. Res.*, **7**:170-175, 1965.
53. Dingell, J. V. and Sanders, E.: Methylation of desmethylimipramine by rabbit lung in vitro, *Biochem. Pharmacol.*, **15**:599-605, 1966.
54. Dingell, J. V., Sulser, F., and Gillette, J. R.: Species differences in the metabolism of imipramine and desmethylimipramine (DMI), *J. Pharmacol. Exp. Ther.*, **143**:14-22, 1964.
55. Douglas, B. H. and Hume, A. S.: Placental transfer of imipramine, a basic, lipid-soluble drug, *Am. J. Obstet. Gynecol.*, **99**:573-573, 1967.
56. Duhm, B., Maul, W., Medenwald, H., Patzschke, K., and Wegner, L: Untersuchungen mit ^{14}C-markiertem noxiptilin, *Arzneim. Forsch.*, **19**:858-870, 1969.
57. Eschenhof, E. and Rieder, J.: Untersuchungen über das schicksal des antidepressivums amitriptylin im organismus der ratte and des menschen, *Arzneim. Forsch.*, **19**:957-966, 1969.
58. Ervik, N., Walle, T., and Ehrsson, H.: Quantitative gas chromatographic determination of nanogram levels of desipramine in serum, *Acta Pharm. Suec.*, **7**:625-634, 1970.
59. Evreux, J. C., Demiaux, J. P., Magnien, J. M., Faucon, G., and Badinand, A.: Évolution des taux tissulaires d'imipramine au cours d'un traitement prolongé, *C.R. Soc. Biol. (Paris)*, **162**:721-725, 1968.
60. Evreux, J. C., Magnien, J. M., Demiaux, J. P., Fauçon, G., and Badinand, A.: Évolution des taux d'imipramine dans divers organes après une injection veineuse, *C.R. Soc. Biol.* (Paris), **162**:1529-1533, 1968.
61. Facino, R. M. and Corona, G. L.: Identification and evaluation of amitriptyline and its basic metabolites by thin-layer chromatography in rabbit organs, *J. Pharm. Sci.*, **58**:764-765, 1969.
62. Facino, R. M., Santagostino, G., and Corona, G. L., Presence of an acid metabolite of amytriptyline in rabbit urine, *Biochem. Pharmacol.*, **19**:1503-1505, 1970.
63. Faigle, J. W. and Dieterle, W.: The metabolism and pharmacokinetics of clomipramine, *J. Int. Med. Res.*, **1**:281-290, 1973.
64. Faragó, A.: Toxicological certification of fatal melipramine poisoning in a child, *Arch. Toxikol.*, **21**:30-37, 1965.
65. Faurbye, A., Jacobsen, O., Kristjansen, P., and Munkvad, I.: Imipramine-N-oxide: Preliminary investigation of a new antidepressive drug, *Am. J. Psychiatry*, **120**:277-278, 1963.
66. Fishman, V. and Goldenberg, H.: A new metabolite of imipramine, *Proc. Soc. Exp. Biol. Med.*, **110**:187-190, 1962.
67. Gillette, J. R., Dingell, J. V., Sulser, F., Kuntzman, R., and Brodie, B. B.: Isolation from rat brain of a metabolic product, desmethylimipramine, that mediates the antidepressant activity of imipramine (Tofranil), *Experientia*, **17**:417-418, 1961.
68. Gram, L. F., Kofod, B., Christiansen, J., and Rafaelsen, O. J.: Imipramine metabolism: pH-dependent distribution and urinary excretion, *Clin. Pharmacol. Ther.*, **12**:239-244, 1971.
69. Gram, L. F. and Overo, K. F.: Drug interaction: inhibitory effect of neuroleptics on metabolism of tricyclic antidepressants in man, *Br. Med. J.*, **1**:463-465, 1972.
70. Gruvstad, M.: Plasma levels of antidepressants and clinical response, *Lancet*, **1**:95-96, 1973.

71. Häfliger, F.: Chemistry of tofranil, *Can. Psychiatr. Assoc. J.*, **4**:69-74, 1959.
72. Hammar, C. G., Alexanderson, B., Holmstedt, B., and Sjöqvist, F.: Gas chromatography-mass spectrometry of nortriptyline in body fluids of man, *Clin. Pharmacol. Ther.*, **12**:496-505, 1971.
73. Hammer, W. M., and Brodie, B. B.: Application of isotope derivative technique to assay of secondary amines: Estimation of desipramine with H^3-acetic anhydride, *J. Pharmacol. Exp. Ther.*, **157**:503-508, 1967.
74. Hammer, W., Idestrom, C. M., and Sjöqvist, F.: Chemical control of antidepressant drug therapy, *in* Garattini, S. and Dukes, M. N. G., editors: *Proceedings first international symposium on antidepressant drugs,* Excerpta Med. Foundation, Amsterdam, 1967, pp. 301-310.
75. Hammer, W., Martens, S., and Sjöqvist, F.: A comparative study of the metabolism of desmethylimipramine, nortriptyline and phenylbutazone in man, *Clin. Pharmacol. Ther.*, **10**:44-49, 1969.
76. Hammer, W. and Sjöqvist, F.: Plasma levels of monomethylated tricyclic antidepressants during treatment with imipramine-like ompounds, *Life Sci.*, **6**:1895-1903, 1967.
77. Harris, S. R., Gaudette, L. E., Efron, D. H., and Manian, A. A.: A method for the measurement of plasma imipramine and desmethylimipramine concentrations, *Life Sci.*, **9**:781-788, 1970.
78. Haydu, C. G., Dhrymiotis, A., and Quinn, G. P.: Plasma imipramine level in syndromes of depression, *Am. J. Psychiatry,* **119**:574-575, 1962.
79. Haydu, G. G., Dhrymiotis, A., and Quinn, G. P.: Two varieties of plasma, imipramine curves in psychotic depressions and normal controls, *Am. J. Psychiatry,* **124**:257-260, 1967.
80. Herrmann, B.: Quantatative methoden zur untersuchung des stoffwechsels von tofranil, *Helv. Physiol. Acta.,* **21**:402-408, 1963.
81. Herrmann, B.: Untersuchungen über den stoffwechsel von 4-[3-(5H-dibenzo [b, f] azepin-5-yl)-propyl]-1-(2-hydroxy-äthyl)-piperazin dihydrochlorid, *Arzneim. Forsch.*, **14**:219-221, 1964.
82. Herrmann, B.: Aspects of the metabolism of imipramine, *in* Brill, H., editor: *Neuro-Psycho-Pharmacology,* 5, Excerpta Medica Foundation, 1967, pp. 347-351.
83. Herrmann, B. and Pulver, R.: Des stoffswechsel des psychopharmakons tofranil, *Arch. Int. Pharmacodyn Ther.*, **126**:454-469, 1960.
84. Herrmann, B., Schindler, W., and Pulver, R.: Papierchromatographischer nachweis von stoffwechselprodükten des tofranil, *Med. Exp.*, **1**:381-385, 1959.
85. Hobbs, D. C.: Distribution and metabolism of doxepin, *Biochem. Pharmacol.*, **18**:1941-1954, 1969.
86. Hucker, H. B.: Metabolism of amytriptyline, *Pharmacologist,* **4**:171, 1962.
87. Hucker, H. B. and Porter, C. C.: Studies on the metabolism of amytriptyline, *Fed. Proc.,* **20**:172, 1961.
88. Hume, A. S. and Douglas, B. H.: Placental transfer of desmethylimipramine, *Am. J. Obstet. Gynecol.,* **101**:915-917, 1968.
89. Ishitani, R., Saito, K., and Kitagawa, H.: The pharmacological studies on dimetacrine. I. Studies on the absorption, distribution and excretion of H^3 labeled dimetacrine in the rat, *Jap. J. Pharmacol.,* **20**:432-438, 1970.

90. Junod, A. F.: Accumulation of ^{14}C-imipramine in isolated perfused rat lungs, *J. Pharmacol. Exp. Ther.,* **183**:182-187, 1972.
91. Keberle, H., Riess, W., Meyer-Brunot, H. G., and Schmid, K.: Species differences in absorption, metabolism, and excretion illustrated by reference to new psycho-active drugs from the dibenzo-bicyclo-octadiene series, *The present status of psychotropic drugs, Proceedings of the 6th international congress of the Collegium Internationale Neuro-Psychopharmacologicum,* Excerpta Medica Found., Amsterdam, 1969, pp. 123-127.
92. Knapp, D. R., Gaffney, T. E., McMahon, R. E., and Kiplinger, G.: Studies of human urinary and biliary metabolites of nortriptyline with stable isotope labeling, *J. Pharmacol. Exp. Ther.,* **180**:784-790, 1972.
93. Krogh-Sorensen, P., Åsberg, M., and Eggert-Hansen, C.: Plasma-nortriptyline levels in endogenous depression, *Lancet,* **1**:113-115, 1973.
94. Kuhn, R.: Untersuchung über mögliche zusammenhange zwischen metabolitenausscheidung and kronkheitsverlauf depressiver zustände unter imipramin medikation, *Psychopharmacologia,* **8**:201-222, 1965.
95. Lehner, H., Gauch, R., and Michaelis, W.: Zum stoffwechsel von 5-methly-10-β-dimethylaminoäthyl-10, 11-dihydro-11-oxo-5h-dibenzo-[b, e] [1, 4]-diazepin HCl III: Isoliering und identifizierung von im urin ausgeschiedenen metaboliten bei mensch und tier, *Arzeneim. Forsch.,* **17**:185-189, 1967.
96. McMahon, R. E., Marshall, F. J., Culp, H. W., and Warren, M. M.: The metabolism of nortriptyline-N-Methyl-^{14}-C in rats, *Biochem. Pharmacol.,* **12**:1207-1217, 1963.
97. Michaelis, W.: Zum stoffwechsel von 5-methyl-10-β -dimethylamino-äthyl-10, 11-dihydro-11-oxo-5H-dibenzo [b, e] [1, 4]-diazepin HCl II: Resorption, verteilung in den organen und ausscheidung der mit ^{14}C markierten substanz beim tier, *Arzneim. Forsch.,* **17**:181-185, 1967.
98. Minder, R., Schnetzer, F., and Bickel, M. H.: Hepatic and extrahepatic metabolism of the psychotropic drugs, chlorpromazine, imipramine, and imipramine-N-oxide, *Arch. Pharmakol.,* **268**:334-347, 1971.
99. Moody, J. P., Tait, A. C., and Todrick, A.: Plasma levels of imipramine and desmethylimipramine during therapy, *Br. J. Psychiatry,* **113**:183-193, 1967.
100. Nagy, A. and Trieber, L.: Quantitative determination of imipramine and desipramine in human blood plasma by direct densitometry of thin layer chromatograms, *J. Pharm. Pharmacol.,* **25**:599-603, 1973.
101. Oberstig, J. im and Bäumler, J.: Suicid mit dem psychopharmakon tofranil, *Arch. Toxikol.,* **19**:339-344, 1962.
102. Populaire, P., Terlain, B., Pascal, S., Lebreton, G., and Decouvelaere, B.: Resporption, excrétion et biotransformation de la triméprimine (7162 R. P.) chez le chien et le lapin. Contribution à l'identification de plusieurs métabolites. Biotransformation chez l'homme, *Prod. Probl. Pharm.,* **25**:632-645, 1970.
103. Remy, D. C., Von Saun, W. A., Engelhardt, E. L., and Arison, B. H.: Amitriptyline metabolites. Synthesis of (R, S)-Z- and (R, S)-(E)-N-

methyl (10,11-dihydro-10-hydroxy-5H-dibenzo [a, d] cycloheptene-$\Delta^{5\gamma}$-propylamine, *J. Org. Chem.*, **38**:700-703, 1973.

104. Rizzo, M., Pantarotto, C., Riva, E., Giannelli, A., Morselli, P. L., and Garattini, S.: Interactions of tricyclic antidepressants with other drugs, *Proceedings 5th international congress on pharmacology*, San Francisco, 1972, p. 193.
105. Rowland, M.: Application of clearance concepts to some literature data on drug metabolism in the isolated perfused liver preparation and in vivo, *Eur. J. Pharmacol.*, **17**:352-356, 1972.
106. Schatz, F., Jahn, U., Andrian, R. W., and Molnar, I.: Untersuchungen über resorption und metabolismus des antidepressivums 9, 9-dimethyl-10-(3-dimethylaminopropyl)-acridan-hydro-gentartrat, *Arzneim. Forsch.*, **18**:862-871, 1968.
107. Schneider, G. and Schneider, G.: Über die aufnahme des psychopharmakons imipramine in das rattenhirn und seinen metabolismus bei einmaliger and bei chronischer gabe des medikamentes, *Psychopharmacologia*, **14**:74-82, 1969.
108. Schneider, G., Schneider, G.: and Bickel, M. H.: Über das auftreten von desmethylimipramin im gehirn der ratte nach gabe von imipramin in abhängigkeit von der injektionsart, *Psychopharmacologia*, **16**:156-160, 1969.
109. Sideropoulos, D. and Bickel, M. H.: Eine todliche vergiftung mit imipramin in kleiner dosis bein einem kleinkind, *Schweiz. Med. Wochenschr.*, **101**:851-854, 1971.
110. Sjöqvist, F., Bergfors, P. G., Borgå, O., Lind, M., and Ygge, H.: Plasma disappearance of nortriptyline in a newborn infant following placental transfer from an intoxicated mother: Evidence for drug metabolism, *J. Pediatr.*, **80**:496-500, 1972.
111. Sjöqvist, F., Berglund, F., Borgå, O., Hammer, W., Anderson, S., and Thorstrand, C.: The pH-dependent excretion of monomethylated tricyclic antidepressants, *Clin. Pharmacol. Ther.*, **10**:826-833, 1969.
112. Sjöqvist, F., Hammer, W., Borgå, O., and Azarnoff, D. L.: Pharmacological significance of the plasma level of monomethylated tricyclic antidepressants *in* Cerletti, A. and Bove, F. J., editors: *The present status of psychotropic drugs, Proceedings of the 6th international congress of the Collegium Internationale Neuro-Psychopharmacologicum*, Excerpta Medica Found., Amsterdam, 1969, pp. 128-136.
113. Viala, A., Gola, C., Cano, J.-P., and Gouezo, F.: Methode de recherche des antidepresseurs imipraminiques dans l'urine par chromatographie en phase gazeuse et par chromatogrphie sur couche mince, *Ann. Pharm. Fr.*, **30**:445-457, 1972.
114. Walter, C. J. S.: Clinical significance of plasma imipramine levels, *Proc. R. Soc. Med.*, **64**:282-285, 1971.
115. Weder, H. H. and Bickel, M. H.: Separation and determination of imipramine and its metabolites from biological samples by gas-liquid chromatography, *J. Chromatogr.*, **37**:181-189, 1968.
116. Whitnack, E., Knapp, D. R., Holmes, H. C., Fowler, N. O., and Goffney, T. E.: Demethylation of nortriptyline by the dog lung, *J. Pharmacol. Exp. Ther.*, **18**:288-291, 1972.
117. Yates, C. M., Todrick, A., and Tait, A. C.: Aspects of the clinical chemistry of desmethylimipramine in man, *J. Pharm. Pharmacol.*, **15**:432-439, 1963.

118. Zeidenberg, P., Perel, J. M., Kanzler, M., Wharton, R. N., and Malitz, S.: Clinical and metabolic studies with imipramine in man, *Am. J. Psychiatry,* **127**:1321-1326, 1971.

11

Development and Submission of an Antidepressant Compound to the FDA for Evaluation as an Investigational New Drug

W. JOSEPH POTTS, PH.D. and
EMANUELA I. DOBRIN, M.S.

INTRODUCTION

Upon recognition that a compound may have efficacy as an antidepressant agent with possible advantages over marketed products in potency, decreased latency of onset, or fewer side effects, it is entered into a development process which will assure compliance with FDA regulations for filing an Investigational New Drug Application (INDA). Individual companies may vary in their methods of bringing a new compound to clinical trials but the FDA requirements are basically the same for all new drugs. These requirements are stated on the IND application (Form FD 1571) and are seen in the accompanying example (Exhibit A). If parts 2 - 5 of Form 1571 are examined, it should be noted that emphasis in the INDA is placed on controls of raw materials and the new chemical substance. This is done to ascertain that the drug contains a minimal amount of impurities and that the quantitative composition and quality will be consistent. The specific requirements of each section of the INDA will be discussed later in this chapter. The process of development necessary to enable a company to comply with the efficacy, safety, and control requirements will be discussed initially. They will be treated as the path through which an antidepressant drug may be routed prior to compilation for submission according to the INDA guidelines.

PART I—DEVELOPMENT

New drug development occurs in a complex environment of research and development. Any system which is used to aid in new drug development should meet several criteria: It should 1) be flexible enough so that the unique requirements of any particular compound may be evaluated, 2) meet all of the requirements of the FDA for an INDA submission, 3) minimize the time requirements from discovery to human testing, and 4) allow for maximal utilization of limited resources in a planned and logical fashion.

The development path of an antidepressant agent serves as an example of the process of such a system. In our laboratories, the antidepressant actions of an agent are discovered by a mouse screening test to determine whether or not a compound blocks reserpine-induced hypothermia, or by profiling in a battery of neuropharmacological tests. The resulting profile of the new compound is then compared with that of a standard antidepressant agent. Following the discovery that a compound shows potential antidepressant properties, more thorough evaluation begins and in some cases standard agents may be tested in a parallel fashion.

The first series of tests are designed to determine the efficacy, potency, and possible mechanism of action of the agent. The group of neuropharmacological studies which have been used in our laboratories includes re-evaluation of the agent in the reserpine-induced hypothermia model (8), evaluation of the new compound's ability to reverse ptosis induced by RO 4-1284, short-acting reserpine-like compound (11), determination of its interaction with amphetamine (16), evaluation both *in vitro* (17) and *in vivo* (15) of its potential to inhibit monoamine oxidase, and examination of norepinephrine reuptake for possible blockade (12). All of these studies are performed in a dose-response fashion and the *in vivo* tests are conducted using two routes of administration.

Data from these tests are reviewed and a decision is made on whether or not to proceed with further studies with the compound based upon this preliminary information. Usually the scientists making the decision comprise a CNS research committee which has been closely following the development of the drug under consideration. The norepinephrine reuptake data only helps to begin to uncover the mechanism of action. Activity or lack of activity in this particular procedure does not determine if the agent should be developed as an antidepressant candidate, but it does influence the types of tests which will be performed in order to elucidate its mechanisms of action. In our laboratories we are not interested in an antidepressant agent which has significant generalized monoamine oxidase inhibiting (MAOI) properties or one which has a low oral to parenteral potency ratio. If the drug under consideration exhibits a mechanism of action as an MAOI we would not test it further, nor would we continue testing if we did not feel it would have advantages as an oral antidepressant. Should further testing be discontinued, the biological information learned about the compound is utilized by chemists to help develop structure activity relationships and design new compounds.

A greater number of resources must be called upon if at this point a decision is made to proceed with further testing. In this phase an acute LD_{50} determination is made, and a broad spectrum of behavioral, neuropharmacological, and neurobiochemical testing procedures are initiated in several species of animals. The agent is evaluated by several routes of administration in a dose-response fashion, and in several models the agent is administered on a chronic daily basis. When the safety studies and this rather broad spectrum of CNS testing procedures are completed, a review group evaluates the data. This evaluation is designed to determine whether any potential CNS effects would preclude further development of the drug.

Once the decision is made to "go", additional pharmacological, endocrinological, and microbiological tests are initiated. These procedures are primarily designed to determine potential side effects of the drug. In the development of an antidepressant agent specifically, the cardiovascular pharmacology is extensively evaluated in several species, particularly to determine whether or not there are any side effects of the drug on the heart. Cardiovascular effects are known to be potential problems with drugs of this class (3, 4). The other areas of special concern for side effects during this phase of testing an antidepressant are anticholinergic and antihistaminic problems and the possible influence of the compound on the pituitary gland.

At this point in development a detailed summary of the activity of the drug is written. Once it is determined that the therapeutic ratio is acceptable and if the compound has potential advantages over existing marketed antidepressant products, a decision is made to begin animal pharmacokinetic studies, sub-chronic (13 week) (7) safety studies, chemical development, and pharmaceutical development. During this phase, an evaluation is made of the market potential for a drug with the specific anticipated effects.

The animal pharmacokinetic studies usually require radio-labelled material which is provided by the original chemist working in conjunction with the radio-chemistry group. The labelled drug is usually evaluated in 3 species which often includes the monkey. The initial studies are concerned with the t-½ (one-half life) and distribution of the drug and its metabolites (9).

Later studies involve the identification and evaluation of the metabolites (5). The purpose of these drug metabolism studies is to determine which animal species would metabolize the antidepressant compound nearest to the way the human would metabolize it.

This type of information can be an invaluable aid in the planning of further pharmacological and safety evaluations (10).

The sub-chronic safety studies are performed in two species, (one has to be a non rodent) over a period of time which is usually to last for 13 weeks (7). The duration of the study and the particular parameters which are evaluated are determined by a planning group consisting of a clinician, a toxicologist/pathologist, a pharmacologist, and a chemist. The protocol for animal safety studies is based on the available biological and chemical data and is designed to meet the requirements of the anticipated clinical studies.

The chemical development group, working with the chemist who originally made the compound, begins to develop procedures for synthesizing the large quantities of compound which will be necessary for pharmaceutical development, safety studies, and clinical studies. The pharmaceutical development operation originates when the chemical development group provides sufficient quantities of drug to start chemical stability studies on the pure compound as well as on the tableted formulation.

The work of the pharmaceutical development group is based upon joint decisions between their scientists and a clinical pharmacologist regarding the dosages needed. They also confer with marketing research people in order to determine the size, color, and appearance of the dosage forms.

When these phases of work are completed and are approved, a physician assigned as a clinical monitor for the compound designs the Phase I protocol. (The Phase I clinical pharmacology studies are concerned with the first introduction of the drug into the normal human. The studies generally undertaken during Phase I include dose-response determinations for safety, tolerance levels, and pharmacokinetic evaluation for metabolism. Some early efficacy studies in patients might be included, but usually these are undertaken in Phase II). The monitor writes the clinical brochure based on the known biology and chemical information which will be used by the cooperating medical investigator in the initial clinical studies. All of this information is then assembled by the regulatory affairs personnel who will make the submission to the Food and Drug Administration's Division of Neuropharmacological Drug Products.

The process described above is obviously a complex, interdependent series of tasks. These tasks are all monitored by means of a critical path method (CPM) (13). The CPM is constructed in a manner similar to a "flow diagram" and outlines sequentially and in parallel the tasks which must be performed. A general CPM has been constructed which includes all of the tasks that are required for any INDA. From this general CPM, highly individualized CPMs are constructed for each drug under study. The individual CPM often does not end at the INDA stage, since additional animal research is continuing to be conducted either internally or on grants to outside academic institutions or research organizations. This information is also submitted to the regulatory affairs group for collation with the internally generated data which comprises the INDA submission.

The CPM technology allows flexibility so that the unique characteristics of any particular drug may be evaluated while permitting all of the FDA requirements to be met. The sequential nature of the CPM makes it possible to plan the use of limited resources for maximal benefit and thus minimizes unnecessary and unplanned delays.

PART II—PROCEDURE FOR SUBMISSION

It is the function of the Regulatory Affairs Department of a pharmaceutical company to insure that the submission of an INDA (or NDA) complies with the requirements of the regulations of the Food, Drug, and Cosmetic Act for the development of a new drug. As stated previously, these requirements are set forth in a general statement in Form FD-1571 for the INDA. The development process of an individual drug must be planned to provide evidence of well controlled studies of safety and indicate efficacy in an animal model for a specific class of drug (e.g., antidepressant). The studies must be particularly designed to show safety for that particular compound in order to begin studies in humans.

The development system for a new drug should be organized and standardized in such a way that when the data are submitted to the FDA for evaluation, chemical, biological, and clinical personnel of the FDA will be able to agree with the sponsor that it is safe to administer the drug to humans. This safety, aside from the more obvious sub-acute and (if available) chronic animal studies, must include assurance that the compound will be stable in the dosage form to be used for human testing and that the qualitative and quantitative composition will be adequate to ascertain that it has the identity, strength, quality, and purity it is purported to have by the sponsor.

The directions for assembling an IND application for a new compound are contained in the Code of Federal Regulations, Chapter 1 - Food and Drug Administration, Title 21 of the Food,

Drug and Cosmetic Act (Office of the Federal Register, Washington, D.C.) (2). The pertinent parts may be designated as follows:

Generally pertinent-

Part 310 - New Drugs
Subpart A - General Provisions
Sec.
310.3 Definitions and Interpretations

Specifically pertinent-

Part 312 - New Drugs for Investigational Use
Subpart A - Exemptions From Section 505(a)
Sec.
312.1 Conditions for exemption of new drugs for investigational use.

[Section 505(a) refers to the Federal Food, Drug, and Cosmetic Act as is defined in § 310.3]

In § 312.1 the regulations which define the procedures to be met for filing the INDA with the Food and Drug Administration are clearly stated as follows:

(a) A shipment or other delivery of a new drug shall be exempt from section 505(a) of the act if all the following conditions are met:

1) The label of such drug bears the statement "Caution: New drug—Limited by Federal (or United States) law to investigational use."

2) The person claiming the exemption has filed with the Food and Drug Administration a completed and signed "Notice of Claimed Investigational Exemption for a New Drug" in triplicate, with the information shown below in form FD-1561; and not less than 30 days have elapsed following the date of receipt of the notice by the Food and Drug Administration; and the Food and Drug Administration has not, prior to expiration of such 30-day interval, requested that the sponsor continue to withhold or to restrict use of the drug in human subjects. The 30-day delay requirement may be waived by the Food and Drug Administration upon a showing of good reason for such a waiver.

As the Regulatory Affairs Department gathers material from the research areas of the company, the material is organized into the format which is required in Form FD 1571. Each numbered part of this form contains specific information which the Neuropharmacology Division of the Office of Scientific Evaluation, of the Bureau of Drugs, at the FDA will require in order to make its assessment of the antidepressant agent. Data pertinent to each numbered part of the IND application is held in a regulatory file until the Notice is submitted. The numbering system, the specific requirements for each part, and the particular type of data meaningful to each part of the INDA form are discussed below. (Also see *Guidelines:* Manufacturing and Controls for INDA's, FDA Papers June, 1973 (6). Although these guidelines may be updated again in the near future, they are the most recent explanations of the INDA regulations.)

1. (See Exhibit A, Form FD 1571, Part 1.)

This part requires a description of the name of the drug and the chemical structure of the new drug substance, and how it is to be administered. Generally, pharmaceutical companies have their chemical compounds well protected by patents and therefore this revelation poses no problem. The nomenclature and structure should be defined with reference to a common source such as the Chemical Abstracts.

2. (See Exhibit A, Form FD 1571, Part 2.)

This part requests a list of the components of the drug. In this instance the drug means the finished dosage form which is to be utilized in the initial clinical trials, i.e.—tablets, or capsules. This information would include the drug substance itself and any excipients such as starch or coloring matter used in the preparation of the tablets or capsules including any moistening or drying agent which might be used and subsequently removed. The components must be listed for each potency level of drug. For instance, if 1, 5, and 10 mg tablets are to be used, each dose level must have its own list of components revealed.

3. (See Exhibit A, Form FD 1571, Part 3)

The quantitative composition of the components listed in Part 2 must be described in this part. Any reasonable variations or ranges in composition that may be expected should be indicated. If new or additional dosage forms are generated, then the quantitative composition of the new forms must be described in subsequent amendments.

4. (See Exhibit A, Form FD 1571, Part 4.)

This part of the INDA requests information concerning the preparation of the new drug substance. A chemical flow diagram showing structural formulas of each substance used in the preparation is acceptable but should include catalysts, reagents, solvents, and conditions (such as temperature) which are required for the preparation of the drug. If the new drug substance is not prepared by the sponsor, the name and address of the supplier should be given.

5. (See Exhibit A, Form FD 1571, Part 5.)

This section is by far the most demanding of all the chemical and quality control requirements. It is usually subdivided into several subparts which show that stringent standards are being met to assure the identity, strength, quality, and purity of the new drug. This part should contain:

A. A description of an interim reference standard to which different lots of new drug used in various biological tests may be compared. This reference standard should be pure and well characterized for identity and strength. Any new method of preparation of the reference standard should be included here. Considerations such as physical properties, odor, description of appearance, color, physical constants, optical effects as well as formulas, molecular weights, etc. should confirm the structure of this standard.

B. Data on any analytical tests such as U.V., N.M.R., I.R., and mass spectroscopy that have been used to identify the new drug and its purity. Various types of chromatography and other resolution studies on the new drug substance should also be included for confirmation of its purity. Specifications should be established for all subsequent batches of the new drug. The rationale for establishing the specifications and interpretations of the analytical data should also be given. By Phase III of the INDA all these must be firmly established.

C. Specifications for the excipients utilized in the dosage forms must also be included.

D. Description of the preparation of the finished dosage forms should also be revealed. Amounts of ingredients, equipment used in packaging and labeling procedures and containers must be described in this section.

E. All assay methods used in the laboratories should be defined in detail to assure the reviewing FDA officer of the high quality control standards met by the testing laboratories. If the compound is prepared as an injectable, then an additional description regarding sterility, as well as proof that it contains no pyrogens and other safety considerations must be offered. Placebos must also be identified and their quality and quantity should be described.

F. Although information on the stability of the compound is not specifically required in the INDA regulations, submission of stability data is usually requested by FDA personnel reviewing the Notice. The stability of the compound should be ascertained by stringent testing procedures at various temperatures and under different conditions. This information should be updated as further studies are done with subsequent dosage forms. This will occur as the compound moves towards the NDA stage. All control numbers must be identified.

6. (See Exhibit A, Form FD 1571, Part 6.)

The preclinical biological studies described previously in the development section of this chapter should be completely revealed and interpreted in this section of the INDA. Published as well as unpublished information should also be included. In addition, if clinical studies were conducted with the new drug in countries other than the U.S.A., such information should be a part of this section. If the drug is a combination of a well known drug or drugs, all pre-existing information and publications pertinent to the experience related to the components described should be included.

Antidepressant compounds are usually single drugs and so the instructions for a combination may not apply. However, the preclinical data may be scientifically demonstrated with reference to the efficacy and safety of other well known types of antidepressant agents, such as tricyclic compounds and/or monoamine oxidase inhibitors.

Part 7 introduces the clinical requirements into the INDA. The regulations described in the following part of this chapter are current but are undergoing scrutiny for possible restatement in the future. New and more stringent regulations may be introduced for the Notice of Claimed Investigational Exemption (INDA) which appear to bring it closer to meeting the demands imposed by the NDA.

7. (See Exhibit A, Form FD 1571, Part 7.)

Copies of all informational material supplied to each investigator must be included in the INDA. This would include samples of the labels for each dosage form to be used by the clinical investigators as well as the clinical brochure. This brochure usually consists of a summation of the available animal data, and of any clinical studies conducted previously (if, for instance, studies were made on the compound in a country other than the U.S.A). The brochure cannot make a claim that efficacy has been established for the use of the drug in the disease state for which it is intended e.g. depression). Generally, at the end of this section, conclusions are offered based on the scientific information which is available about the compound. It is also necessary that all warnings as well as any known or anticipated contraindications about the new drug be included in the brochure. In the case of an antidepressant, the warnings generally should include information pertinent to the class of the compound on trial, such as tricyclic drugs or monoamine oxidase inhibitors. One warning especially pertinent to tricyclic antidepressant compounds concerns the known potential of these drugs to affect the cardiovascular system. At the end of the clinical brochure, appropriate references should be given.

8. (See Exhibit A, Form FD 1571, Part 8.)

This part concerns the qualifications which the sponsor considers essential for clinical investigators who will evaluate the drug. It should take into consideration their medical background and any specialty area in which the investigators are boarded. Research experience considered relevant to conducting such a study may be cited in this part in order to establish the specifications deemed necessary to qualify the clinician.

9. (See Exhibit A, Form FD 1571, Part 9.)

Part 9 requests the names and a summary of the training and experience of each investigator and of the individual charged with monitoring the progress of the investigation. In other words, this section establishes evidence that all the responsible personnel who are to be concerned with the investigations conducted with the antidepressant are well trained and competent to conduct such studies. The sponsor of the INDA must also state in this section that forms FD 1572 (Exhibit B) or FD 1573 (Exhibit C) (Statement of Investigator forms) have been provided by the investigators and are on file in the company. These forms include statements concerning the background education, pertinent training and research experience, and information on the location where the studies will be conducted, including approval by an Institutional Review Committee where indicated. This evidence should demonstrate to the medical officers at the FDA that the sponsor has chosen reliable and well equipped research physicians to perform the investigations.

In addition, it is in this section that the clinical investigator assures, by submission of the signed Forms FD 1572 and FD 1573 to the sponsor, that he will give the drug to subjects under his own supervision or the supervision of co-investigators. He also assures the sponsor that the subjects used will only be included in the study if they have given their informed consent to participate. The investigator also should indicate that he will maintain his records for two years following the approval of the NDA for the new drug (14).

10. (See Exhibit A, Form FD 1571, Part 10.)

The responsibility for the information contained in this part of the Notice of Claimed Investigational Exemption lies within the clinical department of the sponsoring company. This section must contain an outline of the planned clinical investigations. For an initial INDA submission it is only necessary to provide a plan for the first Phase I clinical study which should determine safety and dose-response of the antidepressant in healthy humans. However, if possible, it is desirable to submit an additional outline for planned subsequent studies in human subjects. If the development process discussed earlier in this chapter has been carefully planned, designs for safety testing will be included which will support the proposed clinical studies even beyond the first clinical trial of the drug. It is essential to demonstrate that no clinical study will take place without a supportive animal safety study occurring in proper sequence *prior* to the onset of human testing. For example, if a human pharmacokinetic study is indicated in the outline for future Phase I studies, then it should be absolutely clear to the reader of the submission that this will not take place until a proper supporting animal pharmacokinetic study has occurred in an appropriate animal species.

Part 10 of the INDA submission should also include case report forms and assurance of the investigator(s) capacity to conduct such a study. Evidence should also be given that if the study is conducted within, or affiliated with, an institution, the clinical investigator has obtained permission from an Institutional Review Committee to conduct such a study. The requirements for this committee are defined within this segment of the INDA form (FD 1571 Part 10, c) and a statement is made that by signing of this Form FD 1571 the sponsor has assurance that the study has been approved by an Institutional Review Committee, if that is necessary.

The assurance offered by the outside clinical investigator for approval by the Institutional Review Committee and for guarantee of his/her qualifications and plans for conducting the study as described can be given by the clinical investigator by signing Form FD 1572 (Exhibit B), for the earlier clinical pharmacology studies with the compound or Form FD 1573 (Exhibit C) for the clinical efficacy studies. These forms are sent to the sponsor by the investigator and kept on record in their files. The sponsor's signature on the FD1571 ascertains to the FDA officers that the Statement of Investigator forms are on file within the company and are available for inspection.

Part 10 of Form FD 1571 also gives requirements for further Phase II and III studies which will be conducted in patients with the disease for which the drug is claimed to have utility (e.g. depression. It is indicated within this section that often, animal studies will continue to be ongoing even though the antidepressant is being administered to patients. Sometimes Phase I and II studies will overlap. Phase I and Phase II generally are considered to consist of clinical pharmacology studies, whereas Phase III usually consists of the clinical trials for determination of efficacy of the new compound on a larger number of patients and with additional investigators.

Additionally, this section indicates the more specific requirements for Phase III studies in patients. These must be well controlled and statistically evaluated studies and wherever ethically possible, double-blind trials should be performed in order to ascertain true efficacy of the compound as an antidepressant agent. Long term animal safety studies are often still being conducted even though Phase III clinical trials have begun.

A discussion of these advanced phases of clinical testing is not warranted here since we are primarily considering the initial submission of an INDA, but more extensive Phase II and III clinical testing procedures for antidepressant drugs are discussed in another chapter of this book.

11. (See Exhibit A, Form FD 1571, Part 11.)

This part requires a statement that the sponsor will notify the Food and Drug Administration if the investigation of the antidepressant compound is discontinued and what the reasons are for this cessation of the study.

12. (See Exhibit A, Form FD 1571, Part 12.)

This part requires a statement which assures the FDA that the sponsor will notify each investigator involved in studies with the drug if a New Drug Application for the compound is approved or if the investigation of the compound is discontinued.

13. (See Exhibit A, Form FD 1571, Part 13.)

This section contains a statement made by the sponsor of the INDA that the new drug under consideration will not be sold commercially until a New Drug Application has been approved by the FDA.

14. (See Exhibit A, Form FD 1571, Part 14.)

This final statement in the INDA submission confirms that no studies will be initiated by the sponsor in humans prior to 30 days after receipt of the Notice by the Food and Drug Administration. It assures the FDA that the sponsor of the Notice will withhold or restrict clinical studies at their request prior to the expiration of the 30 day time limit set above. The statement also confirms that no studies will be conducted in institutionalized patients until after the planned studies have been approved by an Institutional Review Committee.

15. (Under the new CFR) (See Exhibit A, Form FD 1571, Part 15.)

When requested by the agency, an environmental impact analysis report pursuant to § 6.1 of this chapter should be submitted.

The INDA notice may be updated by amendment or supplement as experience is gained with the new drug. This can be done through progress reports.

In Section 312.1, statements 3 and 4 inform the sponsor to make shipment or delivery of the new drug according to his commitments in the Notice of Claimed Investigational exemption, and to keep records concerning date of shipments, who the recipients of shipments are, amounts, batch numbers, and identifying code marks for 2 years after an NDA is approved for the drug. These records must be available for inspection by FDA officers on request.

Statement 5 of this section requests the sponsor to monitor the progress of investigations and to submit annual progress reports on the studies.

In Section 312.1, statements 6 and 7 of the Code, instructions are covered which request the sponsor of a Notice of Claimed Investigational Exemption to promptly inform the FDA and all investigators who are conducting studies with the new drug about any adverse effects of the drug. If the adverse effects are very serious, the study must be stopped until the findings are evaluated and assurance can be given that it is safe to proceed with further human testing of the compound. If this assurance cannot be given, all studies with the drug must be stopped and all outstanding supplies of the drug are to be recalled. The FDA officers will meet with the sponsor, if necessary, concerning this serious matter.

Statement 8 of this section of the Code requests that the new drug substance be recalled from a particular investigator, if the investigator has failed to make reports or records of his studies available.

Statement 9 constitutes a request for submission of an NDA once the safety and efficacy of a new drug have been established under the INDA.

Statement 10 asks the sponsor for affirmation that he will not advertise the new drug while it is still under study to establish efficacy and safety, and Statement 11 requests that no commercial distribution or test marketing of the drug will be conducted prior to NDA approval.

Statements 12 and 13, of Section 312.1 of the Code, primarily describe in detail the Form FD 1572 and Form FD 1573, which must be submitted by the investigators who are conducting studies with the new antidepressant.

FINAL RECOMMENDATIONS ON THE INDA

Prior to the submission of the above information for all parts of the INDA to the Regulatory Affairs Group, it is imperative that each department, e.g., Biology, Chemistry, Chemical Development, Development, Packaging, Quality Control, and Clinical, build a system of checks and double checks for accuracy and consistency of the data being submitted. The time from initiation of a project to completion is sometimes so long, (months, and possibly even years) that conditions, specifications, and testing procedures may change without the realization of all the parties involved. It is a good practice to have a Project Coordinator assigned who sees that all the data which are needed for the IND submission are turned in on time (for example—according to Critical Path Method dates) and have been thoroughly examined and approved by the scientific investigators, departmental directors, and a regulatory affairs monitor who is responsible for filing the Notice.

Previously in this chapter, it was stated that the FDA officers who are reviewing an IND submission must be satisfied that the drug is safe and of good and consistent quality before they will approve it for testing in human subjects. It is the responsibility of the sponsor to make certain that these highly ethical standards are met in their INDA submission. This can be accomplished through mutual cooperation between the research groups and the Regulatory Affairs Department of the sponsoring company. Together, these groups should see that all parts of Form FD 1571 are completely and carefully compiled in the Notice of Claimed Investigational Exemption for a New Drug. Finally, this team must be certain that the data being submitted on the new antidepressant are consistent and of such quality and safety that the high standards of all parties concerned will be met.

NDA PLANS

This chapter is not intended to enter into a full description of the advanced planning that must go into the submission of the New Drug Application. However, it will suffice to state that as is described in Form FD 1571 many more extensive clinical tests must be conducted on a wide basis for an NDA submission, and as Phase III is entered, efficacy of the compound must be proven by well controlled clinical trials with the new antidepressant drug. The INDA is the major foundation in the building of an NDA submission.

Simultaneously with an extensive increase in clinical testing, there is a greater research effort generated to attain more rigid chemical and quality specifications with the finalized dosage forms, and to conduct large scale animal safety studies. Included in the animal experiments are more extensive pharmacological examinations as well as teratology, mutagenicity, and carcinogenecity studies. In addition, the compound is examined on a long term basis in animal species which have been shown to metabolize the drug as defined in humans (e.g., 3 year studies in dogs (1) and primates) and continuous data is generated from these chronic animal studies with regard to blood chemistry and organ changes. At the termination of these safety studies the animals are sacrificed and autopsied, and tissues are removed and examined so that gross and microscopic histopathological determinations may be made (10).

While chemical, animal, and clinical studies are being conducted, further work is undertaken to plan proper labelling, package insert information and design of containers, etc. for marketing purposes. Marketing plans are also usually made with regard to the education of physicians to the product's assets as well as to its possible side effects. Production facilities are geared up for the manufacture of large quantities of the finished product. When a compound such as an antidepressant nears NDA approval, Food and Drug Administration inspectors will visit the sponsoring company to make certain that the company is adhering to Good Manufacturing Practices.

Many visits will also be made to FDA headquarters by the company's regulatory, scientific, and clinical personnel at specified intervals to meet with FDA officers for discussion of study results, labelling, and other pertinent matters.

All of these multitudinous activities may culminate in the approval of a New Drug Application. However, this take years of efforts by both the industrial sponsor and FDA officers. It is absolutely necessary to ascertain that the new drug is a quality product with efficacy in the disease of depression and can safely be offered to the medical profession for their treatment of this significant psychiatric disease.

REFERENCES

1. Ambrose, A. M., Larson, P. S., Borzelleca, J. F., and Hennigar, G. R., Jr.: Toxicologic studies on 3′ 4′ - dichloropropionanilide, *Toxicol. & Applied Pharm.,* **23**:650-659, 1972.
2. *Code of Federal Regulations,* Title 21, Parts 310.3, 312, 312.1, Office of the Federal Register, Washington, D.C.
3. Editorial: Cardiovascular complications from psychotropic drugs, *Brit. Med. J.,* **1**:3, January-March, 1971.
4. Editorial: Cardiovascular complications of tricyclic antidepressants, *New Zealand Med. J.,* **74**:390-391, 1971.
5. Eschenhof, E. and Rieder, J.: Studies on the fate of amitriptyline, an antidepressant, in the organism of the rat and of man, *Arzneim. Forsch.* **19**:(6) 957-966, 1969. (German).
6. *FDA Papers,* June 1973 Guidelines: Manufacturing and controls for IND's and NDA's.
7. King, W. R., Michael, W. R., and Coots, R. H.: Feeding of succistearin to rats and dogs, *Toxicol. & Appl. Pharm.,* **18**:26-34, 1971.
8. Lapin, I.: Simple pharmacological procedures to differentiate antidepressants and cholinolytics in mice and rats, *Psychopharmacologia,* **11**:79-87, 1967. (Berlin).
9. Michael, W. R., King, W. R., and Wakim, J. M.: Metabolism of disodium ethane-1-hydroxy-1,1-diphosphonate (disodium etidronate) in the rat, rabbit, dog and monkey, *Toxicol. & Appl. Pharm.,* **21**:503-515, 1972.
10. Peck, H. M.: An appraisal of drug safety evaluation in animals and the extrapolation of results to man. In *Importance of fundamental principles in drug evaluation,* p. 449-471. Proceedings of a Symposium. Ed. D. H. Tedeschi and R. E. Tedeschi, Raven Press, 15 W. 84th Street, New York, New York, 1968.
11. Rubin, B., Malone, M., Waugh, M., and Burke, J.: Bioassay of Rauwolfia roots and alkaloids, *J. Pharmacol. & Exp. Therap.,* **120**:125-136, 1957.

12. Schildkraut, J. J., Winokur, A., Draskoczy. P., and Hensle, J.: Changes in norepinephrine turnover in rat brain during chronic administration of imipramine and protriptyline: a possible explanation for their delay in onset of clinical antidepressant effects, *Amer. J. Psychiat.,* **127**:72-79, 1971.
13. Shaffer, L. R., Ritter, J. B., and Meyer, W. L.: *The critical path method,* McGraw-Hill Book Company, Inc., New York, 1965.
14. Taber, Ben Zion: *Proving new drugs: A guide to clinical trials,* Geron-X, Box 1108, Los Altos, California, 1969.
15. Tedeschi, D. H., Tedeschi, R. E., and Fellows, E. J. The effects of tryptamine on the central nervous system including a pharmacological procedure for the evaluation of iproniazid-like drugs, *J. Pharmacol. & Exp. Therap.,* **126**:223-232, 1959.
16. Weissman, A., Koe, B. K., and Tenen, S. S.: Antiamphetamine effects following inhibition of tyrosine hydroxylase, *J. Pharmacol. & Exp. Therap.,* **151**:339-352, 1966.
17. Wurtman, R. J. and Axelrod, J.: A sensitive and specific assay for the estimation of monoamine oxidase, *Biochemical Pharmacol.,* **12**:1439-1441, Dec. 1963.

DEPARTMENT OF HEALTH, EDUCATION, AND WELFARE
PUBLIC HEALTH SERVICE
FOOD AND DRUG ADMINISTRATION

Exhibit A

Form Approved
OMB No. 57-R0030

NOTICE OF
CLAIMED INVESTIGATIONAL EXEMPTION
FOR A NEW DRUG

Name of Sponsor ______________________________

Address ______________________________

Date ______________________________

Name of Investigational Drug ______________________________

Commissioner
Food and Drug Administration
Bureau of Drugs (BD-26)
5600 Fishers Lane
Rockville, Maryland 20852

Dear Sir:

The sponsor, ______________________________, submits this notice of claimed investigational exemption for a new drug under the provisions of section 505(i) of the Federal Food, Drug, and Cosmetic Act and §130.3 of Title 21 of the Code of Federal Regulations.

Attached hereto, in triplicate, are:

1. The best available descriptive name of the drug, including to the extent known the chemical name and structure of any new-drug substance, and a statement of how it is to be administered. (If the drug has only a code

preclinical data before a clinical trial is undertaken, the Department will notify the sponsor to submit the complete preclinical data and to withhold clinical trials until the review is completed and the sponsor notified. The Food any reasonable alternates for inactive components.

3. Complete statement of quantitative composition of drug, including reasonable variations that may be expected during the investigational stage.

4. Description of source and preparation of, any new-drug substances used as components, including the name and address of each supplier or processor, other than the sponsor, of each new-drug substance.

5. A statement of the methods, facilities, and controls used for the manufacturing, processing, and packing of the new drug to establish and maintain appropriate standards of identity, strength, quality, and purity as needed for safety and to give significance to clinical investigations made with the drug.

6. A statement covering all information available to the sponsor derived from preclinical investigations and any clinical studies and experience with the drug as follows:

a. Adequate information about the preclinical investigations, including studies made on laboratory animals, on the basis of which the sponsor has concluded that it is reasonably safe to initiate clinical investigations with the drug: Such information should include identification of the person who conducted each investigation; identification and qualifications of the individuals who evaluated the results and concluded that it is reasonably safe to initiate clinical investigations with the drug and a statement of where the investigations were conducted and where the records are available for inspection; and enough details about the investigations to permit scientific review. The preclinical investigations shall not be considered adequate to justify clinical testing unless they give proper attention to the conditions of the proposed clinical testing. When this information, the outline of the plan of clinical pharmacology, or any progress report on the clinical pharmacology, indicates a need for full review of the

vestigated (e.g. outside the United States), complete information about such distribution or investigation shall be submitted, along with a complete bibliography of any publications about the drug.

c. If the drug is a combination of previously investigated or marketed drugs, an adequate summary of preexisting information from preclinical and clinical investigations and experience with its components, including all reports available to the sponsor suggesting side-effects, contraindications, and ineffectiveness in use of such components: Such summary should include an adequate bibliography of publications about the components and may incorporate by reference any information concerning such components previously submitted by the sponsor to the Food and Drug Administration. Include a statement of the expected pharmacological effects of the combination.

7. A total of three copies of all informational material, including label and labeling, which is to be supplied to each investigator: This shall include an accurate description of the prior investigations and experience and their results pertinent to the safety and possible usefulness of the drug under the conditions of the investigation. It shall not represent that the safety or usefulness of the drug has been established for the purposes to be investigated. It shall describe all relevant hazards, contraindications, side-effects, and precautions suggested by prior investigations and experience with the drug under investigation and related drugs for the information of clinical investigators.

8. The scientific training and experience considered appropriate by the sponsor to qualify the investigators as suitable experts to investigate the safety of the drug, bearing in mind what is known about the pharmacological action of the drug and the phase of the investigational program that is to be undertaken.

FD FORM 1571 (5/71) PREVIOUS EDITIONS ARE OBSOLETE.

9. The names and a summary of the training and experience of each investigator and of the individual charged with monitoring the progress of the investigation and evaluating the evidence of safety and effectiveness of the drug as it is received from the investigators, together with a statement that the sponsor has obtained from each investigator a completed and signed form, as provided in subparagraph (12) or (13) of this paragraph, and that the investigator is qualified by scientific training and experience as an appropriate expert to undertake the phase of the investigation outlined in section 10 of the "Notice of Claimed Investigational Exemption| for a New Drug." (In crucial situations, phase 3 investigators may be added and this form supplemented by rapid communication methods, and the signed form FD 1573 shall be obtained promptly thereafter.)

10. An outline of any phase or phases of the planned investigations and a description of the institutional review committee, as follows:

a. Clinical pharmacology. This is ordinarily divided into two phases: Phase 1 starts when the new drug is first introduced into man--only animal and in vitro data are available--with the purpose of determining human toxicity, metabolism, absorption, elimination, and other pharmacological action, preferred route of administration, and safe dosage range; phase 2 covers the initial trials on a limited number of patients for specific disease control or prophylaxis purposes. A general outline of these phases shall be submitted, identifying the investigator or investigators, the hospitals or research facilities where the clinical pharmacology will be undertaken, any expert committees or panels to be utilized, the maximum number of subjects to be involved, and the estimated duration of these

iv. The estimated duration of the clinical trial and the intervals, not exceeding 1 year, at which progress reports showing the results of the investigations will be submitted to the Food and Drug Administration.
(The notice of claimed investigational exemption may be limited to any one or more phases, provided the outline of the additional phase or phases is submitted before such additional phases begin. This does not preclude continuing a subject on the drug from phase 2 to phase 3 without interruption while the plan for phase 3 is being developed.)

Ordinarily, a plan for clinical trial will not be regarded as reasonable unless, among other things, it provides for more than one independent competent investigator to maintain adequate case histories of an adequate number of subjects, designed to record observations and permit evaluation of any and all discernible effects attributable to the drug in each individual treated, and comparable records on any individuals employed as controls. These records shall be individual records for each subject maintained to include adequate information pertaining to each, including age, sex, conditions treated, dosage, frequency of administration of the drug, results of all relevant clinical observations and laboratory examinations made, adequate information concerning any other treatment given and a full statement of any adverse effects and useful results observed, together with an opinion as to whether such effects or results are attributable to the drug under investigation.

c. Institutional review committee. If the phases of clinical study as described under 10a and b above are conducted on institutionalized subjects or are conducted by an individual affiliated with an institution which agrees to assume responsibility for the study, assurance must be given that an institutional review committee is responsible for initial progress reports on these early phases, or in the development of the plan for the clinical trial, phase 3. The first two phases may overlap and, when indicated, may require additional animal data before these phases can be completed or phase 3 can be undertaken. Such animal tests shall be designed to take into account the expected duration of administration of the drug to human beings, the age groups and physical status, as for example, infants, pregnant women, premenopausal women, of those human beings to whom the drug may be administered, unless this has already been done in the original animal studies.

b. Clinical trial. This phase 3 provides the assessment of the drug's safety and effectiveness and optimum dosage schedules in the diagnosis, treatment, or prophylaxis of groups of subjects involving a given disease or condition. A reasonable protocol is developed on the basis of the facts accumulated in the earlier phases, including completed and submitted animal studies. This phase is conducted by separate groups following the same protocol (with reasonable variations and alternatives permitted by the plan) to produce well-controlled clinical data. For this phase, the following data shall be submitted:

i. The names and addresses of the investigators. (Additional investigators may be added.)

ii. The specific nature of the investigations to be conducted, together with information or case report forms to show the scope and detail of the planned clinical observations and the clinical laboratory tests to be made and reported.

iii. The approximate number of subjects (a reasonable range of subjects is permissible and additions may be made), and criteria proposed for subject selection by age, sex, and condition.

members of varying background, that is, lawyers, clergymen, or laymen as well as scientists, to assure complete and adequate review of the research project. The membership must possess not only broad competence to comprehend the nature of the project, but also other competencies necessary to judge the acceptability of the project or activity in terms of institutional regulations, relevant law, standards of professional practice, and community acceptance. Assurance must be presented that neither the sponsor nor the investigator has participated in selection of committee members; that the review committee does not allow participation in its review and conclusions by any individual involved in the conduct of the research activity under review (except to provide information to the committee); that the investigator will report to the committee for review any emergent problems, serious adverse reactions, or proposed procedural changes which may affect the status of the investigation and that no such change will be made without committee approval except where necessary to eliminate apparent immediate hazards; that reviews of the study will be conducted by the review committee at intervals appropriate to the degree of risk, but not exceeding 1 year, to assure that the research project is being conducted in compliance with the committee's understanding and recommendations: that the review committee is provided all the information on the research project necessary for its complete review of the project; and that the review committee maintains adequate documentation of its activities and develops adequate procedures for reporting its findings to the institution. The documents maintained by the committee are to include the names and qualifications of committee members, records of information provided to subjects in obtaining informed consent, committee discussion on substantive issues and their resolution, committee recommendations, and dated reports of successive reviews as they are performed. Copies of all documents are to be retained for a period of 3 years past the completion or discontinuance of the study and are to be made available upon request to duly authorized representatives of the Food and Drug Administration. (Favorable recommendations by the committee are subject to further appropriate review and rejection by institution officials. Unfavorable recommendations, restrictions, or conditions may not be overruled by the institution officials.) Procedures for the organization and operation of institutional review committees are contained in guidelines issued pursuant to Chapter 1-40 of the Grants Administration Manual of the U.S. Department of Health, Education, and Welfare, available from the U.S. Government Printing Office. It is recommended that these guidelines be followed in establishing institutional review committees and that the committees function according to the procedures described therein. A signing of the Form FD 1571 will be regarded as providing the above necessary assurances. If the institution, however, has on file with the Department of Health, Education, and Welfare, Division of Research Grants, National Institutes of Health, an "accepted general assurance," and the same committee is to review the proposed study using the same procedures, this is acceptable in lieu of the above assurances and a statement to this effect should be provided with the signed FD 1571. (In addition to sponsor's continuing responsibility to monitor the study, the Food and Drug Administration will undertake investigations in institutions periodically to determine whether the committees are operating in accord with the assurances given by the sponsor.)

11. It is understood that the sponsor will notify the Food and Drug Administration if the investigation is discontinued, and the reason therefor.

12. It is understood that the sponsor will notify each investigator if a new-drug application is approved, or if the investigation is discontinued.

13. If the drug is to be sold, a full explanation why sale is required and should not be regarded as the commercialization of a new drug for which an application is not approved.

14. A statement that the sponsor assures that clinical studies in humans will not be initiated prior to 30 days after the date of receipt of the notice by the Food and Drug Administration and that he will continue to withold or to restrict clinical studies if requested to do so by the Food and Drug Administration prior to the expiration of such 30 days. If such request is made, the sponsor will be provided specific information as to the deficiencies and will be afforded a conference on request. The 30-day delay may be waived by the Food and Drug Administration upon a showing of good reason for such waiver; and for investigations subject to institutional review committee approval as described in item 10c above, an additional statement assuring that the investigation will not be initiated prior to approval of the study by such committee.

Very truly yours,

	INDICATE AUTHORITY

(This notice may be amended or supplemented from time to time on the basis of the experience gained with the new drug. Progress reports may be used to update the notice.)

ALL NOTICES AND CORRESPONDENCE SHOULD BE SUBMITTED IN TRIPLICATE.

3

Exhibit B

DEPARTMENT OF HEALTH, EDUCATION, AND WELFARE
PUBLIC HEALTH SERVICE
FOOD AND DRUG ADMINISTRATION
5600 FISHERS LANE
ROCKVILLE, MARYLAND 20852

STATEMENT OF INVESTIGATOR
(Clinical Pharmacology)

Form Approved
OMB No. 57-R0031

TO: SUPPLIER OF THE DRUG *(Name and address, include Zip Code)*

NAME OF INVESTIGATOR *(Print or Type)*

DATE

NAME OF DRUG

Dear Sir:

The undersigned, ______________________________,
submits this statement as required by section 505(i) of the Federal Food, Drug, and Cosmetic Act and §130.3 of Title 21 of the Code of Federal Regulations as a condition for receiving and conducting clinical pharmacology with a new drug limited by Federal (or United States) law to investigational use.

1. STATE THE EDUCATION AND TRAINING YOU HAVE HAD THAT QUALIFIES YOU FOR CLINICAL PHARMACOLOGY

2. GIVE NAME AND ADDRESS OF THE MEDICAL SCHOOL, HOSPITAL, OR OTHER RESEARCH FACILITY WHERE THE CLINICAL PHARMACOLOGY WILL BE CONDUCTED

3. If the experimental project is to be conducted on institutionalized subjects or is conducted by an individual affiliated with an institution which agrees to assume responsibility for the study, assurance must be given that an institutional review committee is responsible for initial and continuing review and approval of the proposed clinical study. The membership must be comprised of sufficient members of varying background, that is, lawyers, clergymen, or laymen as well as scientists, to assure complete and adequate review of the research project. The membership must possess not only broad competence to comprehend the nature of the project, but also other competencies necessary to judge the acceptability of the project or activity in terms of institutional regulations, relevant law, standards of professional practice, and community acceptance. Assurance must be presented that the investigator has not participated in the selection of committee members; that the review committee does not allow participation in its review and conclusions by any individual involved in the conduct of the research activity under review (except to provide information to the committee); that the investigator will report to the committee for review any emergent problems, serious adverse reactions, or proposed procedural changes which may affect the status of the investigation and that no such change will be made without committee approval except where necessary to eliminate apparent immediate hazards; that reviews of the study will be conducted by the review committee at intervals appropriate to the degree of risk, but not exceeding 1 year, to assure that the research project is being conducted in compliance with the committee's understanding and recommendations; that the review committee is provided all the information on the research project; and that the review committee maintains adequate documentation of its activities and develops adequate procedures for reporting its findings to the institution. The documents maintained by the committee are to include the names and qualifications of committee members, records of information provided to subjects in obtaining informed consent, committee discussion on substantive issues and their resolution, committee recommendations, and dated reports of successive reviews as they are performed. Copies of all documents are to be retained for a period of 3 years past the completion or discontinuance of the study and are to be made available upon request to duly authorized representatives of the Food and Drug Administration. (Favorable recommendations by the committee are subject to further appropriate review and rejection by institution officials. Unfavorable recommendations, restrictions, or conditions may not be overruled by the institution officials.) Procedures for the organization and operation of institutional review committees are contained in guidelines issued pursuant to Chapter 1-40 of the Grants Administration Manual of the U.S. Department of Health, Education, and Welfare, available from the U.S. Government Printing Office. It is recommended that these guidelines be followed in establishing institutional review committees and that the committees function according to the procedures described therein. A signing of the Form FD 1572 will be regarded as providing the above necessary assurance; however, if the institution has on file with the Department of Health, Education, and Welfare, Division of Research Grants, National Institutes of Health, an "accepted general assurance," and the same committee is to review the proposed study using the same procedures, this is acceptable in lieu of the above assurances and a statement to this effect should be provided with the signed FD 1572. (In addition to sponsor's continuing responsibility to monitor the study, the Food and Drug Administration will undertake investigations in institutions periodically to determine whether the committees are operating in accord with the assurances given by the sponsor.)

FD FORM 1572 (5/71)

PREVIOUS EDITION MAY BE USED UNTIL SUPPLY IS EXHAUSTED.

4. ESTIMATE DURATION OF THE PROJECT AND INDICATE THE MAXIMUM NUMBER OF SUBJECTS THAT WILL BE INVOLVED

5. GENERAL OUTLINE OF THE PROJECT TO BE UNDERTAKEN *(Modification is permitted on the basis of experience gained without advance submission of amendments to the general outline, but with the approval of the review committee and upon notification of the sponsor.)*

6. THE UNDERSIGNED UNDERSTANDS THAT THE FOLLOWING CONDITIONS GENERALLY APPLICABLE TO NEW DRUGS FOR INVESTIGATIONAL USE GOVERN HIS RECEIPT AND USE OF THIS INVESTIGATIONAL DRUG

a. The sponsor is required to supply the investigator with full information concerning the preclinical investigation that justifies clinical pharmacology.

names of the subjects need not be divulged unless the records of the particular subjects require a more detailed study of the cases, or unless there is reason to believe that the records do not represent actual studies or do not represent actual results pended or terminated to return to the sponsor any unused supply of the drug.

c. The investigator is required to prepare and maintain adequate case histories designed to record all observations and other data pertinent to the clinical pharmacology.

d. The investigator is required to furnish his reports to the sponsor who is responsible for collecting and evaluating the results, and presenting progress reports to the Food and Drug Administration at appropriate intervals, not exceeding 1 year. Any adverse effect which may reasonably be regarded as caused by, or is probably caused by, the new-drug shall be reported to the sponsor promptly; and if the adverse effect is alarming it shall be reported immediately. An adequate report of the clinical pharmacology should be furnished to the sponsor shortly after completion.

e. The investigator shall maintain the records of disposition of the drug and the case reports described above for a period of 2 years following the date the new-drug application is approved for the drug; or if no application is to be filed or is approved until 2 years after the investigation is discontinued and the Food and Drug Administration so notified. Upon the request of a scientifically trained and specifically authorized employee of the Department, at reasonable times, the investigator will make such records available for inspection and copying. The

only to subjects under his personal supervision or under the supervision of the following investigators responsible to him,

____

____

____

____

and that the drug will not be supplied to any other investigator or to any clinic for administration to subjects.

g. The investigator certifies that he will inform any patients or any persons used as controls, or their representatives, that drugs are being used for investigational purposes, and will obtain the consent of the subjects, or their representatives, except where this is not feasible or, in the investigator's professional judgment, is contrary to the best interests of the subjects.

h. The investigator is required to assure the sponsor that for investigations involving institutionalized subjects the studies will not be initiated until the institutional review committee has reviewed and approved the study. (The organization and procedure requirements for such a committee should be explained to the investigator by the sponsor as set forth in Form FD 1571, division 10, unit c.)

Very truly yours,

____

(Name of Investigator)

____

(Address)

____

Exhibit C

DEPARTMENT OF HEALTH, EDUCATION, AND WELFARE
PUBLIC HEALTH SERVICE
FOOD AND DRUG ADMINISTRATION
5600 FISHERS LANE
ROCKVILLE, MARYLAND 20852

STATEMENT OF INVESTIGATOR

Form Approved
OMB No. 57-R0029

TO: SUPPLIER OF DRUG *(Name and address, include Zip Code)*	NAME OF INVESTIGATOR *(Print or Type)*
	DATE
	NAME OF DRUG

Dear Sir:

The undersigned, ______________________________,
submits this statement as required by section 505(i) of the Federal Food, Drug, and Cosmetic Act and §130.3 of Title 21 of the Code of Federal Regulations as a condition for receiving and conducting clinical investigations with a new drug limited by Federal (or United States) law to investigational use.

1. STATEMENT OF EDUCATION AND EXPERIENCE

a. COLLEGES, UNIVERSITIES, AND MEDICAL OR OTHER PROFESSIONAL SCHOOLS ATTENDED, WITH DATES OF ATTENDANCE, DEGREES, AND DATES DEGREES WERE AWARDED

b. POSTGRADUATE MEDICAL OR OTHER PROFESSIONAL TRAINING *(Indicate dates, names of institutions, and nature of training)*

c. TEACHING OR RESEARCH EXPERIENCE *(Indicate dates, institutions, and brief description of experience)*

d. EXPERIENCE IN MEDICAL PRACTICE OR OTHER PROFESSIONAL EXPERIENCE *(Indicate dates, institutional affiliations, nature of practice, or other professional experience)*

e. REPRESENTIVE LIST OF PERTINENT MEDICAL OR OTHER SCIENTIFIC PUBLICATIONS *(Indicate titles of articles, names of publications and volume, page number, and date)*

FD FORM 1573 (5/71) PREVIOUS EDITION MAY BE USED UNTIL SUPPLY IS EXHAUSTED.

2a. If the investigation is to be conducted on institutionalized subjects or is conducted by an individual affiliated with an institution which agrees to assume responsibility for the study, assurance must be given that an institutional review committee is responsible for initial and continuing review and approval of the proposed clinical study. The membership must be comprised of sufficient members of varying background, that is, lawyers, clergymen, or laymen as well as scientists, to assure complete and adequate review of the research project. The membership must possess not only broad competence to comprehend the nature of the project, but also other competencies necessary to judge the acceptability of the project or activity in terms of institutional regulations, relevant law, standards of professional practice and community acceptance. Assurance must be presented that the investigator has not participated in the selection of committee members; that the review committee does not allow participation in its review and conclusions by any individual involved in the conduct of the research activity under review (except to provide information to the committee) that the investigator will report to the committee for review any emergent problems, serious adverse reactions, or proposed procedural changes which may affect the status of the investigation and that no such change will be made without committee approval except where necessary to eliminate apparent immediate hazards; that reviews of the study will be conducted by the review committee at intervals appropriate to the degree of risk, but not exceeding 1 year, to assure that the research project is being conducted in compliance with the committee's understanding and recommendations; that the review committee is provided all the information on the research project necessary for its complete review of the project; and that the review commit-

taining informed consent, committee discussion on substantive issues and their resolution, committee recommendations, and dated reports of successive reviews as they are performed. Copies of all documents are to be retained for a period of 3 years past the completion or discontinuance of the study and are to be made available upon request to duly authorized representatives of the Food and Drug Administration. (Favorable recommendations by the committee are subject to further appropriate review and rejection by institution officials. Unfavorable recommendations, restrictions, or conditions may not be overruled by the institution officials.) Procedures for the organization and operation of institutional review committees are contained in guidelines issued pursuant to Chapter 1-40 of the Grants Administration Manual of the U.S. Department of Health, Education, and Welfare, available from the U.S. Government Printing Office. It is recommended that these guidelines be followed in establishing institutional review committees and that the committees function according to the procedures described therein. A signing of the Form FD 1573 will be regarded as providing the above necessary assurances; however, if the institution has on file with the Department of Health, Education, and Welfare, Division of Research Grants, National Institutes of Health, an "accepted general assurance," and the same committee is to review the proposed study using the same procedures, this is acceptable in lieu of the above assurances and a statement to this effect should be provided with the signed FD 1573. (In addition to sponsor's continuing responsibility to monitor the study, the Food and Drug Administration will undertake investigations in institutions periodically to determine whether the committees are operating in accord with the assurances given by the sponsor.)

the institution. The documents maintained by the committee are to include the names and qualifications of committee members, records of information provided to subjects in ob- will be used. (If this information has been submitted to the sponsor and reported by him on Form FD 1571, reference to the previous submission will be adequate).

3. OUTLINE THE PLAN OF INVESTIGATION *(Include approximation of the number of subjects to be treated with the drug and the number to be employed as controls, if any; clinical uses to be investigated; characteristics of subjects by age, sex and condition; the kind of clinical observations and laboratory tests to be undertaken prior to, during, and after administration of the drug; the estimated duration of the investigation; and a description or copies of report forms to be used to maintain an adequate record of the observations and tests results obtained. This plan may include reasonable alternates and variations and should be supplemented or amended when any significant change in direction or scope of the investigation is undertaken.)*

4. THE UNDERSIGNED UNDERSTANDS THAT THE FOLLOWING CONDITIONS, GENERALLY APPLICABLE TO NEW DRUGS FOR INVESTIGATIONAL USE, GOVERN HIS RECEIPT AND USE OF THIS INVESTIGATIONAL DRUG

a. The sponsor is required to supply the investigator with full information concerning the preclinical investigations that justify clinical trials, together with fully informative material describing any prior investigations and experience and any possible hazards, contraindications, side-effects, and precautions to be taken into account in the course of the investigation.

b. The investigator is required to maintain adequate records of the disposition of all receipts of the drug, including dates, quantities, and use by subjects, and if the investigation is terminated to return to the sponsor any unused supply of the drug.

c. The investigator is required to prepare and maintain adequate and accurate case histories designed to record all observations and other data pertinent to the investigation on each individual treated with the drug or employed as a control in the investigation.

d. The investigator is required to furnish his reports to the sponsor of the drug who is responsible for collecting and evaluating the results obtained by various investigators. The sponsor is required to present progress reports to the Food and Drug Administration at appropriate intervals not exceeding 1 year. Any adverse effect that may reasonably be regarded as caused by, or probably caused by, the new drug shall be reported to the sponsor promptly, and if the adverse effect is alarming, it shall be reported immediately. An adequate report of the investigation should be furnished to the sponsor shortly after completion of the investigation.

is discontinued. Upon the request of a scientifically trained and properly authorized employee of the Department, at reasonable times, the investigator will make such records available for inspection and copying. The subjects' names need not be divulged unless the records of particular individuals require a more detailed study of the cases, or unless there is reason to believe that the records do not represent actual cases studied, or do not represent actual results obtained.

f. The investigator certifies that the drug will be administered only to subjects under his personal supervision or under the supervision of the following investigators responsible to him,

____

____

____

and that the drug will not be supplied to any other investigator or to any clinic for administration to subjects.

g. The investigator certifies that he will inform any subjects, including subjects used as controls, or their representatives, that drugs are being used for investigational purposes, and will obtain the consent of the subjects, or their representatives, except where this is not feasible or, in the the investigator's professional judgement, is contrary to the best interests of the subjects.

h. The investigator is required to assure the sponsor that for investigations involving institutionalized subjects, the studies will not be initiated until the institutional for a period of 2 years following the date a new-drug application is approved for the drug; or if the application is not approved, until 2 years after the investigation a committee should be explained to the investigator by the sponsor as set forth in form FD 1571, division 10, unit c.)

Very truly yours,

____
(Name of Investigator)

____
(Address)

____

(This form should be supplemented or amended from time to time if new subjects are added or if significant changes are made in the plan of investigation.)

12

Clinical Evaluation of Antidepressant Drugs

HARBANS LAL, PH.D., STUART FIELDING, PH.D.
and JOHN KARKALAS, M.D.

I. GENERAL CONSIDERATIONS

A. Purpose

After completion of appropriate pharmacological and toxicological studies of antidepressant drugs in lower animals, investigations are undertaken to determine their pharmacology, clinical efficacy, and safety in human subjects. Since adequate animal models to test antidepressants are not available, human studies with these drugs are more critical than in several other cases where inference from animal studies can be somewhat more meaningful.

Specifically, there are several pharmacological, clinical, and professional objectives in undertaking clinical evaluation of antidepressant drugs. The pharmacological objectives consist of determining efficacy, pharmacokinetics, and side effects of the test drug. This information is necessary for selection of optimal dose, onset and duration of action, and interaction with other drugs, as well as other biological processes in the body.

The clinical objectives center around the therapeutic value of the drug. A clinician is not only concerned with the information that the drug is active, but is also interested in knowing if it provides improvement over previously available choices for treatment of depression, and whether the test drug has a better safety margin between efficacy and toxicity.

Professional considerations include the designing of experimental protocols which are acceptable to the FDA, investigating teams, practicing psychiatrists, and the profession at large. A foremost consideration is that the new antidepressant provides a more progressive chemotherapy rather than a duplication of what is already available. In addition, researchers also look for clues to evolve new approaches to search for new antidepressants.

B. Methodology

The principles for "adequate and well controlled clinical investigations" published in the May 9, 1970 issue of the *Federal Register*, are applicable to the evaluation of antidepressant. However, difficulty is frequently encountered in establishing an unequivocal diagnosis of depression because quantitative and universally accepted diagnostic criteria are not available. Depression is a subjective symptom which occurs in association with a variety of other types of psychopathology. Therefore, individual studies must describe clearly their operational criteria for selection of patients and each patient should be characterized as to the presence and intensity of various symptoms of depression. This will not only provide more meaningful clinical information but also allow pooling of results from several studies.

Although usual measures and study designs are described in this chapter, the state-of-art in clinical efficacy of antidepressants requires development of new and better techniques. Evidence of clinical efficacy derived from new approaches is given sufficient weight by the FDA in order to encourage further improvements in the tools available to clinical psychopharmacology.

The task of monitoring the progress of clinical investigation rests primarily on the professional staff assigned by the drug company. In carrying out this role, close contact between industry monitors and clinical investigators is maintained. The FDA reviews clinical research plans and assists the project monitors as well as investigators in carrying out various phases of drug evaluation.

Informed consent is needed before a volunteer is included in clinical evaluation. However, severely depressed patients pose a problem in obtaining informed consent. In such a case, the opinion of a second clinician as to the patient's competence to give informed consent and to his understanding of the proposed study should be obtained. Otherwise, permission from the patient's guardian should be obtained. Women with childbearing potential should be included in a study only if results of reproductive and teratologic studies in animals are considered to be satisfactory or where clinical setting provides sufficient insurance against the risk of pregnancy. After safety and efficacy studies are well advanced in adult patients, children and minor adolescents with parental consent may be included in the evaluation. The elderly and patients with a history of drug dependency or patients with cardiovascular, hepatic, renal, or other serious organic diseases, usually should be excluded.

The superiority of existing drugs over placebo is not sufficiently large to exclude placebo controls. Therefore, provision should be made to remove from the study patients whose clinical condition worsens or fails to improve in a reasonable period of time.

II. EARLY CLINICAL PHARMACOLOGY—PHASE I

A. Objective

To provide evidence as to the pharmacological effects, dose-related side effects, and safety in normal volunteers and/or psychiatric patients based upon both single dose and time-limited multiple dose studies. Evidence as to drug absorption, distribution, metabolism, and excretion is desirable if it is technically feasible to obtain it.

B. Subjects

The subjects are prisoners, other confined "normals" or institutionalized patients who are adults of age 21 or over and generally do not require concomitant medication. They are informed volunteers and have normal baseline physical examinations, laboratory tests, and other clinical evaluation. Women of childbearing potential, children, and individuals with serious diseases usually are excluded.

If normal volunteers are used, it must be recognized that the findings may have little relevance when compared with some psychiatric patients, particularly in their ability to tolerate side effects or larger doses of the drug.

C. Setting and Investigator

Usually the setting is a confined one in which provisions are available for close supervision and treatment on a 24-hour basis. The investigator is an especially competent individual with experience in clinical pharmacology, psychiatry, or internal medicine who will conscientiously carry out frequent and thorough evaluation of all study subjects.

D. Design and Assessment

Prior to receiving the test drug, all subjects should receive no other drugs for a period appropriate to insure that there will be no metabolic or symptomatic carryover effects. For example, if the previous drug has a relatively short half-life, the necessary drug-free period may be only several days while for drugs with longer half-life it should be much longer.

Single-Dose Study—It is beyond the scope of this chapter to list the many variations in study designs that may be appropriate for the first trials of a new anti-depressant drug in humans. However, each should encompass the following general principles: First dose in the first subject should be minimal and based on animal toxicity studies (e.g., $^1/_5$ to $^1/_{10}$ of the maximum nontoxic dose in animals); monitoring before and after each dose (hence term single-dose study); determination that each dose level is safe before administering a higher single dose to same or other subjects; interval before repeating same or higher dose in same subject sufficient to insure "washout" (when feasible as determined by animal and evolving human pharmacokinetic and pharmacologic data).

The following, which is to serve only as an example of one possible study design, may be accomplished with approximately six subjects in an open trial. The first subject receives a minimal single dose determined as stated above. The second subject receives the maximum dose given the first subject. Each additional subject then starts at the maximum dose administered to the prior subject. All subjects continue to receive increments of the drug to the maximum tolerated dosage. The subjects are monitored as to laboratory, and when feasible, pharmacokinetic parameters at baseline, prior to receiving increments, and at followup intervals.

Multiple-Dose Study—This is preferably double-blind with placebo control. Numerically balanced or imbalanced parallel group design may be used, e.g., 20 drugs vs 20 placebo, 12 drug vs 8 placebo, or 30 drug vs 10 placebo. Dosages are increased at appropriate intervals (if possible, based on pharmacokinetics of single-dose study). As a precaution, subgroups starting at day or week intervals are used. When treatment emergent symptoms or side effects prohibit further increases, the doses are cut back to maximum tolerated doses and are continued for at least 14 days. By this method, a total duration of approximately six-weeks is usual, although it may often take longer. In any case, the duration of administration should be appropriate to the intended duration of further studies with recognition that additional and longer term safety data will evolve from them.

Safety and/or toxicity are usually assessed by: baseline and repeated extensive physical examinations; vital sign assessments; laboratory tests to assess the hematopoietic, liver, renal, and cardiovascular system. The type, extent, and frequency of testing will depend in part upon the type of drug, the preclinical information available, evolving information, and the eventual intended use of the compound. However, followup data usually should be obtained at least weekly during administration and whenever possible for at least one week after discontinuation of drug.

E. Documentation

Basically all study documentation should include the following:

a. Subject identification, demographic data, pertinent medical history, and vital statistics.
b. Pre-and post-treatment physical examination results.
c. Details of administration of medication and of dosage adjustment.
d. All behavioral and emotional effects observed or reported.
e. All adverse reactions reported or observed, the date, the severity and duration of such reactions, the investigator's judgment of whether drug-related, the control measures utilized, and the results of such measures.
f. All laboratory reports, including normal ranges for particular lab used.

F. Pharmacokinetics

When initial safety studies have been completed, the absorption and half-life of the drug should be determined, if feasible, and the relevancy of such data analyzed as to the evaluation of safety and efficacy.

III. CLINICAL INVESTIGATIONS—PHASE II

A. Objectives

In Phase II the overall objectives are:

1. To identify conditions or symptoms which may be therapeutically responsive to the drug.
2. To estimate the appropriate clinical dosage and duration of effect.
3. To identify adverse effects.

B. Subjects

Early Phase II studies can be conducted with inpatient or outpatient adult males and females who are not pregnant or planning pregnancy in the near future depending on the degree of clinical supervision possible. Other patient categories may be used (children, aged, or females who may become pregnant) when proper animal toxicity studies have been conducted and appropriate dosage for these samples is established by cautious and gradual increments. Patients are continually monitored for safety of the drug, as described in the Phase I.

As determined by comprehensive clinical and laboratory evaluation, patients evaluated early in this phase should require no concomitant medication and have no organic disease that may obscure clinical observations, laboratory tests, or interpretations.

In early Phase II studies, heterogeneous samples are useful to determine range of implications. Later in Phase II, the sample should be as homogeneous as possible, considering the following: age, sex, weight, and socio-occupational group.

Carefully specified criteria for selection of subjects for antidepressant drug trials are desirable for two reasons:

1. The greater the homogeneity of the sample, the greater the likelihood of obtaining reliable and valid results in comparing a new compound with placebo or standard drug.
2. In generalizing the results of clinical trials to therapeutic practice, it is necessary to have an adequate description of the patients' characteristics to provide assurance that they are representative of some clinically relevant population.

C. Target Symptoms

In the evaluation of antidepressant drugs, major problems arise from the semantic confusion associated with the multiple meanings of the term "depression." Depression has different usages in various scientific fields, including physiology, psychology, and psychiatry. In clinical psychiatry, the two uses that are most pertinent to drug investigations are depression as a symptom and as a syndrome. As a symptom, depression may occur in association with a variety of medical and psychiatric disorders. As a syndrome, depression may occur in association with other mental, behavioral, and psychophysiological manifestations in various, and as yet poorly understood, complex combinations.

Failure to clarify the purpose of the study may lead to difficulties in patient selection, in design, in execution of the study, and in unnecessary problems in the interpretation of the data.

1. Depression as a Symptom as a Target for Drug Therapy.

Depression as a symptom occurs in a wide variety of clinical conditions. Antidepressant drug treatment may be useful in such conditions. However, research and clinial experience have not clearly demonstrated that drug treatment of depression as a symptom can be generalized across all states.

We also do not have normative data for distinguishing between the normal depressive state and the pathologic symptom. Research efforts are underway using population survey and epidemiologic techniques to generate such norms.

The following recommendations seem appropriate:

a. Depressive symptoms occur in many transient conditions, such as: post-partum, following coronary disease or long infectious disease, and also as significant accompaniments of many chronic medical ailments of the cardiovascular, rheumatic and arthritic, and gastrointestinal systems. Where a drug is being evaluated for depression in these states, the drug company and the investigators should specify the population, and the criteria for the primary medical diagnoses should be described in detail.

b. Symptoms required to be present at entrance to the study should be specified in the protocol. Two alternative procedures have been used successfully.

They are:

i. Listing of target symptoms, e.g., depression, crying, agitation, insomnia, etc., with a statement as to their frequency in the sample studies, measure of severity, and the duration prior to entrance into the study.

ii. Where established scales are used, pretreatment level should be established below which patients will not be admitted to the study.

c. Where antidepressant drugs are being used for depressive symptoms accompanying other psychiatric conditions, this indication should be specified in the protocol, and the diagnosis criteria identified. In practice, three such populations have been involved in antidepressant drug trials. These are:

i. Alcoholics. Care should be taken to exclude patients who are or have only very recently experienced acute withdrawal symptoms such as tremulousness, or seizures.

ii. Schizophrenic or schizo-affective states. The criteria for the diagnosis should be specified.

iii. Aged patients, including those with CNS disease in whom depression is a frequent concomitant.

2. The Depressive Syndromes and Drug Evaluation

The most common clinical conditions for which antidepressant drugs are evaluated are the various depressive syndromes. Syndrome refers to the temporal coexistence and covariation of related symptoms and behaviors. Patients with a depressive syndrome usually manifest depressed mood (as described below) plus a significant number (4-5) of associated symptoms.

1. Depressed mood characterized by any of the following: sad, low, blue, despondent, hopeless, gloomy
2. Anhedonia—inability to experience pleasure
3. Poor appetite or weight loss
4. Sleep difficulty (insomnia or hypersomnia)
5. Loss of energy; fatigue; lethargy
6. Agitation
7. Retardation
8. Decrease in libido
9. Loss of interest in work and usual activities
10. Feelings of self-reproach or guilt
11. Diminished ability to think or concentrate, such as slowed thinking or mixed-up thoughts
12. Thoughts of death and/or suicide attempts
13. Feelings of helplessness and hopelessness
14. Anxiety or tension
15. Bodily complaints

Since these symptoms will occur together at greater than chance, factor analysis and correlational statistics are useful to identify symptom groupings. Depressive syndromes usually involve various complex patterns or configurations. It is important to acknowledge that there is no one depressive syndrome. There is no agreement as to the bases upon which the various depressive syndromes should be identified and separated. Most investigators currently accept the concept of heterogeneity within the affective disorders and employ various pluralistic or dualistic diagnostic distinctions. The most used pluralistic distinctions are embodied in the official APA-WHO nomenclatures which designate multiple affective states such as manic depressive illness, involutional states, psychoneurotic depression, etc. The dualistic distinctions involve the primary-secondary separation developed by Robins and Guze, the unipolar-bipolar distinctions developed by Peris, Leonhard, and Winokur, and the endogenous-neurotic distinction recently revised by Kiloh, Mendels, Klein, and others. Older distinctions, which have also been used in drug evaluations, are the retarded-agitated typology and the psychotic-neurotic forms.

In addition, there are statistically derived typologies, which utilize computer programs for assignment of patients to multiple groups. The Overall-Hollister typology has been used in antidepressant drug studies. Techniques developed by Paykel, by

Grinker and associates in Chicago, and by Friedman in Philadelphia have not yet been widely applied to drug evaluation.

It is suggested that:

1. The investigator should specify the classification approach used and the criteria for assignment of patients to designated groups.
2. Among the assignment and selection techniques shown to have been effective in drug studies are those developed by Raskin for the NIMH collaborative study, by Overall and Hollister for VA studies, and by Kiloh and Roth for endogenous-reactive types.
3. Investigators usually make use of several scales which have been developed for drug research. For a number of scales, such as the Raskin, Beck, Wittenborn, MMPI, Hamilton, and Zung, information exists as to the range of scores expected in populations, such as outpatient and inpatient, and for grades of severity. These ranges should be compared with new data.
4. The degree of severity of a patient's illness should be described using global scales.
5. The patient's status should be described, i.e., outpatient, day, or inpatient and whether the patient is seen in private practice or in group practice, a clinic, or institutional setting.
6. It is desirable that a variety of socio-demographic and clinical characteristics of the patients be reported. These characteristics include age, sex, racial or ethnic background, social class, previous hospitalization, previous diagnoses of mania or schizophrenia, and previous major therapies, i.e., electroconvulsive therapy, neuroleptics, etc.
7. It is recommended that the criteria for exclusion be identified particularly for patients on the borderline between schizophrenia and the affective diseases.

Sample Size

In early Phase II studies, sample size varies because actual numbers depend on the problems to be investigated and on the magnitude of difference between the treatment and control groups that is to be expected or is actually observed. There should be sufficient numbers of subjects to assure a reasonable likelihood of demonstrating differences if they exist.

In later Phase II or Phase III studies, a minimum of twenty patients per treatment group are necessary if drug-placebo or drug-drug differences are to be demonstrated.

D. Setting and Investigators

In early Phase II studies, an inpatient setting is most often used. If other settings, e.g., outpatient clinic, day hospital, private clinic, or private office are necessary, they should be described and justified.

The investigators should be experienced in evaluating psychiatric drugs and conducting clinical trials; they should have ready access to the appropriate population group for whom the drug may be indicated.

E. Design

Patients are selected so as to provide an unbiased sample of the population of interest and are assigned to treatments at random. Predrug severity of the disorders to be measured are recorded and included as part of the design.

Drug-Free Period

When safe and feasible, each study subject should have a drug-free period for several days prior to receiving the test medication. The number of days would depend upon the prior medication received by the subject and its duration.

There are two reasons for this procedure. One, rapid remitters and placebo responders can be detected and eliminated from the study, thus maximizing the likelihood of establishing drug effect. Second, during the "washout" period, patients who have been taking drugs with potential for dependence or withdrawal will manifest these behaviors.

If patients' symptoms decrease to a level below criteria for entrance into the study during this "washout" period, they should not continue in the study.

Uncontrolled Trials

In early Phase II, several open or uncontrolled trials are desirable to allow investigators sufficient flexibility to explore possible aspects of a new drug's activity and to allow for the determination of an appropriate dosage range for use in double blind studies. It must be kept in mind that information obtained from these early open studies can only form hypotheses which must then be tested in controlled studies. The open studies may be of small sample size; however, it may be desirable for valid clinical measures and selection of patient samples to be consistent among investigators in order to facilitate the interpretation of results.

Controlled Trials

Hypotheses evolved from open studies can be confirmed or refuted only by controlled double-blind studies. In at least some late Phase II studies the investigational new drug is compared to a matching placebo control to establish its efficacy. Other studies include only an active treatment control or both.

Parallel groups, crossover, and other designs are used. The planning of this and other aspects of these studies, whenever feasible, involves extensive consultation with a biostatistician in order to be aware of the advantages, disadvantages, and criteria for validity regarding each possible design before selecting one. Comparisons between two active drugs usually require much larger sample sizes than active drug-placebo comparisons.

Packaging and coding of medications are performed on an individual basis rather than on a treatment group basis. Other psychoactive drugs are avoided. If other drugs are used, this is carefully documented and justified.

F. Dosage and Duration

Open or Uncontrolled Studies

After selection of initial dosage based on all previous data (including pharmacokinetic), dosage in open trials is usually increased until a satisfactory therapeutic response is observed. If adverse effects become a significant problem, further increases are precluded and dosages reduced or discontinued.

Double-blind, Controlled Studies

Dosage may be fixed; however, because of individual metabolism and tolerance, a flexible dosage is often necessary.

A specified range may be used (as determined in earlier trials) within which adjustments are made individually according to specified clinical criteria.

The mode of administration, range, schedule of administration, and criteria for dosage adjustment should be stated in each protocol.

The duration of individual clinical studies in Phase II varies from days to weeks depending on their purpose and the nature of the drug. The therapeutic activity of antidepressant agents usually can be established in trials of approximately four weeks' duration. However, to allow for a further assessment of safety beyond that obtained in Phase II, at least one of the first several Phase II studies should be continued for six weeks with appropriate laboratory monitoring if preliminary data have indicated satisfactory support of efficacy.

G. Assessment

Physical exams and clinical laboratory tests are basically the same as those for Phase I. Appropriate and validated rating scales are used in addition to global assessment. Emergence of symptoms which may represent side effects or possible new uses are recorded. The reliability of the ratings often require more than one rater.

Baseline observations are carried out in all patients immediately before their initiation into the study. The frequency of followup determinations may then vary from days to weeks.

All adverse reactions reported or observed become part of the record. The dose of the drug at the time of appearance of the side effect, the duration of the side effect, severity, judgment as to whether the drug is responsible for the side effect, method of treating the side effect, and the results of the treatment are recorded. If the side effect is severe enough to discontinue the subject from the study, this is documented.

Techniques for Assessment of Change

There are a number of techniques which are applied in the assessment of change with antidepressant drugs. No one technique in itself is considered sufficient, though not all techniques are required. Varying combinations may be employed depending on the phase of investigation and the types of patients.

These techniques include:

1. Global measures. The NIMH and VA studies have used 5-7 point scales. The Menniger Health-Illness Scale may also be used. Categories of improvement (marked-moderate-some-none-worse) are widely used.
2. Clinical Interview Scales. The scales developed by Hamilton, Levi, Overall, Spitzer, Wittenborn, and others are of demonstrated reliability, validity, and sensitivity to drug effects.
3. Self-report techniques. These have gained wide acceptance in outpatient samples. Among those frequently used are the Zung, the Beck, the MMPI, the Symptom Check List (SCL), the Clyde Mood Scale (CMS), and the Adjective Check List.
4. For inpatients and day patients, direct observational approaches to behavior rated by nurses or other personnel have been used. The most common scales are those of Lorr, Burdock, the NOSIE, and the Grosser-Wechsler scales.

5. Social adjustment. Assessment of social adjustment seems most appropriate for drug maintenance trials where patients are followed into the community after discharge from the hospital. In these studies, drug therapy attempts at demonstrating efficacy in the prevention of relapse and recurrence by prophylactic or maintenance therapy. This need occurs in long-term trials with lithium or tricyclics.
6. Psychological techniques, such as projective methods and tests of intelligence, have not been used widely as measures of efficacy. They provide useful associated data, and further research may demonstrate their validity.
7. Verbal sample techniques and content analysis, such as those developed by Gottscalk and associates, have proven sensitive to drug response.
8. Psychophysiological measures, including EEG, pulse rate, blood pressure, EMG, GSR, and pulse volume do not in themselves provide evidence of efficacy but may be useful as associated indices of change. However, pulse, BP, and weight are valuable clinical indicators and are suggested for studies, even though they may not be criteria of efficacy. Specialized psychophysiological methods, such as quantitative EEG analysis, while still in the investigational stage may provide valuable data.

Other techniques, including rating scales, developed by the investigator may be employed provided that evidence for their reliability and validity is available.

Efforts should be made to establish agreement on the use of diagnostic and descriptive terms as well as the handling of assessment instruments. This may be accomplished by investigator meetings or indepth discussion by the monitor with each investigator.

Interpretation

In addition to clinical considerations, the interpretation of studies in this phase involves extensive statistical analysis which often cannot be predetermined. Rather than interpreting studies solely on the material they provide, it is important that all available information concerning a drug be considered, including preclinical studies, before making a final positive or negative conclusion regarding it.

Insofar as possible, it is desirable to demonstrate efficacy within the unit study. However, it may be difficult to obtain enough patients in a unit study to achieve strong statistical evidence of efficacy therein, particularly when two active medications are involved. This may result simply from a scarcity of patients or from particularly strong placebo effects in the type of patient and/or setting involved. Under such circumstances, it is necessary to pool data from several studies to provide convincing statistical evidence of efficacy.

IV. CLINICAL INVESTIGATIONS—PHASE III

By the middle or end of Phase II, sufficient information is available to formulate hypotheses as to the types of patients and the clinical conditions which may respond to the investigational drug. For testing these hypotheses, controlled trials are necessary. This is the major purpose of Phase III studies.

A. Objectives

Extended comparative controlled studies are used to fully confirm the drug's basic antidepressant activity in heterogeneous patient populations and to provide more specific information about symptoms and patient types in which the drug is especially effective. Placebo controlled trials are necessary as are comparisons with standard drugs of established efficacy for the clinical condition.

Long-Term Safety Studies. To establish the safety of a new antidepressant agent when given daily for 3 to 6 months, long-term safety studies are undertaken with particular regard to the nature, incidence, and control of side effects.

B. Subjects

Similar considerations apply as in Phase II. In this phase, patients with the diagnosis of primary depressive syndrome of some form are usually included. Populations with other than primary depressive disorders, such as depression with schizophrenia or in association with anxiety or with medical conditions, may be studied in separate trials.

A greater variety of populations differing as to age, sex, diagnostic categories, social class, treatment setting, previous treatment, etc., are studied. Within each study (or subgroup in studies of sufficient size), patients are selected to be as homogeneous as possible regarding the above variables. In any case, full reporting of patient characteristics is necessary to allow for adequate interpretation of results.

Exclusion should be stated. Exclusion of placebo responders may strengthen a trial. The placebo response for a particular patient population should, at least, be known to the investigator.

Females of childbearing age may be included if results of animal reproductive and teratologic studes are satisfactory.

While it may be possible to demonstrate drug effects in samples as small as twenty patients per treatment group, experience has shown that samples in the range of thirty to fifty patients in each treatment group provide greater assurance.

C. Setting and Investigators

A number of settings may be used, e. g., inpatients, outpatients, and private practice.

Because the extension of claims into other areas involves a variety of types of investigators, it is important to consider the investigator's capability and experience in evaluating and working with patients with depression, his provisions for needed safety precautions, his access to laboratory facilities with suitable controls, and the appropriateness of his clinical setting to allow for valid drug evaluation.

D. Design

Of primary importance during Phase III of a drug's evaluation are controlled studies designed to fully confirm the drug's basic antidepressant efficacy. The design is generally the same as that discussed in Phase II. However, adjustments which do not interfere with validity are made in controls, duration of study, dosage, and design to accommodate greater variations in purpose of studies, settings, investigators, and subjects as discussed under the respective headings in Phase II.

There is wide agreement that a number (preferably three to five) of studies in Phase III should compare the new compound with a placebo and with an established drug of demonstrated efficacy in similar pharmacological class (tricyclic, MAO inhibitor, and psychomotor stimulant). These studies should be double-blind and utilize standard methods of assessment of change.

Crossover designs to control bias have major inherent difficulties because of carryover effect, both pharmacological and psychological, particularly in depressive syndromes (spontaneous remissions, self-limiting, response to attention, etc.).

When it is concluded that the drug's basic antidepressant efficacy has been clearly established by controlled studies, consideration may be given to undertaking further studies on an open trial basis with new populations. Due to the lack of a control group for comparison, these, of course, carry with them the inherent risk of encountering difficulties in interpretation of unexpected findings. However, such findings, as stated previously, can lead to forming hypotheses which must be confirmed or refuted by reviewing already completed controlled studies or by establishing further controlled studies. In providing further experience with the drug (often under conditions of usual medical practice), these studies can be important in providing corroborative support of efficacy demonstrated by well-controlled studies and in adding valuable data regarding safety of the new drug. This is particularly true when a number of investigators working independently obtain similar findings.

Patients may also be evaluated in studies related to other than the major antidepressant claim. For each of these other areas, a number of double-blind studies should be sufficient. Prior to these, it may be necessary to carry out several open studies to familiarize the investigator with the drug's activity and appropriate dosage range in a particular therapeutic situation or special population. In these populations, carefully edited (i.e., they need not include all variables of other studies) clinical pharmacology and therapeutic trials may be carried out to establish tolerance, efficacy, and safety.

Long-term safety studies may be on an open trial basis or may be of a controlled parallel group design.

Data regarding long-term safety may also be obtained from a number of studies rather than from a single formally structured one. For example, provision may be made for patients in therapeutic trials to continue on the drug if it is indicated. Special attention is given to children, elderly patients, and women who are of childbearing potential.

E. Dosage and Duration

It is necessary to establish in dose-response studies the dosage that gives adequate clinical response with a minimum of side effects.

In long-term safety studies, dosage should be of at least the level expected for eventual general therapeutic use. Allowance for adjustments to age, sex, and individual tolerance, of course, must be provided.

The duration of therapeutic trials (Phase III) may vary as in Phase II and, particularly regarding open trials, may often be longer. After baseline determinations in all cases, followup evaluations usually become less frequent as evolving data permit.

The duration of long-term safety studies is usually three to six months. Again, baseline observations should be carried out in all cases and followup evaluations are usually at least monthly.

F. Assessment and Interpretation

This is generally similar to that outlined for Phase II. Valid adjustments are permissible as indicated. Laboratory evaluations are usually not necessary for as many patients as in Phase II on the basis of accumulated data.

Since most Phase III studies involve multiple trials, consideration is given to problems of statistical analysis and interpretation within each trial, among various trials, and when data from a number of trials are grouped or pooled.

G. Maintenance Studies and Long-Term Trials

Currently, there is considerable interest in long-term trials to establish the value of maintenance antidepressant therapy in prevention of relapse or recurrence. Whereas the treatment goal in acute episodes is the reduction of symptoms and the patient's return to a premorbid state; in long-term maintenance therapies, the goals are more ambitious: prevention of relapse of recurrence after an initial episode, facilitation of the patient's social and vocational adaption, relief from minor symptoms, enhancement of personal adjustment, and life satisfaction.

Research methodolgy in these studies is still in the developmental stage and there are many unsolved design and statistical problems.

A major problem is the identification of patients likely to suffer from multiple recurrences. While a significant number of patients with acute depressions are likely to have multiple recurrences, it is difficult on the basis of presenting clinical symptoms to predict which patients experiencing acute depressions are likely to have recurrences. The frequency of recurrence in a large population as well as the duration of intervals between relapse and recurrence is highly variable.

Given this lack of information, investigators have employed different strategies to select samples for long-term maintenance studies. Most investigators advocate selecting patients who have had two or more well-defined episodes and/or hospitalizations. Others have proposed selecting patients with salient symptoms or characteristics such as family history, manic elations, clear-cut retardation, or well-defined periodicity.

In evaluating the efficacy of treatment, the criteria of effectiveness are different from those used in studies of acute treatment. Reduction of mortality, especially from suicide, is a major criterion. Another is prevention or reduction of rehospitalization rates. These effects are more easily identified but occur less frequently than minor relapses or recurrences that may not be of sufficient intensity to require hospitalization. For the detection of such symptomatic change, rating scales and systematic clinical observation are needed.

Moreover, for evaluating criteria in areas such as family and marital functioning, social effectiveness, and vocational performance, new techniques are needed in addition to the established rating scales which assess psychopathology and mood.

Design problems for long-term maintenance studies are considerable. In the absence of established data as to the predictors of relapse and the frequency of rehospitalization and recurrence, a concurrent control group receiving no treatment or placebo is highly desirable. There are significant statistical problems, particularly the need for statistical techniques for repeated measures. Various forms of trend analysis or stochastic models may assume an important role.

A related problem deals with attrition. The longer a trial continues, the greater the likelihood that patients will drop out; the sample finishing the trial is often not identical to that beginning the trial. Life-table methods and other statistical techniques derived from public health morbidity and mortality studies may have applicability in this area.

13

Computer EEG Profiles of Antidepressants: Quantitative Pharmaco-EEG in the Development of New Antidepressive Drugs

TURAN M. ITIL, M.D.

I. INTRODUCTION

Due to lack of knowledge concerning the etiology, physiopathology, and biochemistry of depressive illness, as well as the unknown mode of action of antidepressive drugs, the development of new antidepressive compounds has thus far been exclusively empirical. The basic approach has been a retrospective one. Compounds having chemical and, particularly, pharmacological similarities to existing potent antidepressive drugs, such as tricyclic antidepressants, and to a lesser degree, MAO inhibitors, were selected to be investigated in early clinical trials. Accordingly, clinical pharmacologists and early clinical drug investigators received dozens of so-called "new" compounds, the majority of which are actually only slightly better or worse copies of existing compounds. Serendipity still remains the major factor in the discovery of totally new antidepressive drugs.

Just recently we have developed a method of early detection and classification of psychotropic effects of drugs, using digital computer analyzed, scalp-recorded electroencephalogram (EEG) and a series of sophisticated statistical procedures. This method, called "quantitative pharmaco-electroencephalography" (32-34, 42, 44, 45), was developed on the basis of the following observations:

1. All drugs effective in human psychopathology (psychotropic drugs) produce significant alterations in the scalp-recorded EEG. In our studies with more than 200 experimental and marketed compounds, we observed significant correlations between alterations of human behavior and changes in EEG. To demonstrate the changes in EEG induced by drugs, however, one has to consider

certain factors such as the dosages of the drugs, the type of subjects studied, the time of EEG observations, and the type of EEG evaluations (3, 29, 34). The studies of Fink (7-12, 15) and Goldstein (23-25), as well as our own clearly demonstrated that quantitative evaluation techniques of EEG are inevitable if one is to determine systematic alterations within so-called "normal" variations of the human EEG.

2. The second and perhaps most important observation is the existence of close correlations between the types of EEG alterations and the therapeutic spectrum of psychotropic drugs. It is most surprising that the EEG patterns of all antipsychotic drugs (major tranquilizers), whether they are phenothiazines, thioxanthenes, or butyrophenones, are very similar and are characterized by an increase of slow waves, including slow alpha activity, and decrease of fast waves [chlorpromazine EEG reaction type, (28), or major tranquilizer EEG reaction type, (27)]. The major tranquilizers and the methods effective in treatment of psychosis, such as different kinds of coma treatments and electroshock, produce similar EEG alterations, particularly after 2-3 weeks of treatment (29). In contrast, drugs that produce hallucinatory phenomena in man (hallucinogenic compounds) induce EEG findings almost completely opposite to those of antipsychotic drugs; decrease of slow waves, decrease of slow alpha activity, and increase of desynchronized low voltage fast activity are the characteristic findings of hallucinogenic compounds (14, 30). The drugs effective in anxiety syndromes (anxiolytics or minor tranquilizers) decrease slow waves and increase synchronized higher voltage fast activity. We called these types of EEG alterations "minor tranquilizer" or "anxiolytic EEG reaction type" (27, 32). Drugs effective in depressive syndromes (thymoleptics) produce both slow and fast waves simultaneously, while decreasing alpha activity. We called this kind of EEG phenomenon "promethazine EEG reaction type" (28), or "antidepressant (thymoleptic) EEG reaction type" (27, 29).

3. The third observation is the fact that all classical minor-major tranquilizers, thymoleptics, and CNS stimulants produce EEG alterations after single oral dosages which are very similar to those produced after chronic multiple dosages. The digital computer EEG profiles of single and multiple doses of psychoactive drugs showed extreme similarities (34).

A. Definition of Quantitative Pharmaco-EEG

The process involving the use of digital computer analyzed, scalp-recorded electroencephalogram and a series of statistical procedures for establishing the central effect of a new compound in humans, the prediction of its clinical usefulness, and the effective dosage range and duration of effects after administration of a single, oral dose in normal healthy volunteers has been called "quantitative pharmaco-EEG." Although the conventional electroencephalographical equipment is used and the recorded activity on the paper is a typical conventional electroencephalgram, only 4 of 22 measurements (1.3-3.5, 3.5-7.5, 7.5-13, and 13-20 cps) of digital computer period analysis (49) can be evaluated by the classical "eyeball" evaluation of the records by a clinical electroencephalographer and only 2 of the measurements (1.3-3.5, 3.5-7.5 cps) are actually considered for diagnostic purposes. However, according to our investigations, all 22 computer EEG (CEEG) measurements are important to predict and classify psychoactive drugs. Since these measurements are not the same as those used in conventional electroencephalography, to prevent a misunderstanding, we prefer to call the activities used in quantitative pharmaco-EEG "computerized cerebral bio-potentials" (CCBP) or "computer EEG" (CEEG).

Some of the most important questions asked in quantitative pharmaco-EEG are as follows:

1. Does the drug have any CNS effects?

In order to answer this question the pre-drug and post-drug values of 22 EEG measurements of the total group of subjects studied were compared using either analysis of variance and covariance statistics, or evaluation of the changes from pre-drug values to values after drug administration in terms of analysis of variance or t-test.

2. Does the new compound have any psychotropic use?

This is probably the most important question asked in quantitative pharmaco-EEG trials and to answer it, the most simple, up-to-date, and successful method is the ***CEEG drug profile***. To determine the computer EEG profile of a drug, the pre-drug 22 CEEG measurements for each subject are subtracted from the post-CEEG measurements (1 hour, 3 hours, and/or 6 hours, etc. after drug administration), creating a change mean value for each subject for each of the 22 CEEG measurments. This new set of data is used as input to a one sample t-test, which tests whether the change values are statistically different from zero. The computer t-statistics are then plotted, creating a drug profile. If placebo also is investigated in the same study, CEEG changes induced by placebo are subtracted from the changes induced by active drug. The difference is considered to be the "real" drug effect. According to our studies there are no substantial differences between the drug profiles and drug minus placebo profiles, indicating non-significant effects of placebo. The obtained computer EEG profiles of a new drug are then compared with the available CEEG profiles of more than 60 drugs previously studied using visual means, discriminant analysis, cluster techniques, and/or correlation statistics. Depending on the similarity of the new compound to the previously investigated compounds whose type of clinical effectiveness is known, a prediction is made about the psychoactive properties of the new compound. Obviously, our prediction of the type of psychotropic effects of a new compound based on computer CEEG profiles is also a retrospective one. However, should a new compound not show any similarity to the profiles of previously studied compounds, we may find that it is effective on brain function and that it is a new profile with new clinical applications, which are also important aspects of our method.

3. Does the compound produce time- and dose-related alterations in brain function?

In order to answer this question, pre- and post-drug administration computer EEG measurements are compared using regression statistics.

Using the methods of quantitative pharmaco-EEG in recent years we were able not only to accelerate the evaluation of psychotropic drugs by receiving important information during Phase I trials, but also to predict the antidepressive (thymoleptic) properties of some drugs which could not be determined with the methods of classical animal pharmacology.

II. EEG PATTERN OF ANTIDEPRESSANTS

A. Visual (Eyeball) Evaluation

As early as 1961 we described, among the psychoactive phenothiazines, a group of substances which produce EEG alterations different from those of "promethazine" and "chlorpromazine" type of drugs. We observed that after i.v. injection of these substances, there occurs instant dissolution of the alpha rhythm, accompanied by simultaneous occurrence of low voltage slow waves and superimposed low voltage fast elements (28, 29). Occasionally dissolution of the alpha rhythm may be preceded by a temporary activation of short duration. We observed that levomepromazine produced the most characteristic of these changes and so we called this kind of drug-induced EEG alteration "levomepromazine reaction type" (28). We classified thioridazine, imipramine, amitriptyline, and levomepromazine, as well as some experimental compounds such as KS-75 Sandoz, a piperidyl phenothiazine, and WH 1219 Bayer, a strong anticholinergic phenothiazine, in the same group of drugs based on the type of EEG alterations produced (29). We also observed that the EEG alterations of these compounds after chronic multiple dose oral administration are similar to those after single dose i.v., most commonly with a decrease of alpha and an increase of slow waves with superimposed fast activity. The effectiveness of all of these drugs on depressive syndromes (thymoleptic effect) led us to call this kind of drug-induced alteration the "thymoleptic EEG reaction type" (27).

Whereas in general the EEG alterations with increase of slow waves after tricyclic antidepressants such as amitriptyline and imipramine were observed by the majority of investigators, the alterations after antidepressive MAO inhibitors were not well described (13). It was reported that the MAO inhibitors have few defined EEG effects. Borenstein et al (4) found no significant frequency or amplitude changes but only changes in response to activation after MAO inhibitors. After nialimide a decrease in percentage of time spent in alpha was observed (26), while after phenelzine (48), isocarboxazide (2), iproniazid (19), and nialimide (21) no systematic EEG changes were found.

B. Analog Frequency Analyzer

Using analog frequency analyzer, Fink (8) described the differences in EEG alterations between chlorpromazine, a major tranquilizer, and imipramine, an antidepressant. Later in a well-designed study, he showed that chronic multiple dose administration of chlorpromazine combined with procyclidine increases slow waves with slight decrease of fast activity and slight increase of alpha waves, while imipramine produces, in addition to slow waves, a decrease of alpha activity and an increase of fast beta activity (7). In investigations with acute intravenous administration, we observed that basic characteristics of imipramine-induced alterations are an increase of power in slow frequencies and decrease of alpha and slow beta frequencies, with an increase of faster activities (Fig. 1) (39). The chlorpromazine-induced alterations in normal volunteers were similar to imipramine in all time periods (15-20, 35-40, 55-60 minutes), except 5-10 minutes after i.v. administration. Chlordiazepoxide produced EEG alterations based on analog frequency analyzer that were very different from those induced by chlorpromazine and imipramine. Similar findings were obtained when imipramine and chlorpromazine were intravenously administered in a group of schizophrenic patients (43).

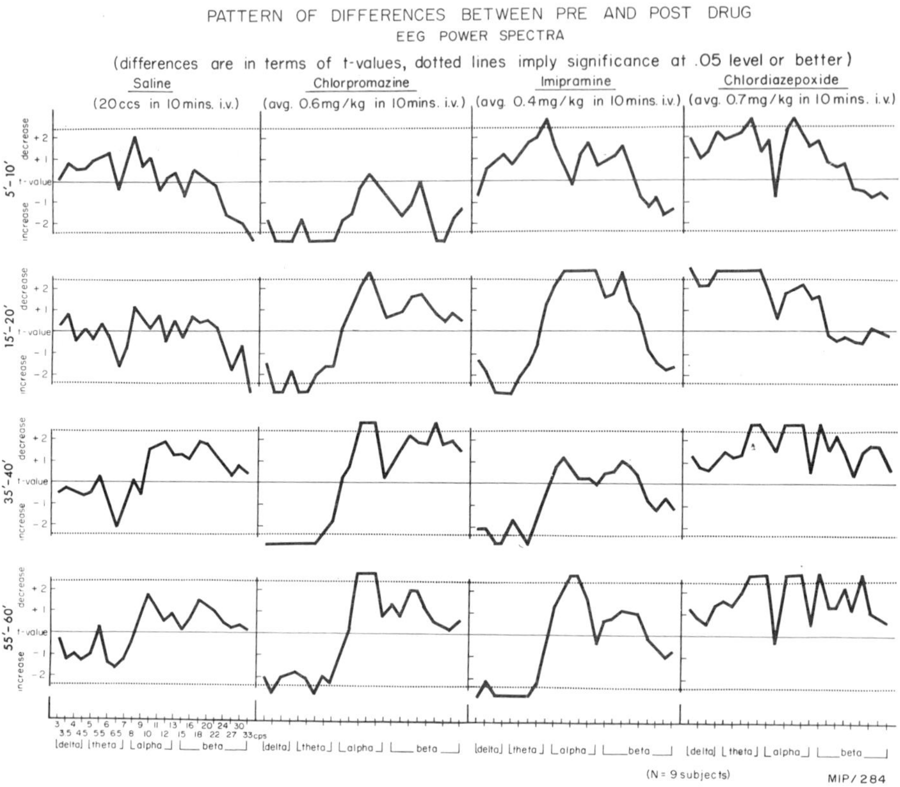

FIGURE 1 *EEG Drug Profiles of Chlorpromazine, Imipramine, and Chlordiazepoxide Based on Analog Power Spectra*—The abscissa shows the frequency ranges of analog frequency analyzer, the ordinate, the differences between pre and post drug (4 different time periods) in terms of t-values. Downward deflection is increase of values and upward decrease of values in comparison to pre-drug measurements. After saline i.v. injection, only 1 of 24 frequency bands showed in 2 of 4 time periods statistically significant changes in comparison to pre-drug values (increase of 33 cps activity). After 0.6 mg/kg chlorpromazine (administered in 10 minutes i.v.), a statistically significant increase of delta and theta frequencies in all time periods was observed. Fast activity increased only during 5-10 minutes after administration, while fast alpha activity decreased in 3 of the 4 time periods. After imipramine (0.4 mg/kg in 10 minute i.v.) slow waves also statistically increased, and there was an increase of fast activities (without reaching the level of statistical significance) in all four time periods. Chlordizepoxide (administered 0.7 mg/kg in 10 minute i.v.) showed significantly different EEG profiles from those of imipramine and chlorpromazine. Slow waves and alpha activity decreased and fast waves showed some increase in the first two time periods. (From Itil, T. M., et al.: *Agressologie* 9(2):267-280, 1968)

C. Digital Computer Period Analysis (Quantitative pharmaco-EEG data) with antidepressants

1. *Computer EEG Profiles of Drugs Known to be Antidepressants:*

a. *Tricyclic Antidepressants:*

(1.) *Amitriptyline:* According to a series of studies, after single oral dosages of 10-75 mg, amitriptyline produced statistically significant alterations in EEG within 1 hour after oral administration which lasted up to at least 6 hours. The computer EEG profile of amitriptyline is characterized by an increase of slow waves (1.3-3.5 and 3.5-7.5 cps bands), decrease of alpha activity (7.5-13 cps), and increase of fast waves over 20 cps (Fig. 2). The first derivative measurements (superimposed activities on top of the primary wave) show a decrease of activities up to 16 cps and increase up to 90 cps. There is a decrease of zero cross average frequency and average absolute amplitude, along with an increase of zero cross frequency deviation, first derivative average frequency and frequency deviation, and amplitude variability (Drohocki). Whereas the changes in frequency bands reach the level of statistical significance, the last 6 measurements are not always significant and their value for the CEEG profiles is still questionable. The computer EEG profiles of amitriptyline show remarkable similarities at different time periods after administration (Fig. 3) and after different dosages (Fig. 4). Also, in different studies (populations) amitriptyline computer EEG profiles showed outstanding similarities (Fig. 5). The consistency of the quality as well as quantity of CEEG profiles after some dosages of amitriptyline indicates that this method is a very useful tool to determine the bioavailability of psychotropic drugs at the CNS level, as reported by Fink (5) and by us (34). It was found that amitriptyline-induced CEEG changes are significantly different not only from those of placebo but also from those of diazepam, as well as from similar antidepressive compounds, such as protriptyline and imipramine (Fig. 6). Amitriptyline produces statistically significant dose-related alterations in up to 9 of 20 CEEG measurements during the first hour after administration, in up to 15 measurements during the third hour, and in up to 7 measurements during the sixth hour after oral administration.

During chronic multiple oral dose administration, the computer EEG profile of amitriptyline is similar to that of single dose, except that instead of an increase, a decrease of fast activities was observed.

(2.) *Imipramine:* According to our studies, imipramine CEEG

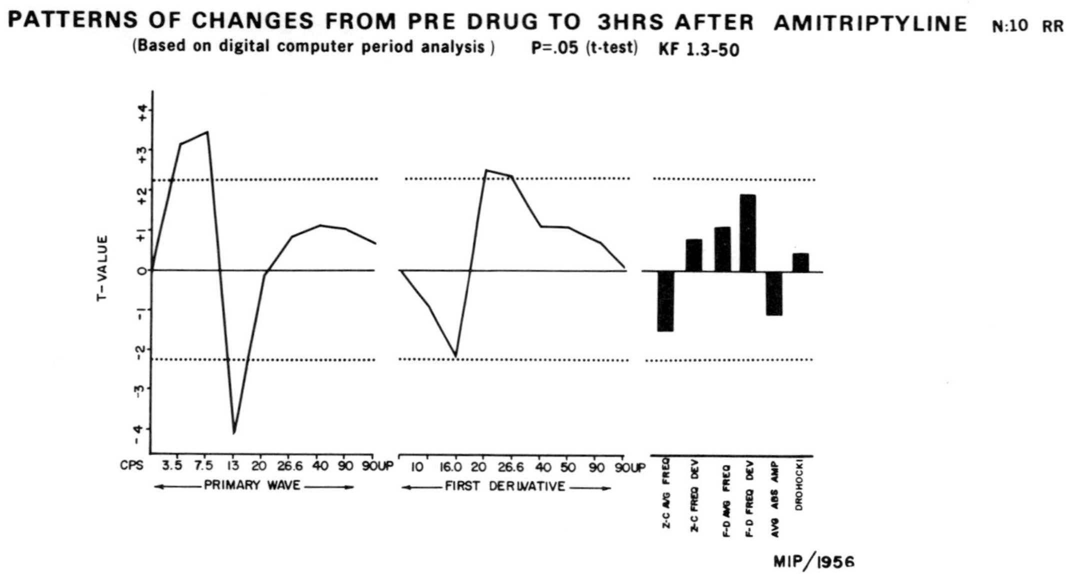

FIGURE 2 *Computer EEG Profiles of Amitriptyline*—The abscissa shows 21 computer EEG measurements, the ordinate, t-values of drug-induced changes from pre to 3 hours. The dotted line indicates P = .05. After 50 mg. amitriptyline, there is an increase of theta and delta waves, as well as fast activities over 26.6 cps and a decrease of alpha activity in the primary wave measurements. In the first derivative measurements there is a decrease of activity up to 16 cps and increase of waves over 20 cps.

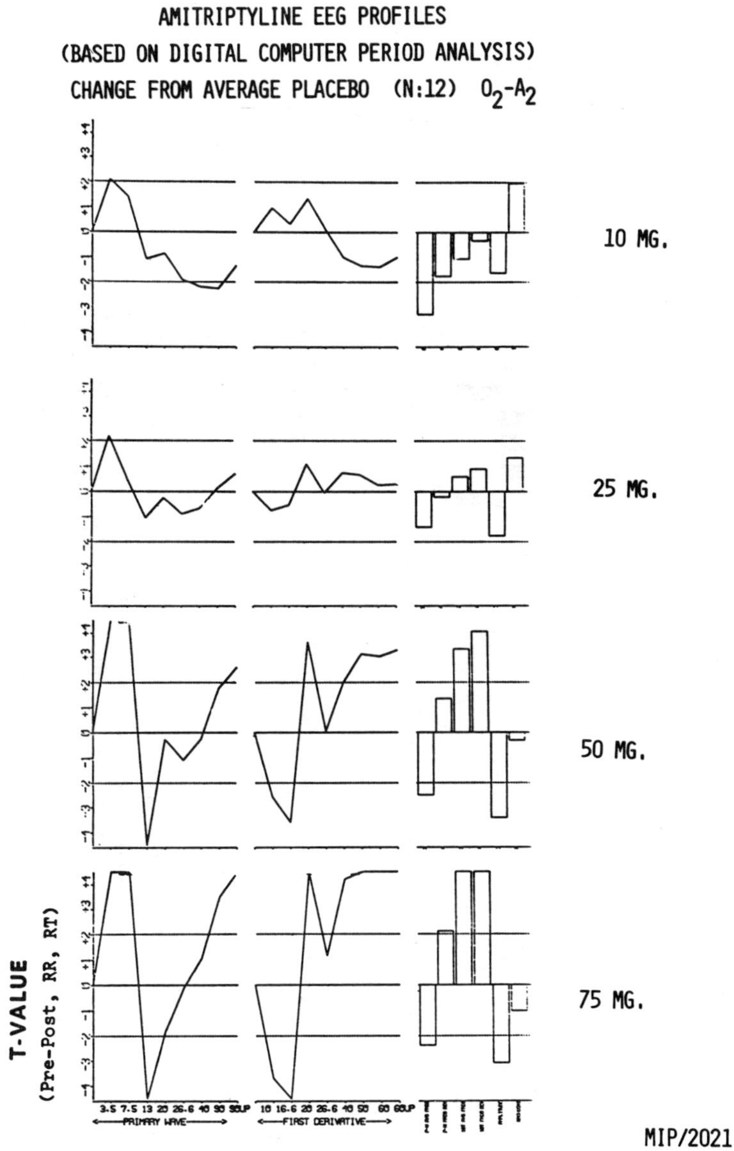

FIGURE 3 *Amitriptyline Computer EEG Profiles at Different Time Periods*—The abscissa and ordinate are the same as in Figure 1. As seen, amitriptyline-induced changes are very similar during the 1st, 3rd, and 6th hours after oral administration. (From Itil, T. M.: *Psychotropic Drugs and the Human EEG,* S. Karger A. G., Basel, New York.)

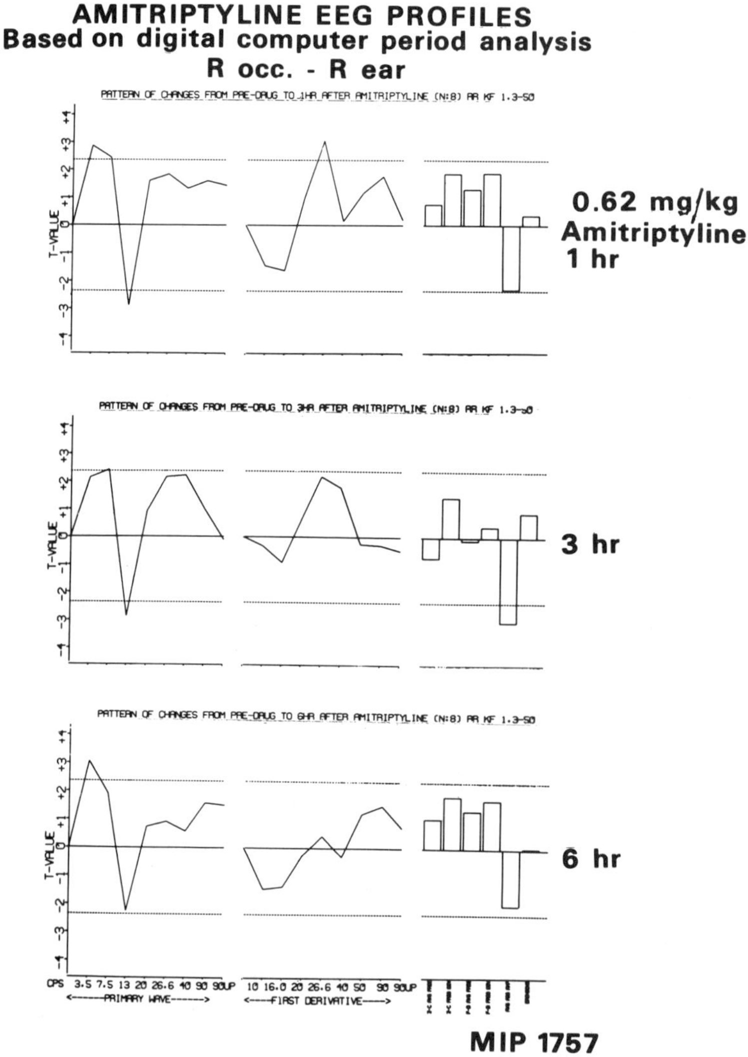

FIGURE 4 *Computer EEG Profiles of Amitriptyline After Different Dosages*—The abscissa and ordinate are the same as in Figure 1. The changes in CEEG measurements after 50 and 75 mg reached the level of statistical significance, and computer EEG profiles showed almost identical changes. After 10 and 25 mg amitriptyline, slow waves increased but fast activity did not.

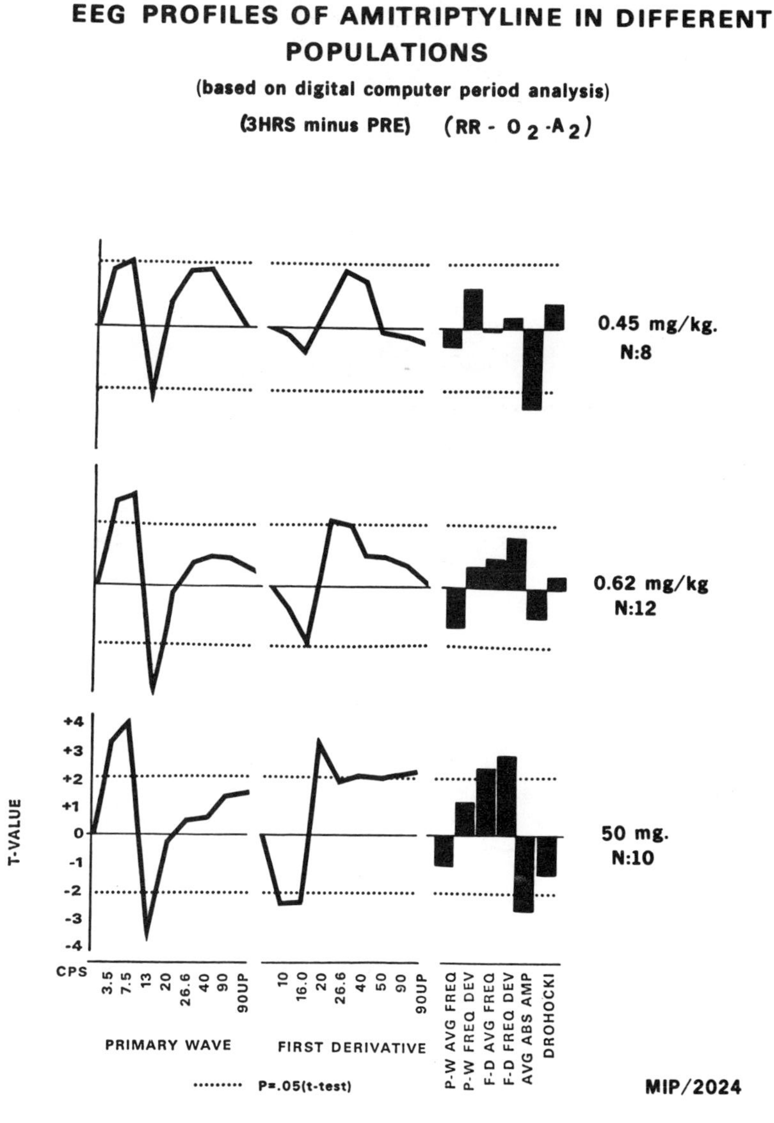

FIGURE 5 *Computer EEG Profiles of Amitriptyline in Different Populations*—The abscissa and ordinate are the same as in Figure 1. Although there are some differences in dosages, amitriptyline produces very similar CEEG profiles in different populations.

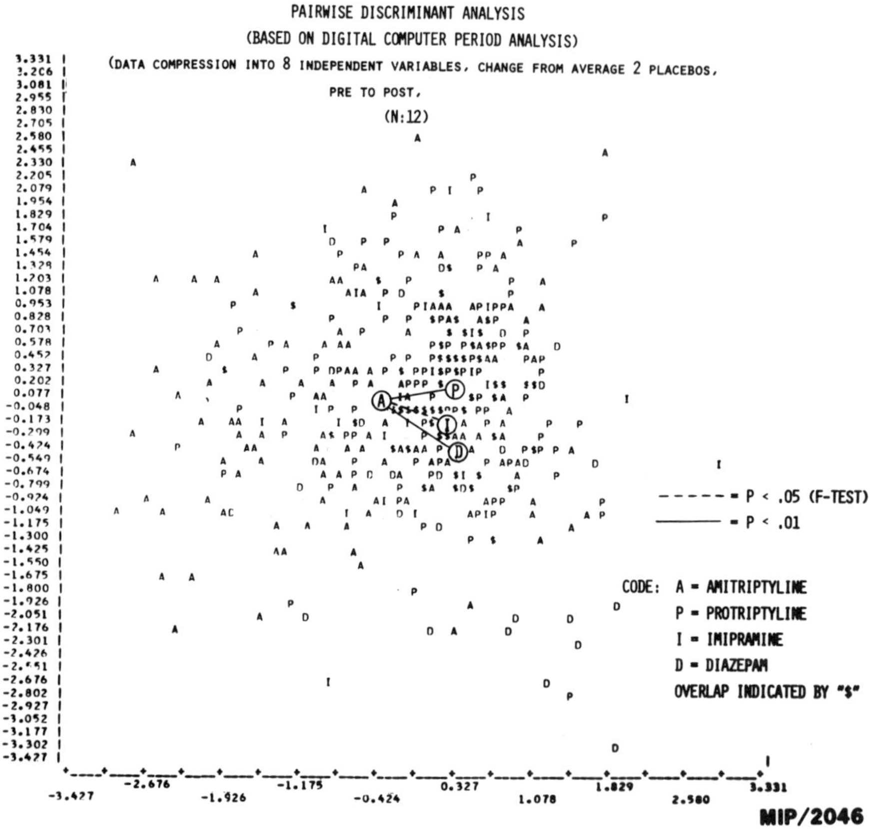

FIGURE 6 *Discrimination of Amitriptyline from Protriptyline, Imipramine, and Diazepam Based on Digital Computer Period Analysis Measurements*—After placebo-induced alterations are subtracted from drug-induced alterations, amitriptyline could be significantly differentiated from protriptyline and diazepam at the level of P<.01, and from imipramine at the level of P<.05.

profiles are very similar to those seen with amitriptyline. Imipramine also produces an increase of slow waves as well as fast beta activity and a decrease of alpha waves in the primary wave measurements, along with a decrease of slow and an increase of fast activity in the first derivative measurements (Fig. 7). In comparison to amitriptyline, however, we observed in various studies that imipramine in some populations decreases, not increases, very slow activity (1.3-3.5 cps), while increasing fast activities. CEEG profiles of imipramine are also similar at different time periods (Fig. 8). In general, the changes lessen during the 6 hours after oral

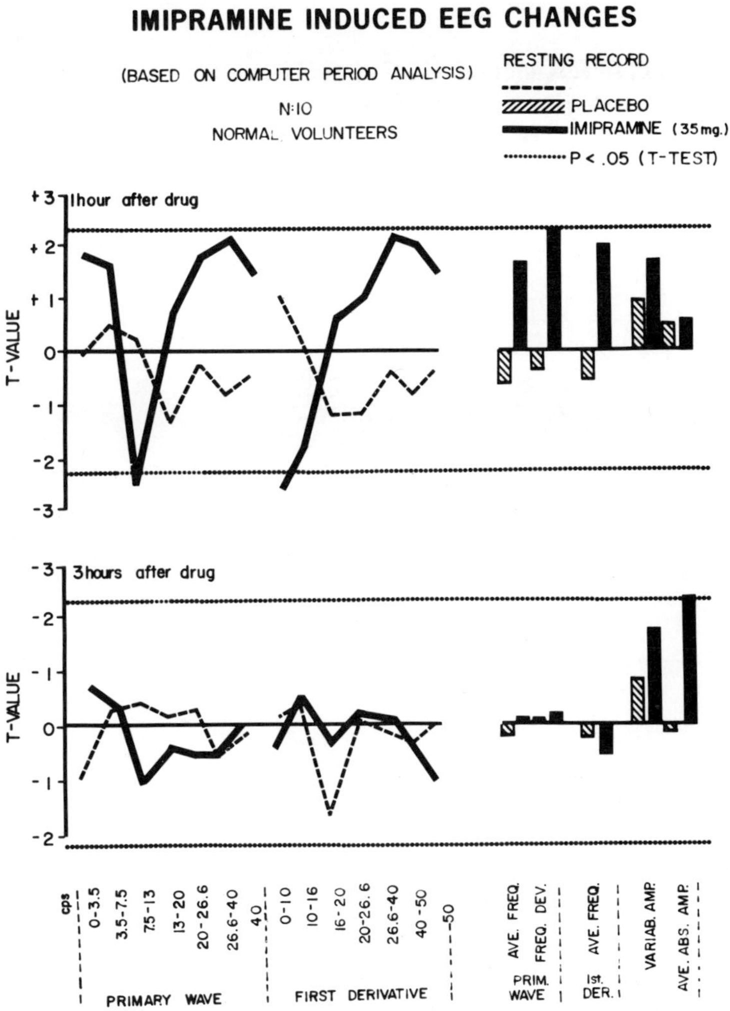

FIGURE 7 *Imipramine Computer EEG Profiles*—The abscissa and ordinate are the same as in Figure 2. One hour after 35 mg imipramine there was an increase of slow and fast waves and decrease of alpha activity in the primary wave measurements. Decrease of slow waves and increase of fast activity occurred in the first derivative measurements. Placebo-induced changes did not reach the level of statistical significance. Changes after 3 hours are negligible.

drug administration. In different populations, there are some obvious similarities of CEEG profiles of imipramine (Fig. 9), which again indicate that CEEG is a very accurate method of determining the bioavailability of antidepressive compounds at the CNS

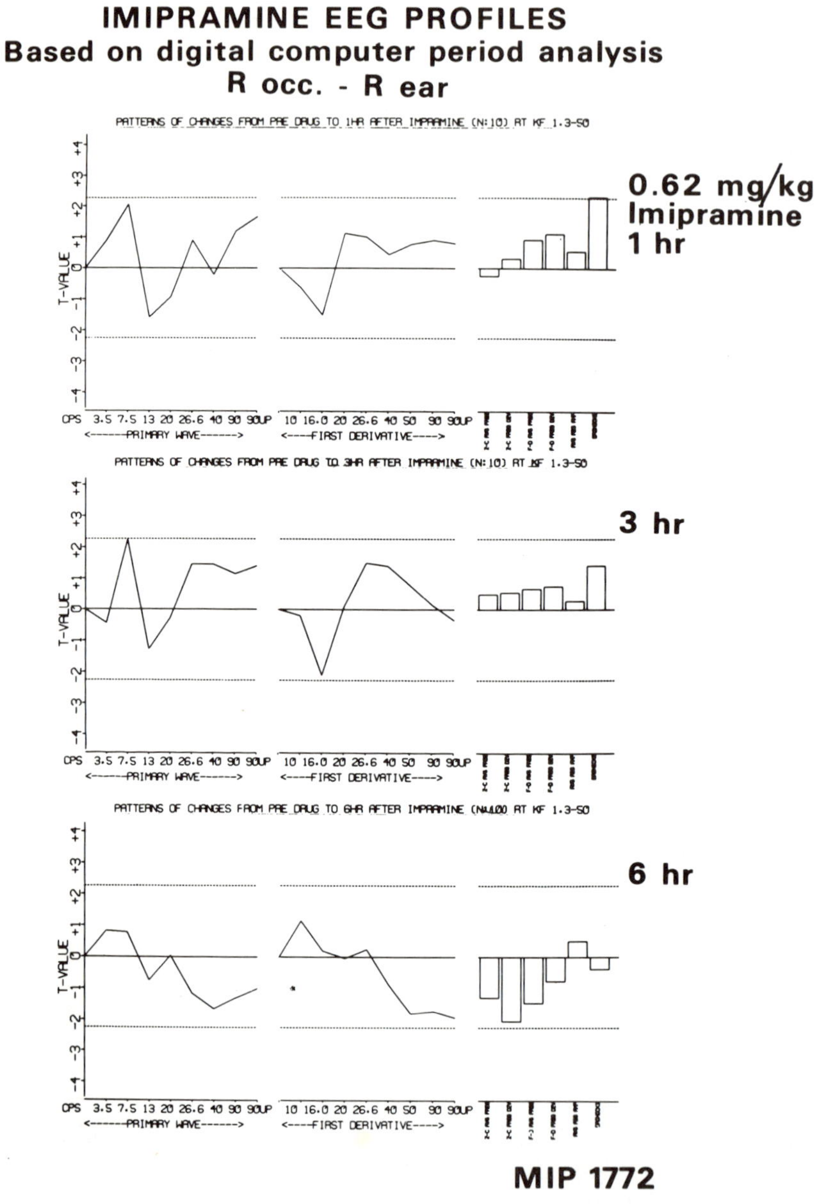

FIGURE 8 *Computer EEG Profiles of Imipramine at Different Time Periods*—The most characteristic computer EEG profile of imipramine is seen after 1 hour. After 3 hours very slow waves decrease. After 6 hours, changes do not reach the level of statistical significance.

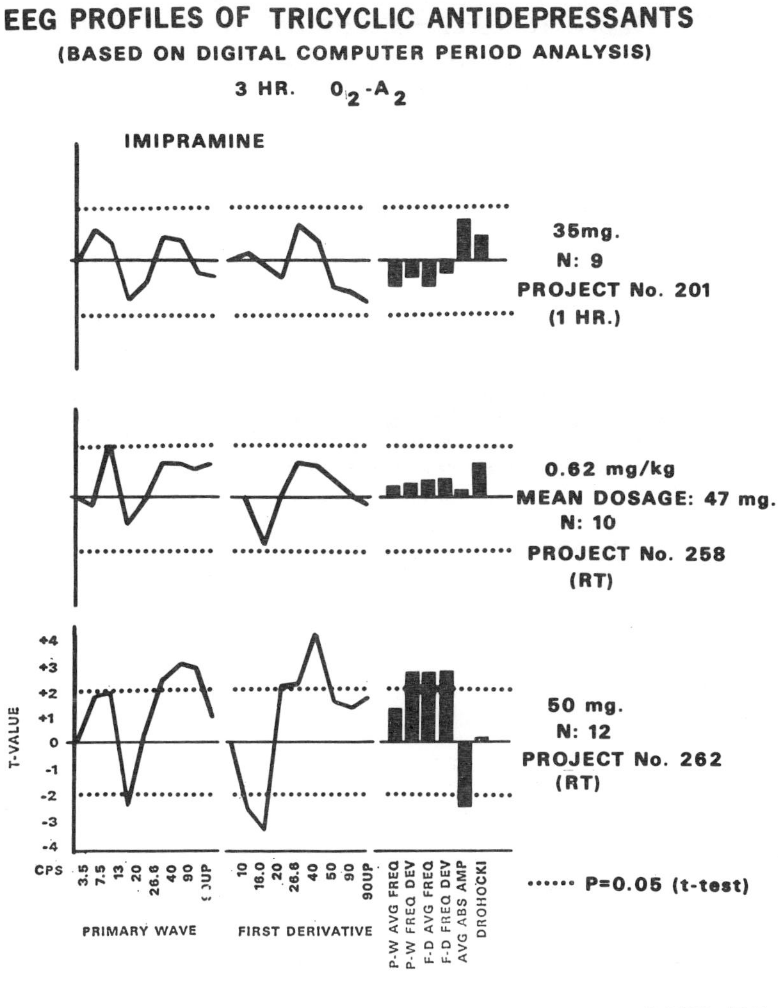

FIGURE 9 *Computer EEG Profiles of Imipramine in Different Populations*—In all 3 populations, imipramine produced an increase of slow waves and fast activity, a decrease of alpha waves in the primary wave measurements, and decrease of slow waves and increase of fast activity in the first derivative measurements. However, in Project #258 very slow waves did not increase but slightly decreased, and in the population of Project #201 in the first derivative measurements, very fast activity decreased instead of increased. As seen, the higher the dosages the better the computer EEG profiles after imipramine.

level. As mentioned above, CEEG alterations induced by imipramine could be statistically discriminated not only from diazepam, but also from amitriptyline. Imipramine compared mg per mg to amitriptyline produces fewer slow waves but more fast activities, supporting the clinical findings that imipramine has more "stimulatory" and fewer "sedative" properties than does amitriptyline.

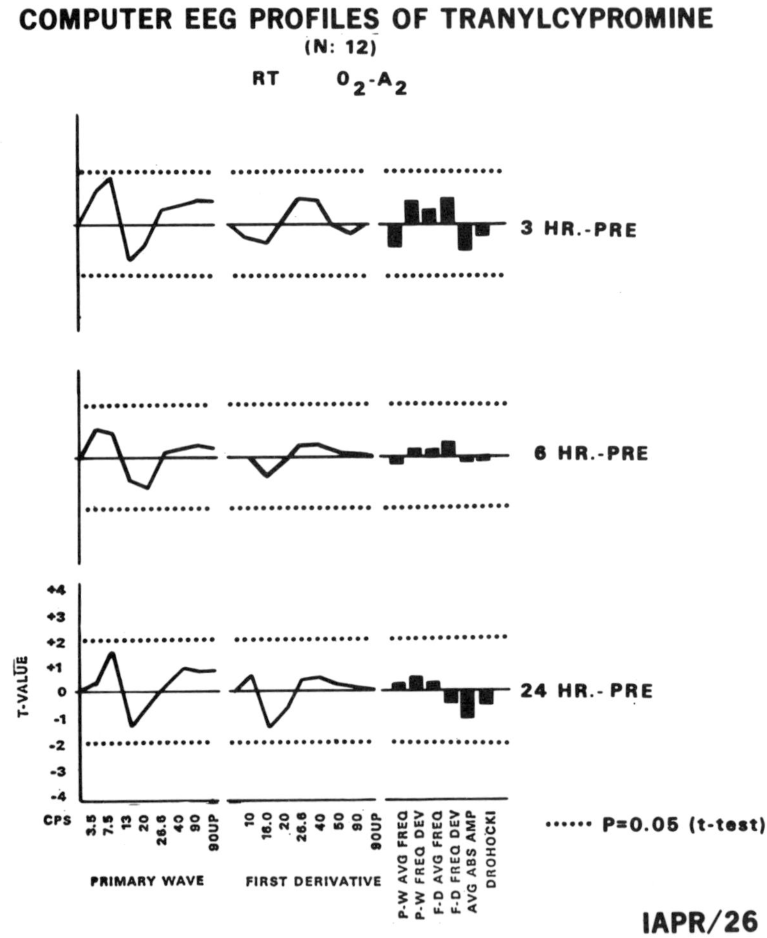

FIGURE 10 *Computer EEG Profiles of Tranycypromine*—Ten mg oral tranylcypromine produced computer EEG profiles characteristic of tricyclic antidepressants with increase of slow and fast waves and decrease of alpha activities. As seen, changes in this population did not reach the level of statistical significance in any of the time periods. However, even 24 hours after a single dose oral administration, there is a typical CEEG profile, similar to 3 and 6 hours after drug administration.

(3.) *Protriptyline:* Similar dosages of amitriptyline and imipramine produce almost identical CEEG profiles even in different populations such as U.S. and Turkish subjects (34), indicating not only extreme sensitivity of the method but also relative "specificity" of these tricyclic antidepressants as far as their effect on brain function is concerned. However, protriptyline's CEEG profile depends very much on the types of subjects studied (biological variability). Our investigations demonstrated that subjects with fast beta EEGs before protriptyline administration showed different CEEG profiles than did those subjects with alpha or slow EEGs. Accordingly, based on two studies (10 subjects in each) we could not determine a "typical" CEEG profile for protriptyline. We found that protriptyline's CEEG profile in low dosages (5-10 mg) seems to resemble imipramine (fewer slow waves and more fast activity than imipramine), while in higher dosages (20 and 40 mg) protriptyline's profile shows more similarity to dextroamphetamine-like compounds (decrease of slow waves, increase of alpha and slow beta activity). Protriptyline-induced CEEG changes are most marked during 1 hour (with amitriptyline during 3 hours) after oral administration. Statistically significant dose-related alterations (dose response curves) with protriptyline were seen only at 1 hour after oral administration and only in up to 4 of 22 EEG measurements. In dosage ranges of 5-40 mg (mean 18.7 mg) protriptyline could be significantly differentiated from amitriptyline (dose ranges 10-75 mg, mean 40 mg) but not from imipramine (50 mg).

(4.) *Doxapine:* We have not done studies with doxapine. However, according to a detailed study by Fink (5) with quantitative EEG, doxapine produces CEEG alterations similar to imipramine. Since this compound also produces alterations in frequency ranges of diazepam and other anxiolytic compounds, Fink predicted that doxapine would have some anxiolytic properties in addition to antidepressive ones. This is in accordance with the clinical findings of depressive patients with anxiety (50).

b. MAO inhibitors:

(1.) *Tranylcypromine:* Of the MAO inhibiting antidepressants, tranylcypromine has CEEG profiles most similar to the tricyclic antidepressants. After the administration of 10 mg tranylcypromine to a group of normal healthy volunteers, typical EEG alterations were observed 3 hours after oral administration and lasted up to 24 hours. Computer EEG profiles of tranylcypromine are characterized by an increase of slow waves, decrease of alpha, and increase of fast activities in the primary wave measurements and decrease of slow and increase of 20-40 cps activities in the first derivative measurements (Fig. 10).

(2.) *Isocarboxazid:* Our investigations demonstrated that isocarboxazid produces statistically significant EEG alterations after single oral dosages of 0.5 mg/kg. The CEEG profiles of isocarboxazid are characterized by an increase of the 13-20 cps activties but decrease of slower and faster frequencies in the primary wave measurements (Fig. 11). The superimposed activities up to 16 cps showed an increase and at the higher frequencies, a decrease. According to CEEG profiles, isocarboxazid does indeed show alterations more similar to the central stimulant compounds than to the tricyclic antidepressants or the other antidepressant MAO inhibitor, tranylcypromine.

c. Psychomotor stimulants:

As is known, some of the stimulant compounds, such as dextroamphetamine and methylphenidate, have been reported to have mood elevating properties. Accordingly, these substances have been used in patients with mild psychic depression.

(1.) *Dextroamphetamine:* Our series of investigations have clearly shown that dextroamphetamine, after single oral dosages of 10-20 mg, produces statistically significant alterations in the brain function of normal healthy volunteers. The CEEG profiles of dextroamphetamine are characterized by a decrease of slow waves, an increase of activities in the ranges of 13-26 cps, and a decrease of faster frequencies in the primary wave measurements (Fig. 12). The CEEG alterations in general are more obvious in the primary wave measurements than in the first derivative. The effects of dextroamphetamine are seen within 1 hour after oral administration and last at least up to 6 hours.

(2.) *Methylphenidate:* The CEEG profiles of methylphenidate in dosages of 0.45 mg/kg are very similar to those seen after dextroampetamine (Fig. 12). In comparison to 0.3 mg/kg dextroamphetamine, methylphenidate in this dosage produces more alpha activity and slow beta waves, but a lesser degree of theta and delta activity. The marked effects of methylphenidate on computer EEG are seen relatively late (6 hours after oral administration).

d. Miscellaneous antidepressive drugs:

There are three compounds which are primarily not accepted as antidepressants but are reported as having antidepressive properties.

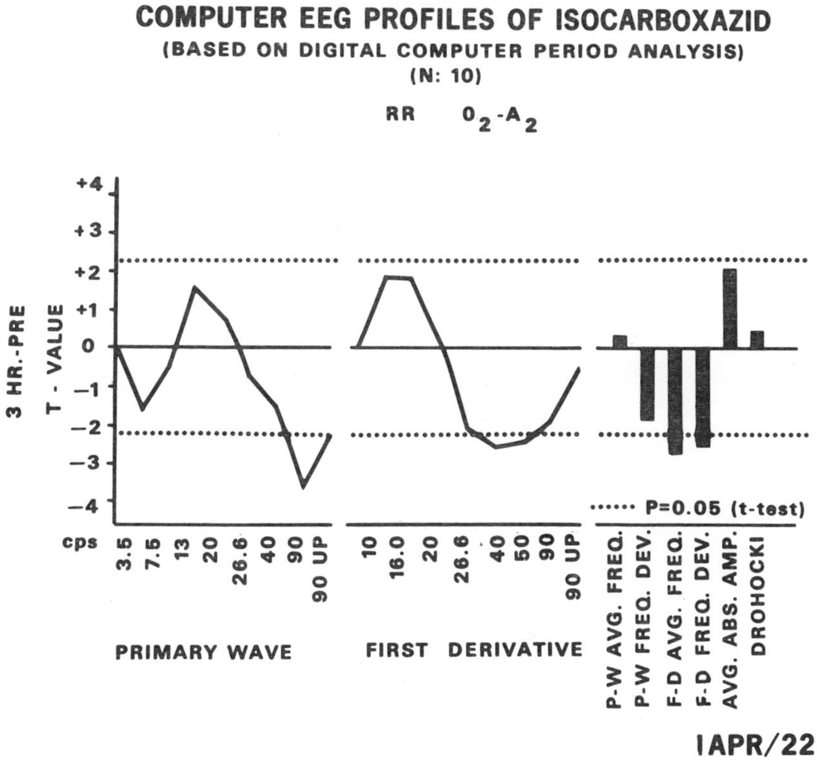

FIGURE 11 *Computer EEG Profile of Isocarboxazid*—A single oral dosage of 0.5 mg/kg isocarboxazid produced an increase of activities in 13-20 cps in both primary wave and first derivative measurements. There was a decrease of very slow waves in the primary wave measurements and a decrease of very fast activity in both primary wave and first derivative measurements. Isocarboxazid, although an MAO inhibitor, showed computer EEG profiles similar to psychomotor stimulants (see Fig. 12).

(1.) *Lithium:* We could study the EEG effects of lithium only with analog frequency analyzer and in manic patients. It was established that lithium produces marked alterations in brain function in daily dosages of 800 mg. Lithium-induced EEG alterations are characterized by a decrease of alpha activity and an increase of slow waves with superimposed fast activites. These EEG findings resemble those seen after anticholinergic thymoleptics and, particularly, anticholinergic hallucinogens (35). As major differences from anticholinergic drugs, we found a marked increase of epileptic potentials and increase of synchronization and

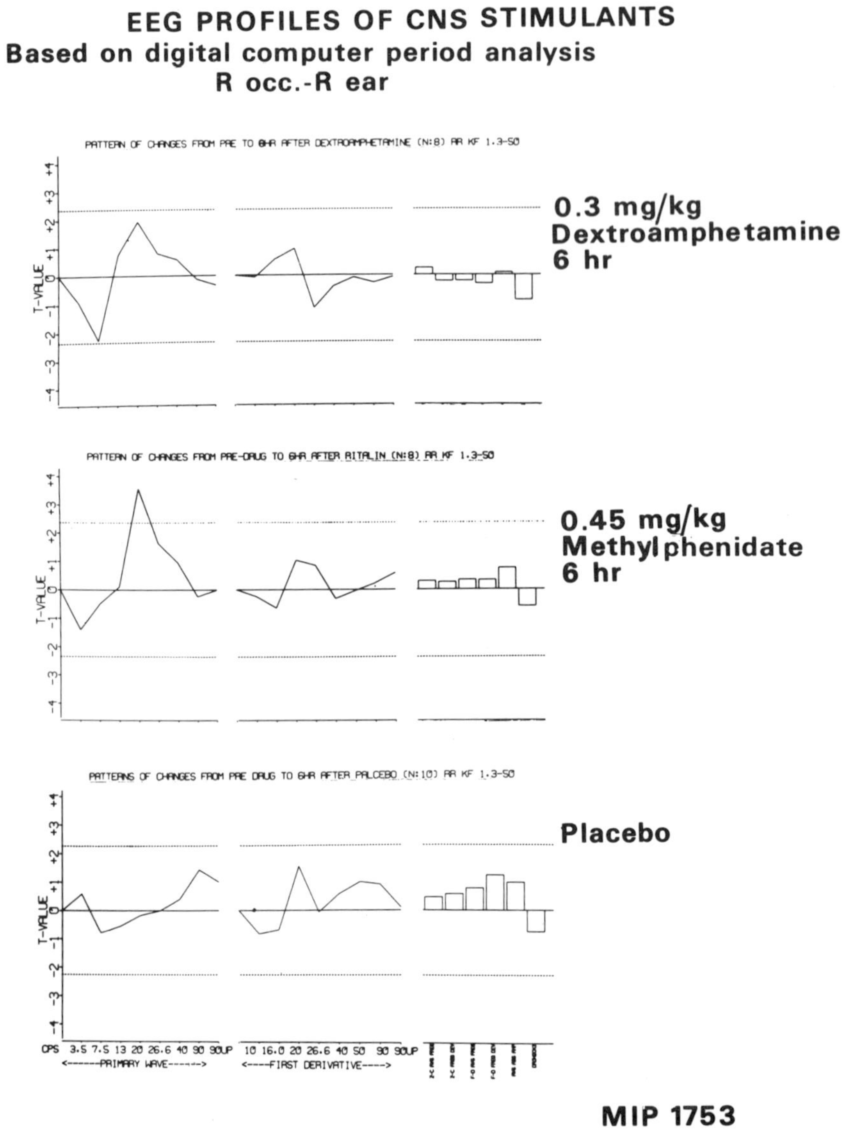

FIGURE 12 *Computer EEG Profiles of CNS Stimulants*—Both dextroamphetamine (0.3 mg/kg) and methylphenidate (0.45 mg/kg) produced very similar computer EEG profiles, particularly in the primary wave measurements. These are characterized by a decrease of slow waves and increase of activities of 13-20 cps.

rhythmical activity after lithium, which are some of the characteristic changes seen after chlorpromazine.

(2.) *Thioridazine:* Thioridazine, a piperidyl phenothiazine, is known as a potent effective antipsychotic (major tranquilizer) and has been reported to have antidepressive effects on some patients, particularly those with psychotic depression. In our studies after single dosages of 50 mg, the computer EEG profile of thioridazine in primary wave measurements is typical for major tranquilizers (antipsychotics) (34). In the first derivative measurements, however, there are obvious similarities to the thymoleptic drugs with decrease of slow waves and increase of superimposed fast activities. Accordingly, we stated that among the antipsychotic phenothiazines, thioridazine is probably the one which shows the closest similarities in CEEG profiles to those of antidepressant drugs. In an earlier study using thiopental activated EEG, we demonstrated the significant differences between perphenazine and thioridazine (29).

(3.) *Thiothixene:* Thiothixene, a potent antipsychotic, was reported to have central stimulatory properties based on clinical trials. In our investigations using digital computer analysis of the EEG, we reported that thiothixene produces slow activities in addition to superimposed fast activities (similar to tricyclic antidepressants) during resting (40) and sleep EEG (41). Although thiothixene EEG profiles in primary wave measurements are very similar to the major tranquilizers, in the first derivative measurements there is an increase of superimposed fast activities (decrease of fast activity with major tranquilizers).

2. *Computer EEG Profiles in the Prediction of Antidepressive Compounds:*

a. *Drugs predicted by animal pharmacology as antidepressants:*

In recent years we have received a series of compounds for EEG and clinical trials which were predicted to be antidepressants based on animal pharmacology models. The methods of quantitative pharmaco-EEG were not only helpful in investigations to determine whether these compounds have any significant CNS effects on humans, but furthermore, based on CEEG profiles, we could confirm or reject the pharmacological prediction.

(1.) *MK-940:* MK-940 (trans-10, 11-dihydro-5,10-epoxy-5-[3-(methylamino) propyl]-5H-dibenzo [a,d] cyclohepten-11-ol hydrogen maleate) was studied in daily dosages of 2-24 mg in a group of depressive patients. CEEG profiles during the first and third weeks of the treatment demonstrated a decrease of slow waves (less than 7.5 cps), an increase of 13-20 cps activity, and a decrease of very fast waves in the primary wave measurements (in dosages of 8-24 mg daily, fast activity decreased) (20). In the first derivative measurements, an increase of slow waves up to 16 cps and decrease of fast activities are noticeable. According to this study, we stated that MK-940 has marked CNS effects similar to CNS stimulatory compounds, but that its CEEG profile is not "typical" for tricyclic antidepressants. Clinically, MK-940 showed marked central stimulatory effects, which were only to some extent antidepressant, although certainly far less so than those of tricyclic antidepressants. Since the other clinical trials confirmed our findings, MK-940 was withdrawn from further clinical studies.

(2.) *CI-579 and CI-600:* CI-579, a dimethylaminopropyl dibenzodiazepine, and CI-600, a methylaminopropyl dibenzo-diazepine, have been predicted by animal pharmacology to be antidepressants. The CEEG profiles of both compounds showed less similarity to profiles of tricyclic antidepressants than to those of CNS stimulants (42. Clinical investigations confirmed our findings. Because of weak antidepressant properties and strong stimulatory side effects, both compounds were withdrawn from investigations.

(3) *SCH-12,650:* SCH-12,650 is a 2-[p-chlorophenyl-2 (pyridyl)-hydroxy methyl] imidazoline maleate. This compound has been predicted by animal pharmacology to be a potent antidepressant. Computer EEG profiles of SCH-12, 650 after single oral dose in psychiatric populations showed some similarity to those of imipramine with a lesser degree of slow waves and more fast activity. SCH-12,650 was found to have some antidepressive properties with obvious central stimulatory effects.

(4.) *OI-77:* OI-77, a new tricyclic (5-methylaminoacetyl-6-methyl-5,6-dihydro-phenanthridine hydrochloride), was predicted by animal pharmacology to be an antidepressant. Computer EEG profiles based on a quantitative pharmaco-EEG study demonstrated that this compound after 15 mg dosages has a CEEG profile similar to imipramine (25 mg). However, both after single dosages and during chronic administration, OI-77 did show less typical tricyclic antidepressant profiles. The presence of a lesser degree of slow waves and marked fast activity suggested that OI-77 would have more stimulatory effects than imipramine. The subsequent clinical trial in a small group of depressive patients showed that OI-77 indeed acts as an antidepressant. The side effects were similar to those seen after tricyclic antidepressants (37).

(5.) *Amoxapine:* Amoxapine (2-chloro-11-(1-piperazinyl) dibenz (b,f) (1,4) oxazepine), a compound chemically and pharmacologically similar to imipramine and amitriptyline, was predicted to be antidepressant. In a quantitative pharmaco-EEG study, it was found that amoxapine in dosages of 6.25 mg., 12.5 mg, 25 mg, 50 mg, and 75 mg, but particularly in dosages of 25 and 50 mg, showed CEEG profiles similar to those seen after 25 mg imipramine in the same population. However, interestingly, amoxapine did not produce very fast activities in either primary wave or first derivative measurements in any of the dosages between 6.25 and 75 mg. In contrast, the 75 mg amoxapine profile showed alterations very similar to loxapine, a major tranquilizer. Accordingly, based on CEEG profiles, we predict that amoxapine in dosages of 25-50 mg would have imipramine-like clinical effects, while in 75 mg and higher dosages it would act like the major tranquilizers, thioridazine and loxapine.

(6.) *GP-41299:* GP-41299 (NN-dimethyl dibenzo thiepine-10 methylamine hydrochloride), in a quantitative EEG study carried out by Fink (5), showed significant CNS effects, similar to those of tricyclic antidepressants. The clinical antidepressive effects as predicted by Fink were confirmed by clinical trials by Gazianaga et al (22).

(7.) *Thyrotropin Releasing Hormone (TRH):* TRH was found to have therapeutic effects in depression (47) which stimulated us to carry out a study with the hormone. In a group of depressive patients, 1,000 mcg TRH administered i.v. produced noticeable changes (Fig. 13). An increase of the frequencies between 13-26.6 cps and a decrease in faster and slower activities in the primary wave measurements and increase of frequencies up to 10 cps and decrease above 10 cps in the first derivative measurements were seen in CEEG profiles. Five of the 16 CEEG measurements reached the level of statistical significance ($P < .05$). CEEG profiles of TRH resemble protriptyline and, more closely, dextroamphetamine.

b. (2) Drugs not predicted by animal pharmacology as antidepressants:

(1.) *Cyclazocine:* Cyclazocine is a benzomorphan derivative (n-cyclopropyl-methyl analog), which is a long-acting antinarcotic and analgesic. In psychiatric populations, it was established that cyclazocine produced marked EEG alterations with decrease of alpha and increase of very slow and very fast activities (13). Digital computer period analysis of the resting and sleep EEG findings showed that the effects of this compound on the CNS are similar to those reported for ditran (36) and imipramine (6-8, 17). In the

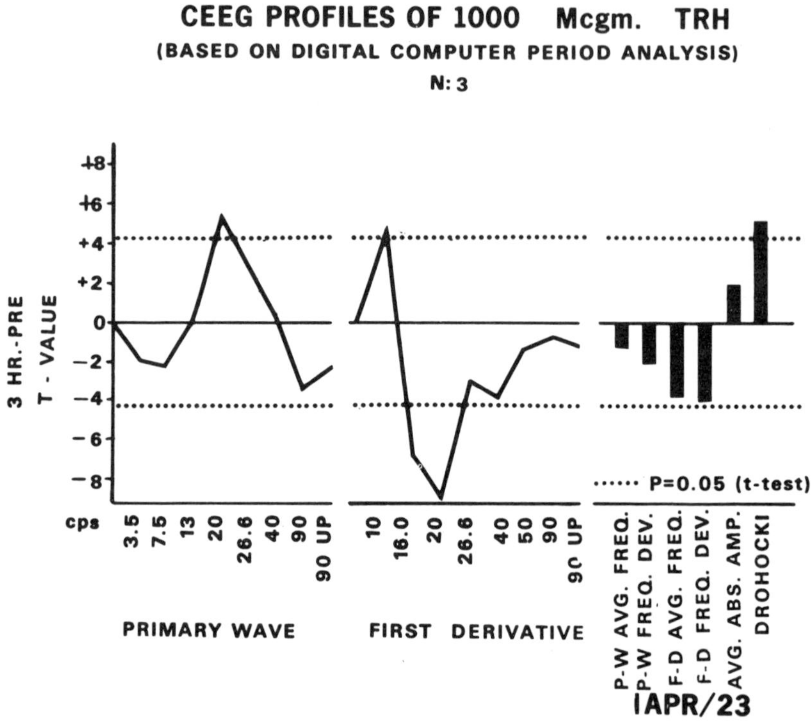

FIGURE 13 *Computer EEG Profiles of Thyrotropin Releasing Hormone*—After 1,000 mcg TRH i.v. produces a decrease of very slow waves, increase of activities in 20-26 cps, and decrease of high frequency activity in the primary wave measurements, as well as an increase of slow waves and decrease of fast activities in the first derivative measurements. CEEG profile of TRH showed some similarity to psycho-stimulants and "stimulatory" tricyclic antidepressants, such as desipramine and protriptyline.

following quantitative EEG investigations carried out by Fink et al (16), the "antidepressant-like" EEG profile of cyclazocine was confirmed. Two subsequent clinical investigations have demonstrated that cyclazocine indeed has antidepressant properties similar to imipramine (1, 18). With half of the dosages used for postwithdrawal narcotic addicts a noticeable improvement was observed in symptoms of depression. Neither the chemical profile nor the pharmacological properties of cyclazocine was predictive for its antidepressant properties.

(2.) *GB-94 (mianserin hydrochloride) and GC-46:* In the search for potent anti-serotonin/antihistamine compounds without side effects to investigate in manic patients, we were offered two compounds which belong to a known group of "tetracyclic" compounds: GB-94 [1, 2, 3, 4, 10, 14b-hexahydro-2-methyl-dibenzo (c,f)-pyrazino-(1, 2-a) azepine monohydrochloride] and GC-46 [2 (N)-methyl-1,3,4, 14b-tetrahydro-2H-pyrazino (1,2,-d) dibenzo (b,f) (1,4) oxazepine]. Based on chemical structures, both compounds have been predicted to be antihistamines and potent antiserotonins; this was confirmed by animal pharmacology. Accordingly, both compounds were investigated in clinical trials in the treatment of allergic conditions, hay fever, asthma, and migraine. Since, however, the clinical testing did not reveal any superiority to existing antihistamines, clinical trials were discontinued.

Before clinical trials in manic patients, we investigated the effects of both compounds in normal volunteers, using the methods of quantitative pharmaco-EEG. In the pilot dose finding trials we were able to determine that both compounds produced noticeable changes in the EEG. Surprisingly, we observed that the types of EEG changes induced by both compounds were similar to those which we described as "antidepressant" EEG reaction type (27, 29). These were characterized by a decrease of alpha activity and an increase of slow waves, with an increase of superimposed fast beta activity. We established that the equivalent dosages of GB-94 were greater than GC-46. Since the increase of slow waves in ratio to the increase of fast activities was much more with GB-94 than GC-46, we predicted the clinical effects of GB-94 would be similar to those of amitriptyline (31, 33). The subsequent double-blind quantitative pharmaco-EEG trial confirmed the findings of the pilot EEG study: both compounds produce computer EEG alterations in brain function that are significantly different from placebo. CEEG profiles of both compounds were similar to those of tricyclic antidepressants (Fig. 14). After 15 mg, GB-94 produced a similar amount of fast activities (superimposed fast activity in the first derivative measurements) as 30 mg GC-46 and a lesser amount of slow waves in the primary wave measurements. Because of its potent CNS effectiveness and greater similarity to amitriptyline, GB-94 was selected for clinical study. A double-blind control study with amitriptyline indicated that GB-94 is indeed a potent antidepressive compound, very similar to amitriptyline in the treatment of depressive syndomes (38). Subsequent clinical trials in five countries confirmed our clinical findings (46). Fink, using his methods of digital computer period analyzed EEG, could also demonstrate that GB-94 produces alterations in brain function similar to antidepressant thymoleptics (10). The onset of the therapeutic effects of GB-94 is faster than that of amitriptyline, although not at the level of statistical significance. To date,

THE EFFECTS OF GB-94 AND GC-46 EEG PROFILES
(BASED ON DIGITAL COMPUTER PERIOD ANALYSIS)

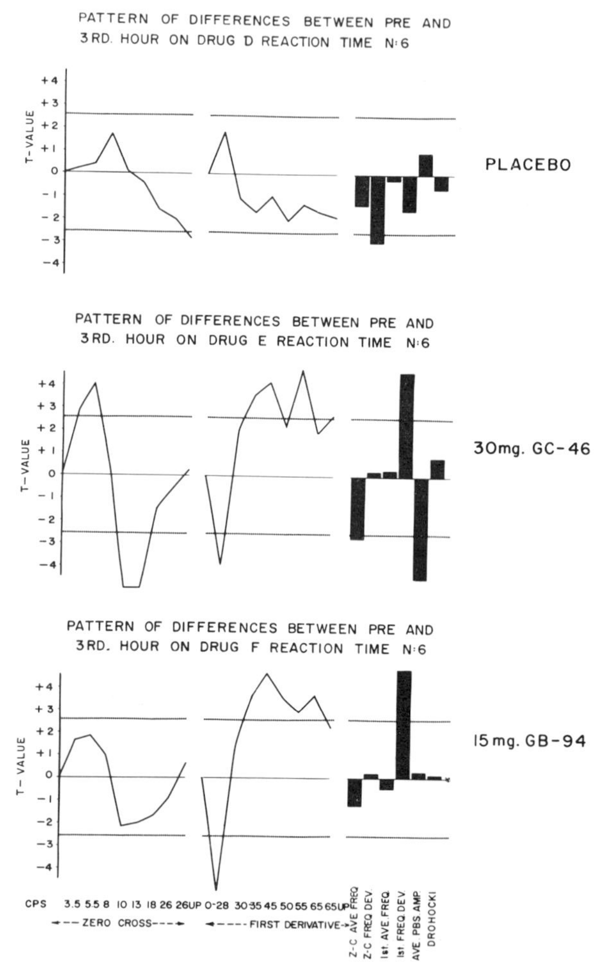

MIP/1659

FIGURE 14 *Computer EEG Profiles of GB-94 and GC-46*—GB-94, after 15 mg single oral dosage, and GC-46, after 30 mg single oral dosage, produced computer EEG profiles similar to tricyclic antidepressants. Particularly in the first derivative measurements, half the dosage of GB-94 produced more changes than twice the dosages of GC-46.

no pharmacological or biochemical properties of GB-94 have been found to explain its antidepressive effects (51).

In an open pilot clinical trial the antidepressive effects of GC-46 were also observed. GC-94, another tetracyclic, which showed only limited CNS effects and no typical CEEG profiles, was found to be not an effective tranquilizer or antidepressant, but a mild stimulant in clinical trials.

(3.) *Mesterolone:* Mesterolone, an androgenic hormone (17-hydroxy-1-methyl-5-androstane-3-1) was predicted to have psychotropic properties because of clinical observations of increase of mental alertness, mood elevation, and improvement of memory and concentration. Quantitative pharmaco-EEG trials demonstrated that mesterolone in single oral dosages of 100-1600 mg has noticeable CNS effects, which are different at the level of statistical significance from those of placebo. Computer EEG profile of mesterolone are characterized by an increase of slow waves and fast activities with decrease of alpha waves in the primary wave measurements and decrease of slow and increase of fast activities in the first derivative measurements (Fig. 15). Since these profiles are similar to those of tricyclic antidepressants, we predicted that mesterolone would be effective in depressive syndromes with and without androgen deficiency. Our further investigations showed that mesterolone indeed has significant CNS effects, even after 10 mg single oral dosage, which has less endocrinological effect. Preliminary clinical trials demonstrated that mesterolone has indeed antidepressive effects in some depressive patients.

III. DISCUSSION AND CONCLUSION

Based on computer analysis of EEG, not only can the CNS effects of a new compound be determined in an objective and relatively easy way in humans, but it is also possible to predict the clinical effectiveness of a new compound according to its CEEG profile. These determinations certainly promise to be an important development in the evaluation of new antidepressive drugs. As is known, chemical development and pharmacological profiling of new compounds require relatively little time and can be objective, while establishment of the clinical effectiveness of a compound is time-consuming, costly, and, overall, full of subjectivity. Recent and proposed future governmental requirements concerning "safer" drugs and issues such as "protection" and "rights" of patients have and will further delay the development of better psychotropic drugs. Despite the favorable changes in psychiatric

COMPUTER EEG PROFILES OF ALL DOSAGES MST COMBINED AS COMPARED WITH PLACEBO

(BASED ON DIGITAL COMPUTER PERIOD ANALYSIS)

N:12 RR

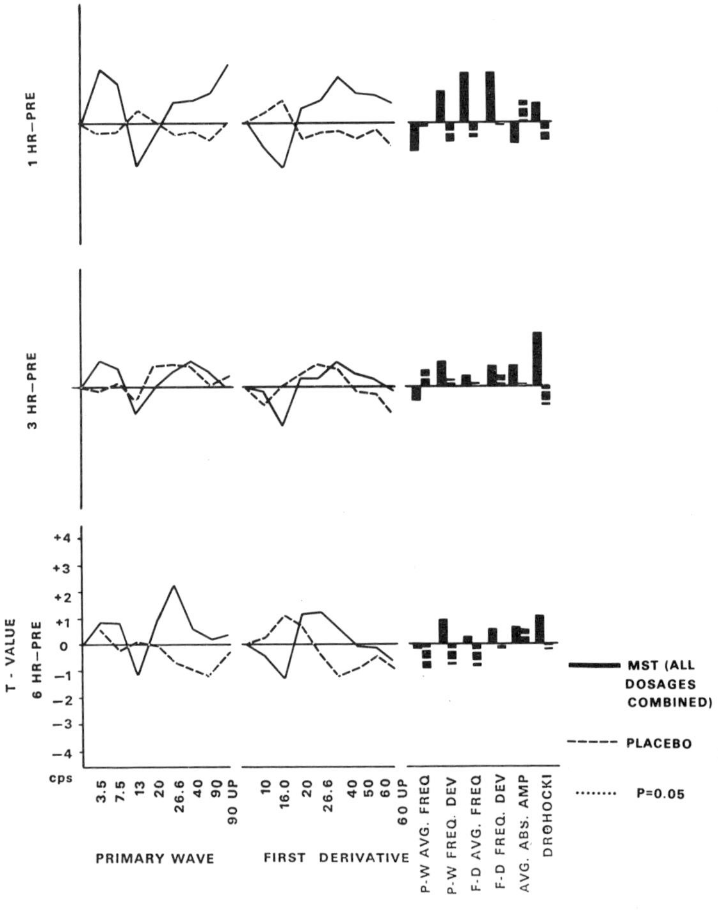

MIP/2366

FIGURE 15 *Computer EEG Profiles of Mesterolone*—In dosages of 100-1600 mg. (mean 620 mg) mesterolone produced computer EEG profiles similar to tricyclic antidepressants. Particularly during the 1st hour and 6th hour after single oral dose administration, the mesterolone-induced EEG changes are significantly different from those induced by placebo. Because of the increase of fast activity more than increase of slow waves (particularly during the 6th hour), the mesterolone CEEG profiles are more similar to imipramine than amitriptyline.

hospitals as a result of the use of drug therapy developed in the last 20 years, we are well aware that we are far from having a cure for psychiatric illness or from being able to apply an etiological treatment. Facing such serious problems as late side effects of major tranquilizers in terms of tardive dyskinesia, certain "addictive" properties of minor tranquilizers, and inadequate and delayed effects of antidepressants, we obviously need better and faster acting new psychiatric drugs. Our methods of quantitative pharmaco-EEG may be very appropriate in answering these needs. The establishment of the CNS effects of a new compound and the prediction of its eventual psychiatric use in humans in an objective way without being dependent on the patient's verbal response or on a clinical model of "trial and error", are major advantages of our method. One might be surprised at the sensitivity of the technique, particularly if one considers the fact that our computer EEG profiles are based on only 22 measurements, that the recordings are being done from 1 or 2 scalp electrodes, and the conventional system of electroencephalography permits recording only up to 70-80 cps waves (although bioelectrical potentials were recorded in cats' brains up to 1300 cps and in humans up to 4,50 cps). Our preliminary investigations with high frequency recordings and analysis (up to 1,000 cps) already suggest that the effects of 1 mg oral dosage of diazepam can be determined with the new technique, while not with the conventional recording and analysis. Only a few years ago we could not believe that certain, statistically significant alterations in computerized cerbral biopotentials may occur without any subjective feeling on the part of the subjects. However, today our studies with some polypeptides (TRH and MIF) and some steroid hormones (mesterolone and cyproterone acetate) clearly demonstrate that these "body's own" substances produce alterations in human brain function which can be recorded and analyzed even after single oral dosages. This is possible despite tremendous intra- and inter-individual variabilities, methodological problems, and the ability to record and analyze only a very limited percentage of the total brain function so that advances in any of these areas would certainly improve our chances of developing new psychotropic drugs. The recent investigations of Fink (5) and our own studies clearly demonstrate that the computer analysis of the EEG is certainly the easiest, least expensive, and most accurate method to determine the bioavailability of psychotropic drugs at the CNS level.

IV. SUMMARY

Retrospective and prospective computer EEG studies with known antidepressants, as well as with compounds not predicted by animal pharmacology to be antidepressants, clearly demonstrate that drugs with antidepressive (thymoleptic) properties, after single oral dosages, produce statistically significant alterations in brain function as exhibited by computerized cerebral biopotentials. In general antidepressant drugs with more "sedative" properties increase slow and fast frequencies and decrease alpha activities in the primary wave measurements (typical tricyclic antidepressant CEEG profile), whereas the stimulant thymoleptics decrease slow waves and increase alpha activity, as well as slow beta waves (similar to psychomotor stimulants). Based on the methods of quantitative pharmaco-electroencephalography using computerized EEG measurements, it is possible not only to establish the CNS effects of new compounds, but also to predict their eventual "psychotropic" properties, to determine the dose-response curve, to seek their bioavailability at the CNS level, and to substantiate biological variability of individual responses to psychotropic drugs.

REFERENCES

1. Abuzzahab, F. S.: The antidepressant properties of cyclozacine, *A.J.C.R.,* **1**:9-15, 1970.
2. Benassi, P., and Bertolotti, P.: Serotonina e inhibitori della monoaminosidase: studio EEG negli epilettici, *Riv. sper. Freniat.,* **84**:351-367, 1960.
3. Bente, D. und Itil, T. M.: Zur Wirkung des Phenothiazin körpers Megaphen aud das menschliche Hirnstrombild, *Arnz. Forsch.,* **4**:418-423, 1954.
4. Borenstein, P., Cujo, P., and Chiua, M.: A propos de la Classification des Substances Psychotropes selon leurs effets sur l'Electroencephalogramme, *Ann. Med.-psychol.,* **2**:429-452, 1965.
5. Fink, M.: EEG profiles and bioavailability measures of psychoactive drugs, *in* Itil, T. M., editor: *Psychotropic drugs and the human EEG,* Karger, Basel/New York, 1974, pp. 76-98.
6. Fink, M.: Electroencephalographic and behavioral effects of tofranil, *Canad. Psychiatr. Ass.,* **4**:1665-1715, 1959.
7. Fink, M.: Quantitative EEG and human psychopharmacology. III. Changes on acute and chronic administration of chlorpromazine, imipramine, and placebo (saline), *in* Wilson, W. P.: *Applications of electroencephalography in psychiatry,* Duke Univ. Press, Durham, N.C., 1965.
8. Fink, M.: Quantitative electroencephalography and human psychopharmacology: frequency spectra and drug action, *Med. Exp.,* **5**:364-369, 1961.
9. Fink, M.: Quantitative electroencephalography in human psychopharmacology. II. Drug patterns, *in* Glaser, G. H. *EEG and behavior,* Basic Books, New York, 1963.
10. Fink, M.: Strategies of new psychotropic drugs development. Pre-

sented at the scientific meeting on the occasion of the 50th anniversary of Organon, Amsterdam, Oct. 27, 1971.
11. Fink, M.: The human electroencephalogram: index of clinical activity of new psychoactive agents, *Mod. Probl. Pharmacopsychiat.,* Vol. **2,** Basel/Karger, Basel/New York, 1969.
12. Fink, M. and Itil, T. M.: EEG analysis by digital computer. II: Relation of pentothal-induced changes to resting patterns, *Electroenceph. clin. Neurophysiol.,* **18**:520-521, 1965.
13. Fink, M. and Itil, T.: EEG and human psychopharmacology: clinical antidepressants, *in* Efron, D. H., Cole, J. O., Levine, J., and Wittenborn, R. O., editor: *Psychopharmacology: a review of progress 1957-1967,* Washington, D. C., U.S. Government Printing Office, 1968, pp. 671-682.
14. Fink, M. and Itil, T.: Neurophysiology of phantastica: EEG and behavioral relations in man, *in* Efron, D. H., Cole, J. O., Levine, J., and Wittenborn, R. O., editors: *Psychopharmacology: a review of progress 1957-1967,* U.S. Government Printing Office, Washington, D. C., 1968, pp. 1231-1239.
15. Fink, M., Shapiro, D., and Itil, T.: EEG profiles of fenfluramine, amobarbital and dextroamphetamine in normal volunteers, *Psychopharmacologia, Berl.* **22**:369-383, 1971.
16. Fink, M., Itil, T. M., Zaks, A., and Freedman, A. M.: EEG patterns of cyclazocine, a narcotic antagonist, *in* Karczmar, A. and Koella, W., editors: *Neurophysiological and behavioral aspects of psychotropic drugs,* Charles C. Thomas, Springfield, Ill., 1969, pp. 62-71.
17. Fink, M., Shapiro, D., Hickman, C., and Itil, T.: Quantitative analysis of the electroencephalogram by digital computer methods. III. Applications to psychopharmacology, *in* Kline, N. S. and Laska, E., editors: *Computers and electronic devices in psychiatry,* Grune & Stratton, New York, 1968.
18. Fink, M., Simeon, J., Itil, T. M., and Freedman, A. M.: Clinical antidepressant activity of cyclazocine—a narcotic antagonist, *Clin. Pharmacol. Ther.,* **11**:41-48, 1970.
19. Funderbunk, W. H., Finger, K. F., Drakontides, A. B., and Schneider, J. A.: EEG and biochemical findings with MAO inhibitors, *Ann. N. Y. Acad. Sci.,* **96**:289-302, 1962.
20. Gannon, P., Itil, T. M., Keskiner, A., and Hsu, W.: Clinical and quantitative electroencephalographical effects of MK-940, *Arzneim.-Forsch.* **20**:971-874, 1970.
21. Gayral, L. and Turnin, J.: Notes sur l'activité de quelques hydrazides inhibitrices de la monoamine-oxydase sur l'electroencephalogrammes de l'homme, *Rev. neurol.,* **103**:265-271, 1960.
22. Gazianega, P., Abrams, R., Simeon, J., Jones, T., and Fink, M.: Clinical evaluation of GP-41299, an antianxiety agent of the doxapine type, *Arzneim. Forsch.,* **22**:1903-1905, 1972.
23. Goldstein, L. and Pfeiffer, C. C.: Quantitative EEG analysis of single dose-effect relationships in normal volunteers of capuride (Pacinox) a new antianxiety drug, Biol. Psychiat., **3**:165-172, 1971.
24. Goldstein, L., Murphree, H. B., and Pfeiffer, C. C.: A comparative study of the EEG effects of antihistamines in normal volunteers, *J. clin. Pharmacol.* **3**:42-53, 1968.
25. Goldstein, L., Murphree, H. B., and Pfeiffer, C. C.: Quantitative

electroencephalography in man as a measure of CNS stimulation, *Ann. N. Y. Acad. Sci.,* **107**:1045-1056, 1963.

26. Guillerm, H., Davost, P. H., Grandmontagne, O., and Prudhomme, B.: Efficacité du nialimide dans les états dépressifs, *Ann. med. psychol.,* **118(1)**:972-978, 1960.
27. Itil, T. M.: Electroencephalography and pharmacopsychiatry, in Freyhan, F. A., Petrilowitsch, N. and Pichot, P., editors: *Clinical psychopharmacology, Modern problems of pharmacopsychiatry, Vol. 1.,* Karger, Basel/New York, 1968, pp. 163-194.
28. Itil, T. M.: Elektroencephalographische befunde zur klassifikation neuro und thymoleptischer medikamente, *Med. Exp. (Basel),* **5**:347-363, 1961.
29. Itil, Turan, M.: Elektroencephalographische studien bei psychosen und psychotropen Medikamenten, Ahmet Sait Matbaasi, Istanbul, 1964.
30. Itil, T. M.: Quantitative EEG and behavior changes after LSD and Ditran, in Karczmar, A. and Koella, W., editors: *Neurophysiological and behavioral aspects of psychotropic drugs,* Charles C. Thomas, Springfield, Ill., 1969, pp. 62-71.
31. Itil. T. M. Quantitative pharmaco-EEG—a new approach to the discovery of a psychotropic drug. In press: Proceedings of the C.I.N.P. Meeting, August, 1972.
32. Itil, T. M.: Quantitative pharmaco-electroencephalography in assessing new antianxiety agents, in Vinar, O., Votava, Z. and Bradley, P. B., editors: *Advances in neuro-psychopharmacology.* North-Holland Publishing Co., Amsterdam, 1971, pp. 199-209.
33. Itil, T. M.: Quantitative pharmaco-electroencephalography in the discovery of a new group of psychotropic drugs, *Diseases of the Nervous System,* **33(8)**: 557-559, August, 1972.
34. Itil, T. M.: Quantitative pharmaco-electroencephalography (the use of computerized cerbral biopotentials in drug research), in Itil, T. M., editor: *Modern problems of pharmacopsychiatry, Vol. 8: Psychotropic drugs and the human EEG,* S. Karger AG, Basel/New York, 1974, pp. 43-75.
35. Itil, T. M. and Akpinar, S.: Lithium effect on human electroencephalogram, *Clinical Electroencephalography,* **2(2)**:89-102, 1971.
36. Itil, T. M. and Fink, M.: Anticholinergic drug-induced delirium: Experimental modification, quantitative EEG and behavior correlations, *J. Nerv. Ment. Dis.,* 143:492-507, 1966.
37. Itil, T. M., Cora, R., Hsu, W., Cig, E. and Saletu, B.: Clinical toxicological and electroencephalographical effects of a new tricyclic antidepressant OI-77, *Arzneimittel-Forschung (Drug Research),* **22(12)**:2063-2066, 1972.
38. Itil, T. M., Polvan, N., and Hsu, W.: Clinical and EEG effects of GB-94, a "tetracyclic" antidepressant (EEG model in discovery of a new psychotropic drug), *Curr. Ther. Res.,* **14(7)**:395-413, 1972.
39. Itil, T., Shapiro, D., and Fink, M.: Differentiation of psychotropic drugs by quantitative EEG analysis. *Agressologie,* **9(2)**:267-280, 1968.
40. Itil, T. M., Saletu, B., Coffin, C., and Klingenberg, H.: Quantitative EEG changes during thiothixene treatment of chronic schizophrenics. *Clinical Electroencephalography,* **3(2)**:109-117, 1972.

41. Itil, T. M., Hsu, W., Klingenberg, H., Gannon, P., and Holden, M.: Effect of thiothixene on digital computer sleep prints of schizophrenic patients, *Physicians' Drug Manual (PDM),* **2(9-10)**:118-123, 1971.
42. Itil, T. M., Saletu, B., Gannon, P., Arat, M., and Hsu, W.: Clinical and EEG investigations with CI-579 and CI-600 (Quantitative pharmaco-electroencephalography and "sleep prints"), *Physicians' Drug Manual,* **4(3-4)**:2-10, 1972.
43. Itil, T., Shapiro, D. M., Fink, M., Kiremitci, N., and Hickman, C.: Quantitative EEG studies of chlordiazepoxide, chlorpromazine, and imipramine in volunteer and schizophrenic subjects, *in* Evans, W. O. and Kline, N. S., editors: *The psychopharmacology of the normal human,* Charles C. Thomas, 1969, Springfield, Ill., pp. 219-237.
44. Itil, T., Gannon, P., Cora, R., Polvan, N., Akpinar, S., Elveris, F., and Eskazan, E.: SCH-12,041, a new anti-anxiety agent (quantitative pharmacoelectroencephalography and clinical trials), *Physicians' Drug Manual (PDM),* **3(3-4)**:26-35, 1971.
45. Itil, T. M., Guven, F., Cora, R. Hsu, W., Polvan, N., Ucok, A., Sanseigne, A., and Ulett, G. A.: Quantitative pharmacoelectroencephalography using frequency analyzer and digital computer methods in early drug evaluations, in Smith, W. L., editor: *Drugs, development, and brain functions,* Charles C. Thomas, Springfield, Ill. 1971, pp. 145-166.
46. Kopera, H.: Aspects of clinical pharmacology and clinical experiences with ORG GB-94. Presented at the 50th anniversary meeting Organon, Amsterdam, October 26, 1973.
47. Prange, A. J., Jr., Wilson, I. C., Lara, P. P., Alltop, L. B., and Breese G. R.: Effects of thyrotropin releasing hormones in depression, *Lancet,* **2**:999-1002, Nov. 11, 1972.
48. Raine, A. C. and Thomas, S. F.: Severe brain syndrome following phenelzine overdosage, *Am. J. Psychiatry,* **119**:373-382, 1962.
49. Shapiro, D., Hsu, W., and Itil, T. M.: Period analysis of the EEG on the PDP-12, in Wulfsohn, N. L. and Sances, A., Jr., editors: *The nervous system and electric currents, Vol. 2.* Plenum Press, New York, 1971, p. 59.
50. Simeon, J., Spero, M., and Fink, M.: Clinical and EEG studies of doxepin: interim report, *Psychosomatics,* **10(2)**:14-17, 1969.
51. Van Riezen, H., Behagel, I.R.H., and Chafik, M.: Development of psychotropic drugs. *Psychopharmacology Bulletin,* **11**:2, pp. 10-15, 1975.

14

Prospectives in Antidepressant Research: Serendipity or Evolution?

MAX WILHELM, PH.D.

In attempting to prophesy prospective developments in the treatment of human disease, one is free to speculate about future developments which could lead to a happier and healthier world. The problems to be solved, however, are greater than ever before. Trust in the innovative power of the human mind and hopes and predictions for a better life are common to most cultures. However, every attempt to predict evolutionary processes, be it philosophical, political, or economical, finally comes to the conclusion originally formulated by Julian Huxley in his psychometabolic analysis of man's own interference with the biological function of his mind; "Only scientific method and a massive deployment of scientific manpower can prevent disaster and ensure evolutionary improvement."(1)

Scientific prophesy, however, is somewhat self-contradictory, since it aims at prediction of future developments which, based on current experience and knowledge, are unforeseeable and hence might best be classified as science fiction. Therefore, any evaluation of heuristic scientific statements must be preceded by the supposition that scientific predictions can not be made with certainty and that answers to problems only raise more questions. The most important future issues presently lie beyond the reach of vigorous scientific exploration and, therefore, researchers should be prepared for the unexpected, if significant discoveries are to be made in the future.

The history of drug treatment of depression represents a typical example of unpredicted advances in biological research, medical diagnosis, and therapy. The revolutionary developments in the management of depression seen during the past 20 years have often been cited as classical examples of serendipity in medicine(2). The discovery of the mood-elevating effect of the MAO-inhibitors(3),the thymoleptic action of imipramine (4), and the antimaniacal action of lithium carbonate (5) would seem to support this position. With these facts in mind, it is indeed very daring to postulate future trends. Perhaps the Delphi technique (6), which seeks to supplement objective scientific facts and experience with subjective opinion, has applicability here.

A brief historic review of drug therapy for the treatment of depression reveals an evolution in which the apparently explosive developments of the immediate past represent a short but logically evolved epoch. The roots of today's discoveries reach back to the ancients. An understanding of the evolution of present day therapeutics might stimulate future developments.

Depression is not only one of the most common, but also one of the strangest psychic maladies to which man is prey. As "spleen" or melancholia, depression has occupied the minds of philosophers and artists for centuries; as a mental illness, it has claimed the attention of psychiatrists who studied the symptomatology of depression; and as a pathological condition of the human organism, it has stimulated physiological and biochemical exploration of the depressive syndrome.

Nepenthes, a mixture of Egyptian herbs referred to as the "secrets of the queens," was the first "antidepressant" described in the literature. Homer (7) depicted it as a pharmakon which would release the melancholic from his black gloom. Pathological mood changes were later described and discussed by various authors, including Hippocrates, Celsus, and Galen. The Arabs discovered the euphoria-inducing properties of kat, cannabis, and coffee. The euphoristic action of opium, too, was known long before it was used in medicine.

In the 16th century, depression was treated with purgatives, while in the 18th century, use of hydrotherapy, belladonna, and venesection was common. In the 19th century, more modern methods of treatment had started to emerge, for example, tincture of opium came into use in the management of depression. During the first half of the 20th century, a wide variety of somatic approaches to the treatment of depression rapidly found favor among practicing physicians. Sex hormones were introduced by Werner in 1934, pentetrazole convulsants by Meduha in 1935, amphetamines by Myerson in 1936, and electroshock therapy by Cerleti in 1938. The discovery of the antidepressant effects of iproniazid and imipramine in 1957 marked the beginning of still another chapter in the history of the treatment of depression.

This retrospective review might evoke the impression that evolution in antidepressant research has been and will remain a discontinuous process, that is, years of dramatic progress appear to alternate with long periods of stagnation. Such an impression is correct, if we restrict our discussion to single and very specific aspects of drug research. However, a comprehensive analysis of the interplay among the various scientific disciplines which contributed to the therapeutic evolution, reveals a continuous system within which emphasis and direction (obvious to an outside observer) change periodically (Fig. 1).

Alternation in research patterns is well illustrated by developments of the past 20 years. Subsequent to the serendipitous discovery of imipramine and iproniazid, research efforts were concentrated primarily on the evaluation and therapeutic application of the more recent findings. The age of empirical discoveries has been followed by a period of intense biological research, aimed at exploration of possible biochemical and physiological correlates of depression, and at the evaluation of the mechanism of action of the newer therapeutic agents.

In attempting to extrapolate the interaction between the different branches of science into the near future, one is tempted to predict a less spectacular period of evolution than was witnessed during the era which ended a few years ago. Empirical thinking dominated this latter period, thus making it more prone to serendipity. Future developments will be the result of an analytical, biomolecular approach, and although discoveries will appear to be less progressive they will, in reality, be more fundamental. (Fig. 2).

Since diagnosis and, consequently, psychochemotherapy is still based on a phenomenological and nosological exploration of the patient, the risk of subjective errors in the treatment of depressive illness cannot be overlooked. Quantification of depressive symptoms and syndromes is still rather imprecise. Establishment of a generally accepted classification of depression and the need for causal therapy based on sound biological principles, are two of the most urgent tasks now confronting those engaged in biological research. Improvements in diagnostic technique will also be required, if rapid therapeutic advances are to be anticipated.

Neurochemistry has already furnished fundamental knowledge which seems to indicate a potential solution to the diagnostic problem. Since 1959 when Everett and Toman (8) first postulated that serotonin and catecholamines may be of importance in depression, considerable progress has been made, particularly in the development of methodology to analyze neurotransmitters in body and organ fluids. It is this sophisticated technique which will enable us to explore the body's biochemical reactions, particularly the cyclic processes of the normal nervous system, and to correlate these findings with abnormalities usually associated with the

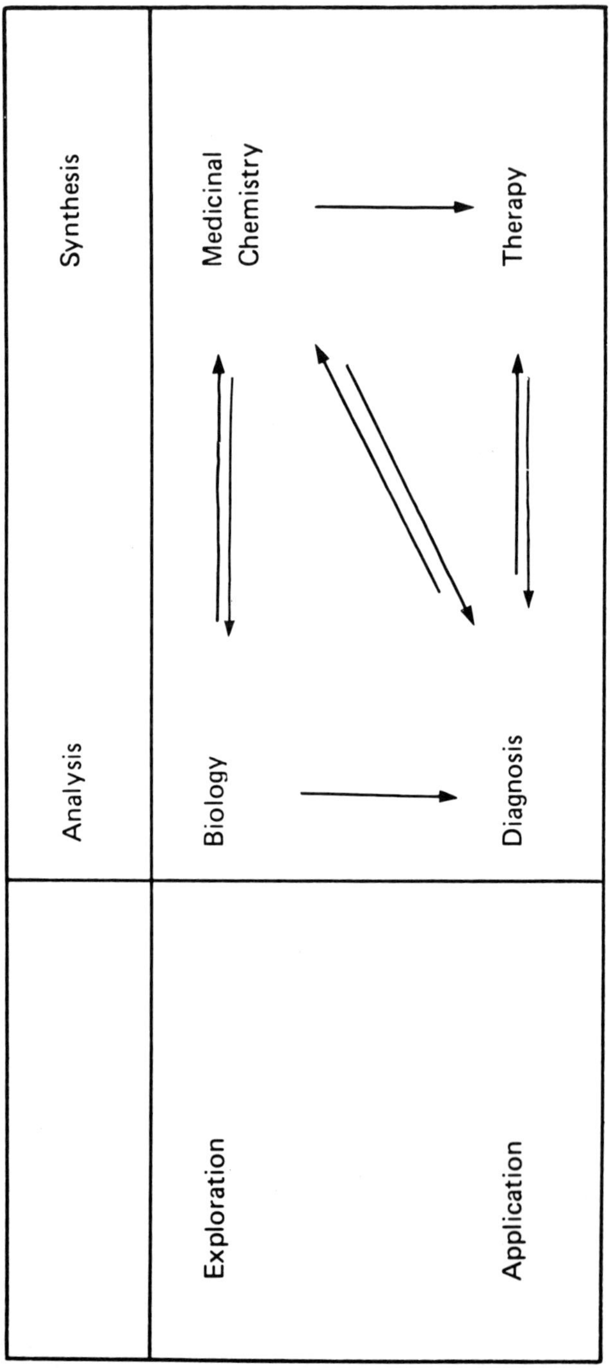

Fig. 1
Evolutionary Fluctuation

TIME	MEDICINAL CHEMISTRY	BIOLOGY	DIAGNOSIS	THERAPY
		Biochem. Classification of Antidepressants	Definition of depressive syndromes	
				Neurotransmitter Precursor Therapy
	Specific NE- and 5-HT Receptor-Blockers	Biochem. Definition of depressive syndromes	Quantitative Symptomatology (Rating scales)	Causal Neuro-Chemotherapy
	Specific Oxidase Inhibitors	Characterization of Neuro-Receptors	Neurochemical Diagnosis	"Biochemical ECT"
		Isolation of specific Amine-Oxidases		
			Quantitative EEG-Analysis	
		Pharmaco-Electroencephalography		

Fig. 2

Evolution in Antidepressant Research

various depressive states. A quantitative analysis of such differences in specific areas of the nervous system may finally result in biochemical classification of depressive disorders (9).

The logical consequence of a biochemical approach to diagnostics is the creation of an equivalent biochemical characterization of the antidepressant drugs, an approach which would make causal therapy feasible. The biochemical profile of many antidepressants has already been explored with respect to their ability to interfere with brain norepinephrine or serotonin metabolism. Most antidepressant drugs presently in use are competitors of both neurotransmitters. The ratio of the interference with the serotonergic and respectively the adrenergic system, is considered to be the determining factor for assessment of evaluating their mood profile (10), Maprotiline®, a specific inhibitor of norepinephrine uptake (11), has a bipolar, antidepressant-anxiolytic profile, a characteristic which underscores the therapeutic value of agents with highly specific biochemical activity. This observation may stimulate chemists to synthesize compounds with a topography similar to that of the neurotransmitters (12). These compounds have the required properties for interaction with neuroreceptors or for competition with neurotransmitters.

A second class of antidepressants that will attract increased attention because of a new perception of enzymatic processes are the enzyme inhibitors. Specific blockers of norepinephrine or serotonin oxidase can be expected to evolve from chemical research as soon as the methodology which differentiates between these enzyme systems is further refined (13) and screening models established.

Speculations have a chance of being proved correct only if certain requirements are met. In the case of drug research, this means the invention and introduction of new methods to take the place of screening procedures that have been in use for many years. Psychopharmacology, in particular, is a field that most urgently needs more discriminatory methods for drug evaluation. The screening methodology now in use yields, at best, basic overview and permits evaluation of drug activity only with reference to activities observed clinically. In the case of antidepressants, information gained from pharmacological research is valuable for prediction of side effects, but scarcely for assessment of antipsychotic properties.

The pharmacological approach presently used in evaluating clinical efficacy is one in which compounds are tested in animal models having chemically-evoked, e.g. reserpine or tetrabenazine, symptoms of human depression. A major criticism of this procedure is the possibility of missing the antidepressant potential of unique compounds which may have a mechanism of action different from that of the test drug. Stimulation of abnormal behavior patterns in animals by induced lesions of specific brain structures may prove to be a method by which evoked states in animal models will correlate more closely with human manifestations of depression and, as such, will be better suited for screening of depression antagonists.

The lack of methodology common to the diagnosis of depressive symptoms in man and to the assessment of drug-induced antidepressant effects in animals explains the serendipitous evolution of research. A quantitative method to measure physiological changes associated with depression would be a valuable tool for evaluation of new antidepressants. The feasibility of such a hypothesis is indicated by Itil's quantitative pharmaco-electroencephalography (14), a methodological technique which, if transferred to animal models will most likely disclose new approaches to the assessment of the antidepressant potential of new drugs.

Research in the area of depression is as old as mankind. It has attracted the most creative philosophers and the most innovative scientists in a mutual effort to explore the power of the human mind and to correct the dread of its distortion. Great progress has been made, but recent accomplishments become minute when compared with the achievements which lie ahead. A continuous evolution of all the faculties of research which have and will continue to contribute to the knowledge of the various aspects of depression can be predicted. It is without doubt that these evolutionary processes will continue well into the future, a future which will witness solutions to many of the perplexing problems related to the treatment of depression.

REFERENCES

1. Huxley, J.: *The Future of Man–Evolutionary Aspects, in Man and HIs Future,* ed. by Wolstenholme, G., Little, Brown and Co., Boston, 1963, p. 22. (A CIBA Foundation Volume)
2. Kline, N. S.: Pharmaceutical agents for treating depression, *Chem. Tech.,* Mar. 1974, p. 141.
3. Kline, N. S.: *Monoamine oxidase inhibitors:* An unfinished picaresque tale, *in Discoveries in Biological Psychiatry,* by Ayd, F., ed. J. B. Lippincot, Philadelphia, 1970, p. 194.
4. Kuhn, R.: Ueber die behandlung der depression mit einem iminodibenzylderivat, *Schweiz. Med. Wochenschr.,* **87**:1135, 1957.
5. Cade, J. F. J.: Lithium salts in treatment of psychotic excitement Med. J. Aust., **2**:349, 1949.

6. Rockwell, M. A.: The Delphi procedure: Knowledge from goat viscera?, *New England J. Med.,* **288**:1298, 1973.
7. Homer: *Odyssey,* Line 219.
8. Everett, G. M. and Toman, J. E. P.: Mode of action of Rauwolfia alkaloids and motor activity, *in Biological Psychiatry,* by Masserman, J. H., editor Grune and Stratton, New York, 1959, p. 75.
9. Schildkraut, J. J.: Norepinephrine metabolites as biochemical criteria for classifying depressive disorders and predicting responses to treatment: Preliminary findings, *Amer. J. Psychiat.,* **130**:695, 1973.
10. Carlsson, A., Corrodi, H., Fuxe, K., and Hokfeld, T.: Effect of antidepressant drugs on the depletion of intraneuronal brain 5-hydroxytryptamine stores, caused by 4-methyl-a-ethyl-meta-tryptamine, *Europ. J. Pharmakol.,* **5**:1969.
11. Maitre, L., Staehelin, M., and Bein, H. J.: Blockade of noradrenaline uptake by 34276-Ba, a new antidepressant drug, *Biochem. Pharmacol.* **20**:2169, 1971.
12. Wilhelm, M.: La chimie des psychotropes polycycliques, *Actualités Chim. Ther.,* **2**:33, 1974.
13. Youdin, M. B. M.: Significance of selective inhibition of multiple forms of monoamine oxidase, *J. Pharmacol.,* **5**(Suppl 1):99, 1974.
14. Itil, T. M., Güven, F., Cora, R., Hsu, W., Polvan, N., Ucok, A., Sanseigne, A., and Ulett, G. A.: Quantitative pharmacoencephalography using frequency analyzer and digital computer methods *in Early Drug Evaluation in Drugs, Development and Cerebral Functions,* by Smith, W. L., ed. C. C. Thomas, Springfield, Ill., 1971, p. 145.

15

Drug Treatments of Depressive Illnesses: A View of the Future

JONATHAN O. COLE, M.D.

At the time of this writing a pessimist could defend the position that ten years hence the drug treatment of depressive disorders will be little advanced from its current status. There is an ominously escalating threat to all research which may well make the future really rather barren. Popular concern over some blatant injustices committed in the name of clinical research (e.g. the Public Health Service Syphilis study or the New York City tumor cell transplant study) is being used by extremist groups to generate highly complex and restrictive regulations governing clinical research. On the other side, the amount of animal toxicology required of drug companies before a new compound is used in man is continually rising in volume and expense, despite the uncertain predictive value of animal safety data for drug actions in man. These factors appear to be inexorably increasing the cost and decreasing the feasability of studying new drug treatments for depression in patients.

An optimist can take the position that, even if all new drug development were to stop tomorrow, we could still learn far more about how to use our current drug therapies without inventing any new drugs at all.

First, if we used proven prophylactic therapies—imipramine for recurrent unipolar depressions and lithium for either unipolar or biopolar depressions—we might substantially reduce the number of depressive states actually requiring treatment with drugs. If we then trained primary care physicians in the proper early treatment of depressive illnesses, subtantial suffering might be prevented. It is possible—but by no means proven—that the surprising efficacy of tricyclic antidepressants like doxepin and imipramine in relatively mildly depressed outpatients may be because potentially more severe depressions are being aborted at an early stage. Otherwise it is hard to reconcile this efficacy with the other firm evidence that tricyclic drugs really work best in retarded endogenous depressions.

One can even fantasy a scheme of the sort informally proposed by Thomas Ban of McGill, where various levels of treatment from primary care physician to psychiatrist's office to general psychiatric ward to research ward for treatment resistant depressions are set up and the treatment personnel at each level are trained to optimally treat appropriate patients and to shunt inappropriate patients up to the next more intensive level of treatment.

What tools could such a system have available at its higher levels? Methods for measuring blood levels of tricyclic compounds and their active metabolites are now available for use in laboratories at a journeyman research level and may be available at the large-scale routine clinical laboratory level soon. Such levels in some studies are relatable to clinical improvement—too low a level being associated with failure to improve and too high a level with toxicity. Checking blood levels in treatment-resistant patients is certainly sensible and technologically feasible on a limited scale already.

Further, it is possible to fantasy—on the basis of existing basic psychopharmacologic data, that there may be some systematic relationship between biochemical abnormalities and depression. Patients low on norepinephrine activity in the brain might be given desipramine as a specific norepinephrine uptake inhibitor. Patients with overactive dopaminergic neurones (e.g. agitated depressions) should specifically respond to a neuroleptic—halperidol or pimozide. Patients with serotonin deficiencies might respond best to chlorimipramine or to some future, even more specific, serotonin reuptake inhibitor. Patients excreting large amounts of methoxyhydroxyphenylglycol (MHPG) in the urine may respond differentially to amitryptaline. If precision in biochemical diagnosis in depression were really greatly improved, studies of the rate of production of amine metabolites in cerebral spinal fluid (CSF) after *probenecid* could be routinely done in more seriously ill or treatment resistant patients.

In fact, in a world deprived of the right to do double-blind, placebo-controlled studies an optimist can take comfort in the fact that we have a variety of credible research procedures which could justifiably be transformed into routine tests in centers of hard-to-treat patients. The quantified EEG and possibly some psychological test procedures could be added to the blood level and biochemical measures suggested above.

The range of safe but unusual drug treatments for depression—particularly treatment resistant depression—(e.g. lithium, l-DOPA, trytophan, MAO inhibitors, the non-MAO tranylcypromineisomer, diphenylhydantoin, LSD) has expanded and most of these would be easy to get through even a rather conservative human rights ethics committee. Also, depressed patients are more likely than most other seriously ill psychiatric patients to be able to give informed consent, of the sort required for treatments with this order of background evidence for safety in man. Many of these drugs can be obtained and given as *treatments,* rather than as *investigational drugs,* under existing law and medical practice assumptions. Again, if clinical investigation is pushed to the wall, it is possible—if not desirable to obtain research information from carefully documented clinical studies using quantitative clinical research methodology but avoiding overt random assignment of patients to treatments.

For example, if one psychiatrist on a clinical unit for treatment of resistant depressions always used an MAO inhibitor first while another always used l-DOPA first and they were assigned alternate admissions, sooner or later a comparison of the two treatments could be made, but doctor personality would be confounded with treatment. If several such units did the same thing and all university-based wards agreed to use the same basic routine clinical assessments, data would eventually emerge which would probably not differ appreciably in conclusions or possible inferences from that obtained from a double-blind, controlled, comparative study. Also, as John Overall has pointed out in the past, large enough samples plus the cussedness and therapeutic eccentricities of a large number of psychiatrists can lead to data which strongly suggest that Drug A is better than Drug B for a given type of patient. It is not proof, but it is a lot better than one doctor's observations on ten patients to demonstrate differential drug effects.

In short, even under adversity and semi-intolerable restrictions, substantial data on efficacy of various newer drugs in depression may be obtained and improvements in predicting which patient will do best on which drug may be attainable.

With respect to the development of really new antidepressant drugs, I have a proposal which might help us find really useful new drugs with less cost and, I hope, less risk.

First, I contend that we have enough current drugs that relieve 70% of acute depressions in 5-21 days. We do not need any more like that unless they operate on a biochemical principal of importance to our understanding of the pathophysiology of depression, (e.g. a specific central serotonin reuptake inhibitor which does not influence dopamine or norepinephrine reuptake). Therefore, drugs need only be studied initially in patients for a day or two. If the patients—or some of them—do not feel much better when an adequate dose is given in the first 48 hours, why persist? This practice should decrease the amount of expensive animal toxicology needed before Phase I studies are begun in man and also the amount of work done in prisoner volunteers (or college students if prisoners are overprotected by future regulations!) and should make it possible to test a wider variety of new potentially unique psychoactive drugs for antidepressant activity in man.

I do not have any special notions about how to find such unusual new drugs, but I would bet on unusual compounds with clear but unusual behavioral effects or with specific actions on brain enzymes or as neurotransmitters or blockers or neurosecretory substances like Thyroid Releasing Hormone (TRH). But maybe real animal models of affective depression are becoming available and something better than reserpine-induced behavioral sedation may become routinely available. On purely anthropomorphic grounds, I have always liked Irwin's swimming-time test as a face-valid measure of optimism—the longer you work without giving up the more optimistic you must be—but I have no idea how well it would predict clinical utility.

Index

Index